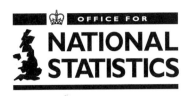

The mental health of children and adolescents in Great Britain

The report of a survey carried out in 1999 by Social Survey Division of the Office for National Statistics on behalf of the Department of Health, the Scottish Health Executive and the National Assembly for Wales

Howard Meltzer
Rebecca Gatward

with

Robert Goodman
Tamsin Ford

'5

D1380073

London: The Stationery Office

↑Y

About the Office for National Statistics

The Office for National Statistics (ONS) is the Government Agency responsible for compiling, analysing and disseminating many of the United Kingdom's economic, social and demographic statistics, including the retail prices index, trade figures and labour market data, as well as the periodic census of the population and health statistics. The Director of ONS is also Head of the Government Statistical Service (GSS) and Registrar-General in England and Wales and the agency carries out all statutory registration of births, marriages and deaths there.

Editorial policy statement

The Office for National Statistics works in partnership with others in the Government Statistical Service to provide Parliament, government and the wider community with the statistical information, analysis and advice needed to improve decision-making, stimulate research and inform debate. It also registers key life events. It aims to provide an authoritative and impartial picture of society and a window on the work and performance of government, allowing the impact of government policies and actions to be assessed.

Information services

For general enquiries about official statistics, please contact the National Statistics Public Enquiry Service:

Telephone	-	020 7533 5888
Textphone (Minicom)	-	01633 812399

Alternatively write to the National Statistics Public Enquiry Service, Zone DG/18, 1 Drummond Gate, London, SW1V 2QQ. Fax 020 7533 6261 or e-mail **info@ons.gov.uk**.

Most National Statistics publications are published by The Stationery Office and can be obtained from The Publications Centre, P.O. Box 276, London, SW8 5DT. Tel 0870 600 5522 or fax 0870 600 5533.

National Statistics can also be contacted on the Internet at **http://www.ons.gov.uk**

ISBN 0 11 621373 6

Contents

                                                                              Page

Authors' acknowledgements   v
List of tables   vi
List of figures   viii
Notes   ix

Summary of the report   1

Part 1: Prevalence of mental disorders

1   Background, aims and coverage of the survey   9
     1.1   Background   9
     1.2   Aims of the survey   11
     1.3   Timetable   12
     1.4   Coverage of the survey   12
     1.5   Content of the survey   13
     1.6   Coverage of the report   14
     1.7   Access to the data   14

2   Concepts and methods used in assessing mental disorders   16
     2.1   Introduction   16
     2.2   Definitions of mental disorder   16
     2.3   Concepts   16
     2.4   Methods of assessing mental disorders   17
     2.5   Single versus multiple informants   19
     2.6   Case vignette assessment   20

3   Sampling and interviewing procedures   22
     3.1   Introduction   22
     3.2   Sample design   22
     3.3   Survey procedures   23
     3.4   Survey response rates   23
     3.5   Interviewing procedures   24

4   Prevalence of mental disorders   26
     4.1   Introduction   26
     4.2   Prevalence of mental disorders by personal characteristics   26
     4.3   Prevalence of mental disorders by family characteristics   27
     4.4   Prevalence of mental disorders by household characteristics   29
     4.5   Prevalence of mental disorders by areal characteristics   30
     4.6   Odds Ratios of socio-demographic correlates of mental disorders   31

5   Characteristics of children with mental disorders   62
     5.1   Introduction   62
     5.2   Characteristics of children with any disorder   62
     5.3   Emotional disorders   63
     5.4   Conduct disorders   63
     5.5   Hyperkinetic disorders   64
     5.6   Less common disorders   64

Part 2: Children and adolescents with specific mental disorders

6	**Mental disorders and physical complaints**		**73**
	6.1	Introduction	73
	6.2	General health	73
	6.3	Physical complaints	73
	6.4	Life threatening illnesses	74
	6.5	Accidents and injuries	75
	6.6	Parent's view of child's mental health	75
7	**Use of services**		**82**
	7.1	Introduction	82
	7.2	Use of health services for any reason	82
	7.3	Use of services for significant mental health problems	83
	7.4	Use of professional and non-professional help	84
	7.5	Socio-demographic correlates of service use	85
	7.6	Trouble with the police	85
8	**Scholastic achievement and education**		**91**
	8.1	Introduction	91
	8.2	Special Educational Needs	91
	8.3	Specific learning difficulties	92
	8.4	Absenteeism from school	93
	8.5	Truancy	93
9	**Social functioning of the family**		**99**
	9.1	Introduction	99
	9.2	Mental health of parent	99
	9.3	Family functioning	100
	9.4	Reward strategies and punishment regimes	101
	9.5	Stressful life events	101
	9.6	Social functioning correlates of mental disorders	102
	9.7	Impact of the child's mental disorder on the family	102
10	**Children's social functioning and lifestyle behaviours**		**119**
	10.1	Introduction	119
	10.2	Friendships	119
	10.3	Help-seeking behaviour	120
	10.4	Smoking, drinking and drug use	121

Part 3: Appendices

A	*Sampling, weighting and adjustment procedures*	133
B	*Statistical terms and their interpretation*	138
C	*Sampling errors*	140
D	*Follow-up findings*	147
E	*Survey documents*	149
F	*Glossary of terms used in the report*	228

Authors' acknowledgements

We would like to thank everybody who contributed to the survey and the production of this report. We were supported by our specialist colleagues in ONS who contributed to the sampling, fieldwork and computing elements for the survey.

A special thank you is extended to Robert Goodman from the Institute of Psychiatry, London, who designed the questionnaire for the assessment of the mental health of children, took on the task of making clinical ratings of over ten thousand completed interviews, gave sound advice on the preliminary analysis of the survey data and not least gave encouragement and support to the whole research team for the past five years.

Great thanks are also due to the 300 interviewers who worked on the survey.

The project was steered by a group comprising the following, to whom thanks are due for assistance and specialist advice at various stages of the survey:

Department of Health
Mrs K Tyson (chair)
Ms A Roberts
Dr R Jezzard
Miss H Jones
Mr A Boucher
Mr D Hird
Mr M Rae
Mr P Smith
Dr P Baldry
Mr J O'Shea (secretariat)

Scottish Office
Dr D Will
Mr G Russell

Welsh Office
Dr S Watkins
Mr J Sweeney

Department for Education and Employment
Mr N Remsbery
Mr R McElheran

Expert advisors:
Prof R Goodman (Institute of Psychiatry, London)
Dr I Frampton (Royal Cornwall Hospital)
Prof I Goodyer (University of Cambridge)
Prof R Harrington (University of Manchester)
Dr T Brugha (University of Leicester)
Prof R Nichol (University of Leicester)
Prof R Jenkins (Institute of Psychiatry, London)
Professor G Lewis (University of Wales)

Office for National Statistics
Ms S Carey
Ms R Gatward
Dr H Meltzer

Most importantly, we would like to thank all the parents, young people, and teachers for their co-operation.

List of tables

Page

3. Sampling and survey procedures
3.1 Response to initial CBC letter 22
3.2 Response to interview 23
3.3 Achieved interviews by type of
     informant 24

4. Prevalence of mental disorders
4.1 Prevalence of mental disorders by age
     and sex 33
4.2 Prevalence of mental disorders by
     ethnicity, age and sex 34
4.3 Prevalence of mental disorders by
     family type, age and sex 36
4.4 Prevalence of mental disorders by
     family structure, age and sex 38
4.5 Prevalence of mental disorders by
     number of children in household,
     age and sex 40
4.6 Prevalence of mental disorders by
     educational qualifications of parent,
     age and sex 42
4.7 Prevalence of mental disorders by
     family's employment, age and sex 44
4.8 Prevalence of mental disorders by gross
     weekly household income, age and sex 46
4.9 Prevalence of mental disorders by
     receipt of disability benefits, age and sex 48
4.10 Prevalence of mental disorders by social
     class, age and sex 50
4.11 Prevalence of mental disorders by
     tenure, age and sex 52
4.12 Prevalence of mental disorders by type
     of accommodation, age and sex 54
4.13 Prevalence of mental disorders by
     region, age and sex 56
4.14 Prevalence of mental disorders by
     ACORN classification, age and sex 58
4.15 Odds Ratios for socio-demographic
     correlates of mental disorders 60
4.16 Odds Ratios for socio-demographic
     correlates of emotional disorders 61

5. Characteristics of the sample
5.1 Number of children with each mental
     disorder by age and sex 67
5.2 Child's personal characteristics by type
     of mental disorder 67
5.3 Family characteristics by type of mental
     disorder 68

Page

5.4 Family's employment status, social class
     and income by type of mental disorder 69
5.5 Household and geographical
     characteristics by type of mental disorder 70

6. Mental disorders and physical complaints
6.1 General health rating by type of mental
     disorder 76
6.2 Type of physical complaint by type of
     mental disorder 77
6.3 Odds Ratios for physical complaints &
     socio-demographic correlates of
     mental disorders 78
6.4 Prevalence of mental disorders by type
     of physical complaint 79
6.5 Experience of a life threatening illness
     by type of mental disorder 79
6.6 Experience of accidents and injuries by
     type of mental disorder 80
6.7 Prevalence of mental disorders by type
     of accident or injury 80
6.8 Parental view of child's mental health
     by clinical assessment of type of mental
     disorder 81
6.9 Clinical assessment of type of mental
     disorder by parental view of child's
     mental health 81

7. Use of services
7.1 Use of health services in the past 12
     months (for any reason) by type of
     mental disorder 86
7.2 Use of services for significant mental
     health problems by type of mental
     disorder 87
7.3 Use of professional and non-professional
     help by type of mental disorder 88
7.4 Use of professional and non-professional
     help by number of mental disorders 89
7.5 Odds Ratios for the socio-demographic
     correlates of service use 89
7.6 In trouble with the police in the past 12
     months by type of mental disorder,
     age and sex 90
7.7 Ever been in trouble with the police by
     type of mental disorder 90

8. Scholastic achievement and education

8.1   Officially recognised special educational needs by type of mental disorder   95

8.2   Level of officially recognised special educational needs by type of mental disorder   95

8.3   Prevalence of mental disorder by level of SEN   96

8.4   Odds Ratios for mental disorder & socio-demographic correlates of SEN   96

8.5   Specific learning difficulties by type of mental disorder   97

8.6   Prevalence of mental disorders by specific learning difficulties   97

8.7   Absenteeism from school by type of mental disorder   97

8.8   Truancy (parent interview) by type of mental disorder   98

8.9   Truancy (young person interview) by type of mental disorder   98

8.10   Truancy (teacher questionnaire) by type of mental disorder   98

9. Social functioning of the family

9.1   Distribution of parent's GHQ-12 scores by type of mental disorder   105

9.2   Distribution of parent's GHQ-12 scores by number of mental disorders   105

9.3   Prevalence of mental disorders by parent's GHQ-12 score   105

9.4   Prevalence of mental disorders by parent's GHQ-12 score (grouped)   106

9.5   Distribution of family functioning scores by type of mental disorder   106

9.6   Distribution of family functioning scores by number of mental disorders   107

9.7   Prevalence of mental disorders by family functioning score   107

9.8   Reward strategies by type of mental disorder   108

9.9   Punishment regimes by type of mental disorder   109

9.10   Prevalence of mental disorders by type of non-physical, parental punishment   110

9.11   Prevalence of mental disorders by type of physical, parental punishment   111

9.12   Stressful life events by type of mental disorder   112

9.13   Number of stressful life events by type of mental disorder   113

9.14   Prevalence of mental disorders by type of stressful life events   113

9.15   Prevalence of mental disorders by number of stressful life events   114

9.16   Odds Ratios for social functioning and socio-demographic correlates of mental disorder   114

9.17   Impact of child's problems on family relationships by type of mental disorder   115

9.18   Impact of child's problems on social life and stigma by type of mental disorder   116

9.19   Impact of child's problems on parent's health by type of mental disorder   117

9.20   Impact of child's problems on parent's health behaviour by type of mental disorder   118

10. Children's social functioning and lifestyle behaviours

10.1   Friendship behaviour by type of mental disorder   123

10.2   Friendship score by type of mental disorder   124

10.3   People asked for help by type of mental disorder   124

10.4   Type of help sought by type of mental disorder   125

10.5   Potential helpers by type of mental disorder   125

10.6   Type of potential help by type of mental disorder   126

10.7   Smoking behaviour by age, survey source and sex   126

10.8   Drinking behaviour by age, survey source and sex   127

10.9   Drug taking by survey source   128

10.10 Prevalence of mental disorders by smoking behaviour   128

10.11 Prevalence of mental disorders by drinking behaviour   129

10.12 Prevalence of mental disorders by use of cannabis   129

List of figures

Page

1. Background aims and coverage of the survey
1.1   Timetable for survey   12

4. Prevalence of mental disorders
4.1   Prevalence of any mental disorder by age and sex   33
4.2   Prevalence of any mental disorder by ethnicity   35
4.3   Prevalence of any mental disorder by family type   37
4.4   Prevalence of any mental disorder by family structure   39
4.5   Prevalence of any mental disorder by number of children in household   41
4.6   Prevalence of any mental disorder by educational qualifications of parent   43
4.7   Prevalence of any mental disorder by family's employment   45
4.8   Prevalence of any mental disorder by gross weekly household income   47
4.9   Prevalence of any mental disorder by receipt of disability benefits   49
4.10   Prevalence of any mental disorder by social class   51
4.11   Prevalence of any mental disorder by tenure   53
4.12   Prevalence of any mental disorder by type of accommodation   55
4.13   Prevalence of any mental disorder by country/region   57
4.14   Prevalence of any mental disorder by ACORN classification   59

5. Characteristics of the sample
5.1   Sex distribution by type of mental disorder   64
5.2   Family's employment situation by type of mental disorder   65
5.3   Gross weekly household income by type of mental disorder   65
5.4   Tenure by type of mental disorder   66
5.5   ACORN classification by type of mental disorder   66

Page

6. Mental disorders and physical complaints
6.1   Percentage of children with a mental disorder by type of physical complaint   74

7. Use of services
7.1   Use of services (for any reason) by type of mental disorder   83
7.2   Contact with primary & secondary health services by type of mental disorder   84
7.3   Use of professional and non-professional help by type of mental disorder   84

8. Scholastic achievement and education
8.1   Officially recognised SEN by type of mental disorder   91
8.2   Prevalence of mental disorder by level of SEN   92

9. Social functioning of the family
9.1   Prevalence of mental disorders by parent's GHQ-12 score   100

10. Children's social functioning and lifestyle behaviours
10.1   Distribution of friendship scores by type of mental disorder   120
10.2   Help seeking behaviour by type of mental disorder   121

Notes

1 Tables showing percentages
The row or column percentages may add to 99% or 101% because of rounding.

The varying positions of the percentage signs and bases in the tables denote the presentation of different types of information. Where there is a percentage sign at the head of a column and the base at the foot, the whole distribution is presented and the individual percentages add to between 99% and 101%. Where there is no percentage sign in the table and a note above the figures, the figures refer to the proportion of people who had the attribute being discussed, and the complementary proportion, to add to 100%, is not shown in the table.

The following conventions have been used within tables showing percentages:
- \-   no cases
- 0   values less than 0.5%

2 Small bases
Very small bases have been avoided wherever possible because of the relatively high sampling errors that attach to small numbers. Often where the numbers are not large enough to justify the use of all categories, classifications have been condensed. However, an item within a classification is occasionally shown separately, even though the base is small, because to combine it with another large category would detract from the value of the larger category. In general, percentage distributions are shown if the base is 30 or more. Where the base is lower, actual numbers are shown in square brackets.

3 Significant differences
The bases for some sub-groups presented in the tables were small such that the standard errors around estimates for these groups are biased. Confidence intervals which take account of these biased standard errors were calculated and, although they are not presented in the tables, they were used in testing for statistically significant differences. Statistical significance is explained in Appendix B to this Report.

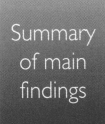

Summary
of main
findings

Summary of main findings

The findings described in this report and summarised here focus on the prevalence of mental disorders among 5-15 year olds and on the associations between the presence of a mental disorder and biographic, socio-demographic, socio-economic and social functioning characteristics of the child and the family. Causal relationships should not be assumed for any of the results presented in this report.

Background, aims and coverage (Chapter 1)

- The primary purpose of the survey was to produce prevalence rates of three main categories of mental disorder: conduct disorders, emotional disorders and hypekinetic disorders based on ICD-10 (International Classification of Diseases, tenth revision) and DSM-IV (Diagnostic and Statistical Manual, fourth revision) criteria.

- The second aim of the survey was to determine the impact or burden of children's mental health. Impact covers the consequences for the child, burden reflects the consequences for others.

- The third main purpose of the survey was to examine the use of health, social, educational and voluntary services among children with mental disorders.

- The surveyed population comprised children and adolescents, aged 5-15, living in private households in England, Scotland and Wales.

- Fieldwork for the survey took place between January and May 1999.

Concepts and methods (Chapter 2)

- This report uses the term, mental disorders, as defined by the ICD-10, to imply a clinically recognisable set of symptoms or behaviour associated in most cases with considerable distress and substantial interference with personal functions.

- The methodological strategy for the survey was a one-stage design with all children eligible for a full interview, i.e., without a screening stage.

- The measures designed for the present study incorporated structured interviewing supplemented by open-ended questions. When definite symptoms were identified by the structured questions, interviewers used open-ended questions and supplementary prompts to get informants to describe the problems in their own words.

- Data collection included information gathered from parents, teachers, and the children themselves (if aged 11-15).

- A case vignette approach was used for analysing the survey data - using clinicians to review the responses to the precoded questions and the transcripts of informants' comments, particularly those which asked about the child's significant problems.

Summary - *continued*

Sampling and survey procedures (Chapter 3)

- The sample was drawn from Child Benefit Records held by the Child Benefit Centre (CBC).

- 14,250 opt out letters were despatched by the Child Benefit Centre on behalf of ONS: 30 letters for each of the 475 postal sectors selected for the survey.

- After subtracting those addresses that opted out or were ineligible, 12,529 addresses were allocated to the ONS interviewers.

- Information was collected on 83% of the children eligible for interview from up to three sources resulting in 10,438 achieved interviews.

- Among the co-operating families, almost all the parents and most of the children took part. Four out of five teachers also returned their questionnaires.

Prevalence of mental disorders (Chapter 4)

- All the rates presented below are based on the diagnostic criteria for research using the ICD-10 Classification of Mental and Behavioural Disorders with strict impairment criteria - the disorder causing distress to the child or having a considerable impact on the child's day to day life.

- 10% of children aged 5 -15 years had a mental disorder: 5% had clinically significant conduct disorders; 4% were assessed as having emotional disorders - anxiety and depression - and 1% were rated as hyperactive.

- As their name suggests, the less common disorders (autistic disorders, tics and eating disorders) were attributed to half a percent of the sampled population.

- Among 5-10 year olds, 10% of boys and 6% of girls had a mental disorder. In the older age group, the 11-15 year olds, the proportions of children with any mental disorder were 13% for boys and 10% for girls.

- The prevalence rates of mental disorders were greater among children:
    - in lone parent compared with two parent families (16% compared with 8%)
    - in reconstituted families rather than those with no step-children (15% compared with 9%)
    - in families with five or more children compared with two-children (18% compared with 8%)
    - if interviewed parent had no educational qualifications compared with a degree level or equivalent qualification (15% compared with 6%)
    - in families with neither parent working compared with both parents at work (20% compared with 8%)
    - in families with a gross weekly household income of less than £200 compared with £500 or more (16% compared with 6%)
    - in families of social class V compared with social class I (14% compared with 5%)
    - whose parents are social sector tenants compared with owner occupiers (17% compared with 6%)
    - in household with a *striving* rather than a *thriving* geo-demographic classification (13% compared with 5%)

Summary - *continued*

Characteristics of children with mental disorders (Chapter 5)

- Children with a mental disorder compared with other children were more likely to be boys, living in a lower income household, in social sector housing and with a lone parent. They were less likely to be living with married parents or in social class I or II households.

Mental disorders and physical complaints (Chapter 6)

- The overall proportion of children with a fair, bad or very bad general health rating was 7%, the corresponding proportion among children with a mental disorder was 20% compared with 6% of those without a disorder.

- The physical illness or health conditions which showed the greatest disparity in prevalence rates between children with a mental disorder and those with no disorder were: bedwetting (12% compared with 4%), speech or language problems (12% compared with 3%), co-ordination difficulties (8% compared with 2%), and soiling pants (4% compared with 1%).

- Among children who had a life-threatening illness, about 1 in 6 were found to have a mental disorder.

- 25% of children who had accidental poisoning had a mental disorder, whereas the corresponding rate among children who had a broken bone was 12%, just above the national average.

Use of services (Chapter 7)

- Almost a half of the children with a mental disorder had been in contact with a GP in the past 12 months for any reason compared with just over a third of children with no disorder.

- Children with a disorder were more likely to have been taken to an Accident and Emergency department than those without a disorder (26% compared with 17%) and on more than one occasion (7% compared with 4%).

- Inpatient stays were slightly more common among children with a disorder than those with no disorder (9% compared with 5%).

- Children with a mental disorder were more likely than other children to have visited an Outpatient Department in the past year (29% compared with 18%.)

- One half of the children with mental disorders had seen someone from the educational services, about one quarter had used the specialist health care services and one fifth had contact with the social services.

- Two thirds of children assessed as having a mental disorder had seen a secondary level service provider in the last year.

- Parents of children with an emotional disorder were the group most likely to have asked family or friends for advice (23%) and the least likely to have sought professional services (63%).

- 25% of 11-15 year olds reported that at one point in their lives they had been in trouble with the police, which included 43% of children with a disorder and 21% of children with no disorder.

Summary - *continued*

Scholastic achievement and education (Chapter 8)

- 1 in 5 children had officially recognised special educational needs - those with a disorder were about three times more likely than other children to have special needs: 49% compared with 15%.

- Among children with officially recognised special educational needs, 28% of those with a disorder and 13% without a disorder had been issued with a statement of SEN by the local authority (Stage 5).

- The prevalence rate of mental disorders ranged from 6% among children who did not have special educational needs to 40% among children who were at Stage 5.

- Given that the rate of specific learning difficulties (SpLD) was set at 5%, children with a mental disorder were three times more likely than those with no disorder to have SpLD: 12% compared with 4%.

- 25% of children with emotional disorders had been absent from school for 11 days or more in the past term compared with 21% of children with conduct disorders and 14% with hyperkinetic disorders.

- According to young people's own reports, those with a disorder were about four times more likely than other children to have played truant: 33% compared with 9%. Children with conduct disorders had the highest rate of truancy at 44%.

Social functioning of the family (Chapter 9)

- 47% of children assessed as having a mental disorder had a parent who scored 3 or more on the GHQ12 (the twelve-item General Health Questionnaire), approximately twice the proportion of the sample of children with no disorder, 23%.

- The proportion of children with GHQ12 screen-positive parents rose from 23% of the no-disorder group to 44% of children with one disorder to 50% of those with two disorders and to 68% of children with three disorders.

- Children with a mental disorder were twice as likely to live in families rated as having *unhealthy functioning* compared with children with no disorder: 35% and 17% respectively.

- Children with mental disorders were far more likely to be frequently punished than children with no mental disorder: 18% compared with 8% were frequently sent to their rooms; 17% compared with 5% were frequently grounded, and 42% compared with 26% were frequently shouted at.

- 50% of children with a mental disorder had at one time seen the separation of their parents, compared with 29% of the sample with no disorder. The corresponding figures for problems with the police were 15% and 5% and for a parent or sibling dying - 6% compared with 3%.

- Two factors associated with the highest prevalence rates of mental disorders were: children (aged 13-15) who had split with a boyfriend or girlfriend (24%) and children whose parents had been in trouble with the police (22%).

- About 1 in 3 of their parents said the child's problem made their relationship more strained.

Summary - *continued*

- 20% of parents with no partner in the household reported that the child's problem was a contributory factor to a previous relationship breaking up.

- One quarter of parents said their children's problems caused difficulties with other family members.

- Eighty seven per cent of parents said their child's problems made them worried and 58% felt that their child's problems caused them to be depressed.

Social functioning of the child (Chapter 10)

- Among 11-15 year olds, 6% had a severe lack of friendship: 9% of those with mental disorders and 5% with no disorder.

- One quarter of young people had felt so unhappy or worried that they asked people for help. Children with a disorder were almost twice as likely, than those without a disorder, to have sought help and advice: 41% compared with 23%.

- 41% of 11-15 year olds who regularly smoked were assessed as having a mental disorder (28% had a conduct disorder, 20% had an emotional disorder and 4% were rated as having a hyperkinetic disorder) compared with the overall rate of 11%.

- 24% of young people who drank alcohol more than once a week had a mental disorder, three times the proportion among the group who had never drunk any alcohol.

- About one half of the 11-15 year olds who frequently used cannabis, i.e., more than once a week, had a mental disorder compared with one fifth of the less than once a month users and one tenth of those who had never used cannabis.

Part 1: Prevalence of mental disorders

Mental health of children and adolescents in Great Britain

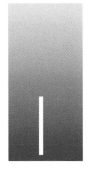

Background, aims and coverage of the survey

1.1 Background

The survey of the mental health of children and adolescents in Great Britain is the sixth major survey of psychiatric morbidity to be carried out by ONS (formerly OPCS) commissioned by the Department of Health, Scottish Health Executive and National Assembly for Wales. All the previous five surveys covered adults aged 16-64 but were distinct in terms of the respondents' place of residence or particular psychiatric problems:

- adults living in private households (Meltzer et al. 1995 a, b, c)
- residents of institutions specifically catering for people with mental health problems: hospitals, nursing homes, residential care homes, hostels, group homes and supported accommodation (Meltzer et al. 1996 a, b, c)
- homeless adults living in hostels, nightshelters, private sector leased accommodation or roofless people using day centres (Gill et al., 1996)
- adults known to have a psychotic disorder (Foster et al., 1996)
- prisoners (Singleton et al., 1998)

The rationale put forward for a national survey of psychiatric morbidity among children and adolescents is exactly the same as for the survey of adults.

"In order to plan mental health services effectively, it is necessary to know how many severely ill people there are, what their diagnoses are, and how far their needs for treatment are being met. The extent of the morbid population in the community needs to be known so that the resources and planning can effectively take this into account."

Official statistics on the mental health of children in Great Britain

Maughan (1995) summarised the official statistics collected on child health problems and the limitations with their interpretation. These included

- Data on psychiatric service use
- Consultations with GPs and others
- Trends in specific problem areas (e.g. substance abuse, delinquency and suicide)

She commented that data on the use of psychiatric services are the most problematic as indicators of prevalence rates of mental health problems among young people because the great majority of psychiatric problems go untreated. This has long been recognised in relation to adult disorders and epidemiological studies suggest that it is also true in childhood. Rutter (1970) found that only about 10% of children in the community with disorders were in contact with specialist services at any one time.

A second difficulty with official statistics is that when children do receive help for psychiatric problems it may come from a range of services: paediatric, education and social services as well as psychiatric services.

Many of the professionals (outside of the psychiatric services) who treat children with mental health problems may not use psychiatric classification systems in their practice. Those within the psychiatric service may use different classification systems.

Thus, official statistics on service use give little indication of the extent of childhood psychiatric disorders.

Review of previous research

Epidemiological surveys in Great Britain which have focused on psychiatric morbidity among children have concentrated on:

- Specific disorders - hyperactivity (Taylor et al., 1991), anorexia nervosa (Crisp et al., 1996), autism (Wing and Gould, 1978)

- Particular age ranges - adolescents (Kashani et al., 1987) ten year olds (Vikan, 1985)

- Comprehensive studies in particular localities - Isle of Wight (Rutter, 1976; Rutter, 1989), Edinburgh and Oxford (Platt et al., 1988) and Inner cities (Rutter, 1975).

Brandenberg et al (1990) reviewed the published reports from eight prevalence surveys of childhood and adolescent disorders carried out in the 1980s in Australia, Canada, Holland, New Zealand, Norway and the USA. She highlighted how the surveys differed in focus (psychiatric disorders), coverage (age, place of residence), sample design (number of stages, sample size, number and type of informants) and instrumentation. Prevalence rates varied from 5% (Vikan, 1985) to 26% (Verhulst et al., 1985) among 8 to 11 year olds.

A more recent review by Bird (1996) also demonstrated that different studies with different methodologies arrive at very varied prevalence estimates, with much higher rates being reported by studies that judge disorders just from symptoms without taking account of resultant social impairment.

Lessons from previous epidemiological surveys

Defining psychiatric disorder solely in terms of psychiatric symptoms can result in implausibly high rates. For example, Bird et al. (1988) estimated from their epidemiological study that about 50% of Puerto Rican children aged between 4 and 16 years met criteria for at least one DSM-III diagnosis. As Bird et al. (1990) noted, many of the children who were eligible for DSM-III diagnoses were not significantly socially impaired by their symptoms, did not seem in need of treatment, and did not correspond to what clinicians would normally recognise as "cases". This underlines the importance of defining psychiatric disorders not only in terms of symptom constellations, but also in terms of significant impact. Including impact criteria can dramatically alter prevalence estimates. For example, in the Virginia Twin Study, the population prevalence of DSM-III-R disorder was 42% as judged by symptoms alone, falling to 11% when impairment criteria were included (Simonoff et al., 1997).

In DSM-IV (American Psychiatric Association, 1994), most of the common child psychiatric disorders are now defined in terms of impact as well as symptoms; operational criteria stipulate that symptoms must result either in *substantial distress* for the child or in *significant impairment* in the child's ability to fulfil normal role expectations in everyday life. This same requirement for impact, in terms of significant distress or social incapacity, characterises the diagnostic criteria employed in the research version of ICD-10 (World Health Organization, 1994).

These findings emphasise the need to use measures of psychiatric disorder that consider not only symptoms but also resultant distress and social incapacity. Failure to do so will result in unrealistically high prevalence rates and will mislead service planners by labelling many children with relatively innocuous symptoms as having psychiatric disorders.

While previous surveys have often used measures of psychiatric disorder that inappropriately included children with many symptoms but little resultant impairment, these same surveys have inappropriately failed to diagnose another group of children who do make considerable and appropriate use of child and adolescent mental health services. Despite having psychiatric symptoms that result in distress and social impairment, these children do not meet the full criteria for an operationalised diagnosis such as hyperkinesis, separation anxiety disorder or oppositional defiant disorder. With clinical judgement, these children can be assigned non-operationalised diagnoses, e.g. anxiety disorder, Not Otherwise Specified (NOS); disruptive behaviour disorder, NOS.

A substantial minority of children with psychiatric disorders seem to "fall between the cracks" of the operationalised diagnostic categories because they have partial of undifferentiated syndromes (Goodman et al, 1996; Angold et al, 1999). This emphasises the need to incorporate clinical judgement into measures of psychiatric disorder so as not to miss children who are severely distressed or impaired by symptoms that do not meet current operationalised diagnostic criteria.

Does it matter if previous surveys have used measures of psychiatric disorder that are simultaneously over-inclusive and under-inclusive? As far as estimating prevalence is concerned, the problems or over-inclusiveness and under-inclusiveness will cancel out to some extent, though the number of children with symptoms but not much impact is substantially larger than the number with impact but relatively few symptoms.

As far as examining the appropriateness of current service provision is concerned, the two types of error add rather than cancel out. Diagnosing children who have symptoms without much impact will make it look as if services are failing to see these children. At the same time, failing to diagnose children who fall between the cracks of the current diagnostic system will make it look as if services are inappropriately (rather than correctly) seeing these children.

1.2 Aims of the survey

Prevalence

The primary purpose of the survey was to produce prevalence rates of three main categories of mental disorder: conduct disorder, hyperactivity and emotional disorders (and their comorbidity), based on ICD-10 and DSM-IV criteria. Where there were sufficient numbers, the survey also aimed to provide prevalence rates of type of problem (e.g., separation anxiety, social phobia etc.) and to investigate the comorbidity or co-occurrence of disorders.

Impact and burden

The second aim of the survey was to determine the *impact* and *burden* of children's mental health problems in terms of social impairment and adverse consequences for others.

The measurement of burden and impact are essential parts of the survey as they fulfil several functions: forming an integral part of diagnostic assessment, acting as measures of severity of the disorder, and helping to describe the problem in its social context. Social impairment is measured by the extent to which each particular mental problem interferes with relations with other family members, forming and keeping friendships, participation in leisure activities, and scholastic achievement. More broadly, impact reflects distress to the child or disruption to others as well as social impairment.

The *burden* of the child's problem is a measure of the consequences of the symptoms in terms of whether they cause distress to the family by making the parents worried, depressed, tired or physically ill. Whereas *impact* covers the consequences for the child, *burden* reflects the consequences for others.

Services

The third main purpose of the survey was to examine service provision. The examination of service use requires the measurement of contextual factors (stressful life events, lifestyle behaviours and risk factors). These factors are alluded to in The Health of the Nation: Key Area Handbook for Mental Illness in describing children's use of and need for services (Sections 3.27, 3.12 and 3.13).

"Particular attention should be paid to identifying the current provision of services dedicated to the needs of children and adolescents." (Section 3.27)

"The needs of children and adolescents are different from those of adults. Psycho-social factors which affect parents can also have distinct and separate effects on their children. In assessing needs, purchasers and providers will need to consider the child **and** the family, the school or college **and** the child's general social network." (Section 3.12)

"Some particular issues to consider when assessing the need for services for children and adolescents are: the rate and effect of changes in family circumstances such as separation, divorce or death of a parent; the level of homelessness and poor living conditions; and drug addiction and alcohol misuse in both children/adolescents and their parents." (Section 3.13)

Emotional and behavioural problems which resolve rapidly and spontaneously are far less relevant for service planning than problems that persist unless help is provided. While it is possible for a cross-sectional survey to ask informants to recall how long symptoms (and resultant impairments) have been present, there are well known biases associated with this sort of retrospective enquiry. The survey aimed to determine the prevalence of persistent disorders by asking a sample of informants about symptoms and resultant impairments on two separate occasions. Therefore, the main survey and its follow up component measure current psychopathology and examine whether help has been provided already, or whether help is provided over the course of the subsequent six months.

1.3 Timetable

Carrying out a national survey of the development and well-being of children and adolescents for the first time in Great Britain required a considerable amount of feasibility and pilot work. The general strategy was to look at various sampling strategies at the same time as designing and developing the interview schedules and interviewer procedures, and to carry out tests on children from the private household population as well as those known to have mental health problems. Comments were sought from experts in child psychiatric epidemiology, as well as those involved in service policy and practice. Figure 1.1 summarises the timetable for the whole programme of research.

1.4 Coverage of the survey

Region

The surveyed population comprised children and adolescents living in private households in England, Scotland (including the Highlands and Islands) and Wales.

Age

The survey focused on the prevalence of mental health problems among young people aged 5-15. Teenagers, aged 16 and above, were included in the previous adult surveys. Children under the age of 5 were excluded primarily because the assessment instruments for these children are different and not so well developed as those for older children.

The feasibility study which took place in January to March 1997 included a questionnaire for parents of 3 and 4 year olds. The questions were based on the Richman questionnaire revised by Nichol for a study of pre-school children (Nichol et al., 1987). Fifty seven families of 3-4 year olds were interviewed. The data were presented in terms of case studies which highlighted the areas where parents expressed concern about their children: eating habits, potty training, bedtime, indoor play etc. Discussions of the report on the feasibility study by an expert group recommended that 3 and 4 year olds should not be included in the main survey because of the problems in finding an appropriately sensitive instrument.

Childhood psychopathology

Though children and teenagers can be affected by many different mental health problems, most of these are rare. The survey concentrated on the three common groups of disorders: emotional disorders such as anxiety, depression and obsessions; hyperactivity disorders involving inattention and overactivity; and conduct disorders characterised by awkward, troublesome, aggressive and antisocial behaviours.

Figure 1.1 Timetable for survey

From	To	Activity
Sep.1994	Dec. 1995	Preliminary discussions between ONS and DH
Jan. 1995	Mar. 1995	Review of the literature, looking at the practicalities and logistics of carrying out a national survey, and evaluating the suitability of published assessment instruments
Jan. 1996	Mar. 1996	Reviewing options for a feasibility study
Apr.1996	Dec. 1996	Designing sample and questionnaires for feasibility study
Jan. 1997	Mar. 1997	Fieldwork for feasibility study
Apr. 1997	Dec. 1997	Analysis, interpretation and report writing of feasibility study and design of pilot survey
Jan. 1998	Mar. 1998	Fieldwork for pilot study
Apr. 1998	Dec. 1998	Analysis, interpretation and report writing of pilot study and design of main stage survey. Carrying out a mini-pilot in October 1998 to finalise survey documents
Jan. 1999	May. 1999	Main stage fieldwork
Apr. 1999	Aug. 1999	Clinical assessment of survey data
Jun. 1999	Jul. 1999	Six month, postal follow-up of respondents in fieldwork during January and February 1999.
Aug. 1999	Mar. 2000	Analysis, interpretation and report writing of main survey.

1.5   Content of the survey

A brief summary of the sections of the questionnaire is shown below, subsumed under the headings of questionnaire content for parents, children and teachers. The rationale behind using three sources of information is described in Chapter 2.

Questionnaire content for parents

This interview schedule for parents was asked of a parent of all selected children. It included the following sections:

- Background characteristics
- General Health
- Strengths and Difficulties Questionnaire(SDQ)
- Post Traumatic Stress Disorder (PTSD)
- Separation anxiety
- Specific Phobias
- Social Phobia
- Panic attacks and agoraphobia
- Compulsions and Obsessions
- Generalised Anxiety
- Depression
- Attention and activity
- Awkward and troublesome behaviour
- Less Common Disorders
- Impact
- Significant problems
- Use of services for significant problems

- Stressful Life Events

- Use of all types of services
- Strengths
- Education and Employment (parent and partner)
- State Benefits (parent and partner)

- Self completion: GHQ12 and Family Functioning

Questionnaire content for children and adolescents

Questions for children aged 11-15, by face to face interview, included the following topics:

- Friendship
- Strengths and Difficulties Questionnaire (SDQ)

- Separation anxiety
- Specific Phobias
- Social Phobia
- Panic attacks and agoraphobia
- Post Traumatic Stress Disorder (PTSD)
- Compulsions and Obsessions
- Generalised Anxiety
- Depression
- Attention and activity
- Awkward and troublesome behaviour
- Less Common Disorders
- Significant problems
- Strengths

The self-completion element for the 11 to 15-year-olds included:

- Chronic fatigue syndrome (M.E.)
- Awkward and troublesome behaviour
- Moods and feelings
- Help from others
- Smoking cigarettes
- Use of alcohol
- Experience with drugs

All children, aged 5-15 were assessed for dyslexia by means of the British Picture Vocabulary Scale (BPVS-II) and the reading and spelling elements of the British Abilities Scale (BAS-II). The rationale behind the choice of instruments and their administration are described in Chapter 8.

Questionnaire content for teachers

A postal questionnaire was sent to teachers covering scholastic achievement as well as assessments of behaviour and emotional well-being:

- Scholastic achievement and special needs
- Strengths and Difficulties Questionnaire (SDQ)
- Emotions
- Attention, activity and impulsiveness
- Awkward and troublesome behaviour
- Other concerns
- Help from school

1.6   Coverage of the report

One of the main purposes of this report is to present prevalence rates for mental disorders among children and adolescents aged 5-15 in England, Scotland and Wales during the first half of 1999. These are presented in Chapter 4.

In order to interpret these results, it is important to have an understanding of the concepts and methods adopted for this study; these are described in Chapter 2. Chapter 3 describes the sampling and interview procedures.

Part 2 of the report contains 6 chapters on specific topics (e.g. physical illness, services or social functioning) for children with all disorders as distinct from chapters on particular disorders.

The final part of the Report contains the technical appendices and has six sections. The first gives details of the sampling design and shows how the data were weighted. The second section describes the statistical terms used in the report and their interpretation. The third section gives examples of standard errors from the prevalence tables. Section 4 presents the results of a 6 month follow up study of a subsample of survey respondents. The last two sections comprise the survey documents and a glossary of terms.

1.7   Access to the data

Anonymised data from the survey will be lodged with the ESRC Data Archive, University of Essex, within 3 months of the publication of this report. Independent researchers who wish to carry out their own analyses should apply to the Archive for access. For further information about archived data, please contact:

> ESRC Data Archive
> University of Essex
> Wivenhoe Park
> Colchester
> Essex CO4 3SQ
>
> Tel: (UK) 01206 872323
> FAX: (UK) 01206 872003
> Email: archive@Essex.AC.UK

References

American Psychiatric Association (1994). *Diagnostic and Statistical Manual of Mental Disorders (4th edn).* Washington, DC: American Psychiatric Association.

Angold, A., Costello, E. J., Farmer, E. M. Z., Burns, B. J & Erkanli, A. (1999) Impaired but undiagnosed. *Journal of the American Academy of Child and Adolescent Psychiatry*, 38, 129-137.

Bird, H. R. (1996) Epidemiology of childhood disorders in a cross-cultural context. *Journal of Child Psychology and Psychiatry*, 37, 35-49.

Bird, H. B., Canino, G., Rubio-Stipec, M., Gould, M. S., Ribera, J., Sesman, M., Woodbury, M., Huertas-Goldman, S., Pagan, A., Sanchez-Lacay, A. & Moscoso, M. (1988). Estimates of the prevalence of childhood maladjustment in a community survey in Puerto Rico. *Archives of General Psychiatry*, 45, 1120-1126.

Bird, H. B., Yager, T. J., Staghezza, B., Gould, M. S., Canino, G. & Rubio-Stipec, M. (1990). Impairment in the epidemiological measurement of childhood psychopathology in the community. *Journal of the American Academy of Child and Adolescent Psychiatry*, 29, 796-803.

Brandenburg, N.A., Friedman, R.M., Silver, S.E., (1990) "The epidemiology of child psychiatric disorder: prevalence findings from recent studies" *Journal of the American Academy of Child and Adolescent Psychiatry*, 29:76-83

Crisp, A.H., Palmer, R.L., Kalucy, R.S., (1976) How common is anorexia nervosa? A prevalence study", *British Journal of Psychiatry* ,128:549-54

Department of Health, (1995) *The Health of the Nation Handbook on Child and Adolescent Mental Health*

Foster K, Meltzer H, Gill B and Hinds K. (1996) *OPCS Surveys of Psychiatric Morbidity in Great Britain, Report 8: Adults with a psychotic disorder living in the community* HMSO: London

Gill B, Meltzer H, Hinds K and Petticrew, M., (1996) *OPCS Surveys of Psychiatric Morbidity in Great Britain, Report 7: Psychiatric morbidity among homeless people*, HMSO: London.

Goodman, R. (1997). The Strengths and Difficulties Questionnaire: A research note. *Journal of Child Psychology and Psychiatry*, 38, 581-586.

Goodman, R. (1999) The extended version of the Strengths and Difficulties Questionnaire as a guide to child psychiatric caseness and consequent burden. *Journal of Child Psychology and Psychiatry*, 40, 791-801.

Goodman, R., Meltzer, H., & Bailey V. (1998) The Strengths and Difficulties Questionnaire: A pilot study on the validity of the self-report version. *European Child and Adolescent Psychiatry*, 7, 125-130.

Goodman, R. & Scott, S. (1999) Comparing the Strengths and Difficulties Questionnaire and the Child Behaviour Checklist: Is small beautiful? *Journal of Abnormal Child Psychology*, 27, 17-24.

Goodman, R., Yude, C., Richards, H. & Taylor, E. (1996) Rating child psychiatric caseness from detailed case histories. *Journal of Child Psychology and Psychiatry*, 37, 369-379.

Kashani, J.H., Beck, N.C., Hoeper, E.W. et al (1987) Psychiatric Disorders in a community sample of adolescents. *Am. J. Psychiatry* 144: 584-589

Maughan, B., (1995) *Mental Health* in (ed.) B. Botting *The Health of Our Children*, London: HMSO

Meltzer H, Gill B, Petticrew M and Hinds, K. (1995a) *OPCS Surveys of Psychiatric Morbidity in Great Britain, Report 1: the prevalence of psychiatric morbidity among adults living in private households.* HMSO: London

Meltzer H, Gill B, Petticrew M and Hinds, K.(1995b) *OPCS Surveys of Psychiatric Morbidity in Great Britain, Report 2: Physical complaints, service use and treatment of adults with psychiatric disorders.* HMSO: London

Meltzer H, Gill B, Petticrew, M and Hinds K. (1995c) *OPCS Surveys of Psychiatric Morbidity in Great Britain, Report 3: Economic activity and social functioning of adults with psychiatric disorders.* HMSO: London

Meltzer H, Gill B, Hinds K and Petticrew M. (1996a) *OPCS Surveys of Psychiatric Morbidity in Great Britain, Report 4 The prevalence of psychiatric morbidity among adults living in institutions,* HMSO: London

Meltzer H, Gill B, Hinds K and Petticrew M. (1996b) *OPCS Surveys of Psychiatric Morbidity in Great Britain, Report 5: Physical complaints, service use and treatment of residents with psychiatric disorders.* HMSO: London

Meltzer H, Gill B, Hinds K and Petticrew M. (1996c) *OPCS Surveys of Psychiatric Morbidity in Great Britain, Report 6: Economic activity and social functioning of residents with psychiatric disorders.* HMSO: London

Nicol, A.R., Stretch, D.D., Fundundis, T., Smith, I and Davidson, I., (1987) The nature of mother and toddler problems - I Development of a multiple criterion screen. *J. Child Psychol. Psychiatry,* **28**:739-754

Platt, S., Hawton, K., Kreitman, N., Fagg, J., Foster, J., (1988) Recent clinical and epidemiological trends in parasuicide in Edinburgh and Oxford: a tale of two cities *Psychological Medicine* **18**:405-18

Rutter, M., Tizard, J., and, Whitmore, K., (1970) *Education, health and behaviour,* Longmans, London

Rutter, M., Cox, A., Tupling, C., Berger, M., Yule, W., (1975), "Attainment and adjustment in two geographical areas I. The prevalence of psychiatric disorder" *Br. J. Psychiatry* **126**, 493-509

Rutter, M., Tizard, J., Yule, W., Graham, P., Whitmore, K., (1976) Research report: *The Isle of Wight Studies* 1964-1974 *Psychological Medicine* **6**:313-32

Rutter, M., (1989) Isle of Wight Revisited: *Twenty five years of Child Psychiatric Epidemiology* American Academy of Child and Adolescent Psychiatry.

Simonoff, E., Pickles, A., Meyer, J. M., Silberg, J., Maes, H. H., Loeber, R., Rutter, M., Hewitt, J. K. & Eaves, L. J. (1997). The Virginia twin study of adolescent behavioral development: influences of age, gender and impairment on rates of disorder. *Archives of General Psychiatry,* **54**, 801-808.

Singleton, N., Meltzer, H., Gatward, R., Coid, J., and Deasey, D. (1998) *Psychiatric morbidity among prisoners in England and Wales* HMSO: London

Taylor, E., Sandberg, S., Thorley, G., Giles, S., (1991) "*The epidemiology of childhood hyperactivity*", Oxford, Oxford University Press

Verhulst, F.C., Berden, G.F.M.G., Sanders-Woudstra, J.A.R., (1985), Mental health in Dutch children: (II) the prevalence of psychiatric disorder and relationship between measures *Acta Psychiatr. Scand. Suppl.* **324**, 1-45

Vikan, A., (1985) Psychiatric epidemiology in a sample of 1510 ten-tear-old children, I. *J. Child Psychol. Psychiatry,* **26**: 55-75

Wing, L., Gould, J., (1978), Systematic recording of behaviours and skills of retarded and psychotic children *J. Autism Child. Schizophr.* **8**, 79-97

World Health Organisation (1993) *The ICD-10 classification of mental and behavioural disorders: diagnostic criteria for research.* World Health Organisation: Geneva

2 Concepts and methods used in assessing mental disorders

2.1 Introduction

This chapter is divided into five sections. In the first of them, the use of the term, mental disorder, in relation to young people is discussed and the definitions of the terms used in this report are outlined. The second section aims to define concepts related to prevalence. This is followed by a discussion of methods of assessment, in particular the choice between one- and two-stage sampling designs and the selection of assessment instruments. The penultimate section examines the advantages of gathering information from multiple informants (parent, teacher and child) and the chapter ends with a description of how a clinical input was added to the interpretation of the survey data.

Estimates of the prevalence of psychiatric morbidity among young people depend on the choice of concepts as well as how they are operationalised. These, in turn, depend on the particular purposes and aims of the study. This point needs emphasising because it means that estimates from this survey will not necessarily be comparable with those obtained from other studies using different concepts and methods or using samples which may not be representative of the total population of children and adolescents aged 5-15.

2.2 Definitions of mental disorder

Although this survey report uses the term, mental disorder, in relation to children, there is a recognition that this terminology can cause concern. (NHS Health Advisory Service, 1995)

"First such terms can be stigmatising, and mark the child as being different. However, unless children with mental health problems are recognised, and some attempt is made to understand and classify their problems, in the context of their social, educational and health needs, it is very difficult to organise helpful interventions for them. The second concern is that the term mental disorder may be taken to indicate that the problem is entirely within the

child. In reality, disorders may arise for a variety of reasons, often interacting. In certain circumstances, a mental or psychiatric disorder, which describes a constellation or syndrome of features, may indicate the reactions of a child or adolescent to external circumstances, which, if changed, could largely resolve the problem."

"It is important to define terms relating to the mental health of children and adolescents because experience shows that lack of terminological clarity leads to confusion and uncertainty about the suffering involved, the treatability of problems and disorders and the need to allocate resources."

Because the questionnaires used in this survey were based on ICD-10 and DSM-IV diagnostic research criteria, this report uses the terms mental disorders as defined by the ICD-10: to imply a clinically recognisable set of symptoms or behaviour associated in most cases with considerable distress and substantial interference with personal functions.

2.3 Concepts

Period prevalence

This survey aims to establish the prevalence of mental disorders during a particular period prior to interview. This time period is not the same for each disorder and is subject to various criteria:

- Criteria imposed by the measurement instrument
- Criteria chosen by the research team
- Criteria contingent on the nature of the disorder itself
- Criteria imposed by the nature of the sample

Co-occurrence of disorders

Instruments used for clinical assessments of psychiatric disorders often allow for several possible diagnoses to be made. Although it would be possible to impose a hierarchy among different disorders, the prevalence rates presented in subsequent chapters of this report do not have a hierarchy imposed on them. Thus, individuals with multiple diagnoses can be represented in several parts of a table. However, Chapter 4 of this report does present data on the co-occurrence of disorders.

2.4   Methods of assessing mental disorders

Two key decisions had to be made in deciding how to measure the prevalence of mental disorders of children and adolescents. The first related to whether to adopt a one- or two-stage design, i.e. ask all questions of all respondents or start off with a short screening instrument applicable to all children followed up with a detailed assessment with all screen positives and a sample of screen negatives. The second crucial question was whether to use or adapt an existing instrument or create a new one afresh from first principles.

We decided on adopting a one-stage design with a questionnaire created anew based on ICD-10 and DSM-IV diagnostic research criteria. The strengths and weaknesses of the options considered are described below.

One- versus two-stage designs

About half of the national surveys that have been carried out in other countries have used the multimethod-multistage approach of Rutter et al. (1970) to ascertain potential cases. In this approach, rating scales completed by children above a certain age and/or parents and/or teachers are used as first stage screening instruments. Subjects with scores above the cut-off score are identified as potential cases and further evaluated. A small sample of individuals with scores below the cut-off threshold are also selected for interview to assess the frequency of false negatives, i.e., those who have problems but whose rating scale scores were below the cut-off score.

In the second stage, children with scores above the cut-off score and a sample of those with scores below this value are interviewed using semi-structured or structured psychiatric interview instruments. At this stage categorical diagnoses are made. The overall prevalence of disorder is determined at the conclusion of this two-stage process.

The other method does not base caseness upon the multimethod-multistage approach. All children and adolescents identified through the initial sampling procedure are eligible for diagnostic assessment. There are many advantages of such an approach:

- Detailed information is collected on all children. A sample distribution can be produced on all subscales even though only those with above-threshold score will have psychopathology.

- Because the survey aims to investigate service use, social disabilities, stressful life events, risk factors and the use of tobacco, alcohol and drugs, it is also important to have this information for all children from which a control sample can be selected.

- With the possibility of a longitudinal element in the survey, there is a large pool of children from which to select controls who could be matched on several characteristics to the children who exhibit significant psychiatric symptoms during the first stage interview.

- A one-stage design is likely to increase the overall response rate compared with a two-stage (screening plus clinical assessment) design.

- A one-stage design reduces the burden put on respondents. Ideally, a two-stage design would require a screening questionnaire to be asked of a parent, a teacher as well as the child, followed up with an assessment interview administered to the child and the parent. A one-stage design only requires an interview with the parent and child and, if possible, the administration of a teacher questionnaire.

- One of the advantages of a one-stage over a two-stage design is that its implementation is cheaper and can be carried out in a far shorter timescale.

Screening instruments

Two rating scales have commonly been used for the first-stage, screening process in community-based studies of children: the Rutter Scales: A and B

(Rutter et al., 1970), the Child Behaviour Checklist (Achenbach and Edelbrock, 1983).

The Rutter Child Scale A and Rutter Child Scale B cover aspects of behavioural and emotional functioning within the past year. These scales were used as first-stage screening instruments in their entirety (Connell et al., 1982), or in an abridged form (Vikan, 1985). The Rutter scales, along with additional items assessing attention deficit disorder and affective disorder, were used to gather supplementary information in the New Zealand study (Anderson et al., 1987).

The Child Behaviour Checklist (CBCL) describes symptoms of emotional and behavioural disturbance over the past 6 months. It is a 138-item scale for use with 4 to 16 year-olds and assesses a wide range of pathological behaviours (118 items) and the child's social competence (20 items). Parent and teacher forms were used to screen subjects in the Netherlands (Verhulst et al., 1985) and Puerto Rico (Bird et al., 1988).

However, the CBCL has often criticised as being unnecessarily long, as having a negative perspective and may not be better than the more quickly-administered instrument like the Rutter scales.

The Strengths and Difficulties Questionnaire

Another brief alternative to the CBCL is the Strengths and Difficulties Questionnaire (SDQ), which is a brief behavioural screening questionnaire that can be administered to the parents and teachers of 4-16 year olds and also to 11-16 year olds themselves. It covers common areas of emotional and behavioural difficulties, also enquiring whether the informant thinks that the child has a problem in these areas, and if so, asking about resultant distress and social impairment. It has been shown to be of acceptable reliability and validity, performing at least as well as the CBCL and Rutter questionnaires (Goodman, 1997; Goodman et al., 1998; Goodman & Scott, 1999; Goodman, 1999). Though originally published in English, it is currently available in over 40 languages, including Welsh, Gaelic and the languages spoken by the main immigrant communities in Britain. The SDQ was used in the 1997 Health Survey for England. (McMann et al., 1996)

Diagnostic instruments

In his review of diagnostic instruments, Angold (1989) makes the distinction between fully-structured and semi-structured diagnostic interviews.

The semi-structured interviews which were reviewed either can not be undertaken by lay interviewers without extensive additional training or do not cover the desired age range:

K-SADS (Schedule for Affective Disorders and Schizophrenia) requires considerable clinical judgement. It is intended for administration by clinically sophisticated interviewers.

ISC (Interview Schedule for Children) requires extensive clinical experience and interview-specific training. The final diagnosis is arrived at in a group conference.

CAS (Child Assessment Schedule) has been used by lay interviewers but is only suitable for children aged 7 to 12.

CAPA (Child and Adolescent Psychiatric Assessment) requires substantial training to produce sufficient familiarity with the instrument especially for those who are clinically inexperienced. It applies to children aged 8-16. One of the advantages that it has over the previous three instruments is that it can produce ICD-10 diagnoses (as well as DSM-III-R).

The two, fully-structured, interview schedules reviewed by Angold (1989) were the DISC (Diagnostic Interview Schedule for Children) and the DICA (Diagnostic Interview for Children and Adolescents).

The DISC is applicable for children aged 6 and above. An interview with the child takes 40-60 minutes and the parent version about 60-70 minutes. Non-clinically trained interviewers require about 2-3 days training. It generates DSM-III-R diagnoses. Diagnostic algorithms for scoring the results of the interview are available

The DICA is applicable to children aged 6 and above. It takes about 40-45 minutes to complete and exists for administration to parents or children. Only a short period of interviewing training is necessary, and interviewers do not need to have had clinical experience. It is can be scored for ICD diagnoses.

Hodges (1993) has also reviewed structured interviews for assessing psychiatric morbidity among children: CAPA, CAS, DICA, DISC, ISC, K-SADS. She looks at what lessons have been learnt from their use and reliability and validity data. Unfortunately, prevalence studies are not covered in the scope of her review.

Constructing a new instrument

The measures designed for the present study were intended to combine some of the best features of structured and semi-structured measures. Using existing semi-structured measures for a large national survey would have been impractical and prohibitively expensive since it would have required recruiting a team of several hundred clinically trained interviewers or providing prolonged additional training and supervision to lay interviewers.

Given the practical and financial imperative to use lay interviewers with relatively little additional training, it was clear that the main interviewing would need to be fully structured. The disadvantage of relying entirely upon existing structured interviews is that the results are far less clinically convincing than the results of surveys based on semi-structured interviewing. When informants answer fully structured interviews, they often over-report rare symptoms and syndromes because they have not really understood the questions. (Brugha et al., 1999) To circumvent this problem, the new measures use structured interviewing supplemented by open-ended questions. When definite symptoms are identified by the structured questions, interviewers use open-ended questions and supplementary prompts to get parents to describe the problems in their own words. The specfic prompts used were:

Description of the problem
Specific examples
What happened the last time?
What sorts of things does s/he worry about?
How often does the problem occur?
Is it many times a day, most weeks, or just once or twice?
Is it still a problem?

How severe is the problem at it's worst?
How long has it been going on for?
Is the problem interfering with the child's quality of life?
If so, how?
Where appropriate, what does the family/child think the problem is do to and what have they done about it?

Answers to these questions and any other information given are transcribed verbatim by the interviewers but are not rated by them. Interviewers are also given the opportunity to make additional comments, where appropriate, on the respondents' understanding and motivation.

A small team of experienced clinicians review the transcripts and interviewers' comments to ensure that the answers to structured questions are not misleading. The same clinical reviewers can also consider clashes of information between different informants, deciding which account to prioritise. Furthermore, children with clinically relevant problems that do not quite meet the operationalised diagnostic criteria can be assigned suitable diagnoses by the clinical raters. There are no existing diagnostic tools that combine the advantages of structured and semi-structured assessments in this sort of way, which is why a new set of measures were specifically designed for this survey.

The new measures and their validity are described in more detail elsewhere. (Goodman et al., 2000)

2.5   Single versus multiple informants

While single-informant investigation characterised nearly all of the early epidemiological studies, more recent studies (within the multi-method multi-stage approach) have broadened data collection to include information gathered from parents, teachers, and the subjects themselves. Hodges (1993) has pointed out that children and adolescents can respond to direct questions aimed at enquiring about their mental status and that there is no indication that asking these direct questions has any morbidity or mortality risks.

A well-established fact is that information from many sources is a better predictor of disorder than just one source. Many experienced clinicians and researchers in child psychiatry believe that information gleaned from multiple informants facilitates the best estimate of diagnosis in the individual case (Young et al., 1987). At the population level, information from multiple informants enhance the specificity of prevalence estimates.

Angold (1989) states:

"In general, parents often seem to have a limited knowledge of children's internal mental states and to report less in the way of depressive and anxiety symptoms than their children would report. On the other hand adults seem to be better informants about externalised or conduct disorder items such as fighting and disobedience. Teachers are good informants about school behaviour and performance, whilst parents are informative about home life."

Hodges (1993) comments that agreement between child and parent has varied depending on type of pathology:

"There appears to be more agreement for behavioural symptoms, moderate agreement for depressive symptoms, and poor agreement for anxiety."

One of the problems of collecting information from various sources is finding the best way to integrate the information which may show a lack of agreement. One method has been to accept a diagnosis irrespective of its source (Bird et al., 1992). Others have promoted "case vignette" assessments where clinical judgements are made on detailed case histories from several sources. (Goodman et al., 1996)

2.6 Case vignette assessment

This case vignette approach for analysing survey data uses clinician ratings based on a review of all the information of each subject. This information includes not only the questionnaires and structured interviews but also any additional comments made by the interviewers, and the transcripts of informants' comments to open-ended questions particularly those which ask about the child's significant problems. The case vignette approach was extensively tested among community and clinical samples in the pre-pilot and pilot phases of the survey.

The clinical raters perform four major tasks. Firstly, they use the transcripts to check whether respondents appear to have understood the fully structured questions. This is particularly valuable for relatively unusual symptoms such as obsessions and compulsions - even when parents or young people say "yes" to items about such symptoms, their own description of the problem often makes it clear that they are not describing what a clinician would consider to be an obsession or compulsion.

Secondly, the clinical raters consider how to interpret conflicts of evidence between informants. Reviewing the transcripts and interviewers' comments often helps decide whose account to prioritise. Reviewing all of the evidence, it may be clear that one respondent gives a convincing account of symptoms, whereas the other respondent minimises all symptoms in a defensive way. Conversely, one respondent may clearly be exaggerating.

Thirdly, the clinical raters aim to catch those emotional, conduct and hyperactivity disorders that slip through the 'operationalised' net. When the child has a clinically significant problem that does not meet operationalised diagnostic criteria, the clinician can assign a 'not otherwise specified' diagnosis such as 'anxiety disorder, NOS' or 'disruptive behaviour disorder, NOS.'

Finally, the clinical raters rely primarily on the transcripts to diagnose less common disorders such as anorexia nervosa, Tourette syndrome, autistic disorders, agoraphobia or schizophrenia. The relevant symptoms are so distinctive that respondents' descriptions are often unmistakable.

The following three case vignettes from the pilot study provide illustrative examples of subjects where the clinical rating altered the diagnosis. In each case the "computer-generated diagnosis" is the diagnosis arrived at by a computer algorithm based exclusively on the answers to fully structured questions. In these three illustrative instances, the computer-generated diagnoses were changed by the clinical raters.

Subject 1: overturning a computer-generated diagnosis. A 13 year-old boy was given a computer diagnosis of a specific phobia because he had a fear that resulted in significant distress and avoidance. In his open-ended description of the fear, he explained that boys from another school had threatened him on his way home on several occasions. Since then, he had been afraid of this gang and had taken a considerably longer route home every day in order to avoid them. The clinical rater judged his fear and avoidance to be appropriate responses to a realistic danger and not a phobia.

Subject 2: including a diagnosis not made by the computer. A 7-year-old girl fell just short of the computer algorithm's threshold for a diagnosis of ADHD because the teacher reported that the problems with restlessness and inattentiveness resulted in very little impairment in learning and peer relationships at school. A review of all the evidence showed that the girl had officially recognised special educational needs as a result of hyperactivity problems, could not concentrate in class for more than 2 minutes at a time even on activities she enjoyed, and had been offered a trial of medication. The clinician concluded that the teacher's report of minimal impairment was an understatement, allowing a clinical diagnosis of ADHD to be made.

Subject 3: both adding to and subtracting from computer generated diagnoses. A 14-year-old girl received computer-generated diagnoses of simple phobia, major depression and oppositional-defiant disorder. The transcripts of the open-ended comments provided by the girl and her mother included convincing descriptions not only of a depressive disorder but also of anorexia nervosa of one year's duration. The supposed phobia was an anorexic fear of food, and the oppositionality had only been present for a year and was primarily related to battles over food intake. Consequently, the clinical rater made the additional diagnosis of anorexia nervosa and overturned the diagnoses of simple phobia and oppositional-defiant disorder.

References

Achenbach, T.M., & Edelbrock, C.S., (1983), *"Manual for the Child Behaviour Checklist and Revised Child Behaviour Profile",* Burlington, Vermont, University of Vermont, Department of Psychiatry.

American Psychiatric Association (1994). *Diagnostic and Statistical Manual of Mental Disorders (4th edn).* Washington, DC: American Psychiatric Association.

Angold, A. (1989) Structured assessments of psychopathology in children and adolescents in (ed) C. Thompson, *The Instruments of Psychiatric Research*, John Wiley & Sons Ltd.

Anderson, J.C., Williams, S., McGee, R. & Silva, P.A. (1987) DSM-III disorders in preadolescent children, *Arch. Gen. Psychiatry*, **44**: 69-76

Bird, H.R., et al, (1988), Estimates of the prevalence of childhood maladjustment in a community survey in Puerto Rico, *Arch. Gen. Psychiatry*, **45**: 1120-1126

Bird, H.R., Gould, M.S. and Staghezza, B. (1992) Aggregating data from multiple informants in child psychiatry epidemiological research. *J. Am. Acad. Child Adol. Psychiatry* **31**, 78-85

Brugha, T.S., Bebbington, P.E., and Jenkins R. (1999) A difference that matters: comparisons of structured and semi-structured psychiatric disgnostic interviews in the general population. *Psychological Medicine,* **29**. 1013-1020

Connell, H.M., Irvine, L., & Rodney, J. (1982) Psychiatric Disorder in Queensland primary schoolchildren. *Aust. Paediatr. J.,* **18**: 177-180

Goodman, R. (1997). The Strengths and Difficulties Questionnaire: A research note. *Journal of Child Psychology and Psychiatry*, **38**, 581-586.

Goodman, R. (1999) The extended version of the Strengths and Difficulties Questionnaire as a guide to child psychiatric caseness and consequent burden. *Journal of Child Psychology and Psychiatry,* **40**, 791-801.

Goodman, R., Meltzer, H., & Bailey V. (1998) The Strengths and Difficulties Questionnaire: A pilot study on the validity of the self-report version. *European Child and Adolescent Psychiatry*, **7**, 125-130.

Goodman, R. & Scott, S. (1999) Comparing the Strengths and Difficulties Questionnaire and the Child Behavior Checklist: Is small beautiful? *Journal of Abnormal Child Psychology*, **27**, 17-24.

Goodman, R., Yude, C., Richards, H. & Taylor, E. (1996) Rating child psychiatric caseness from detailed case histories. *Journal of Child Psychology and Psychiatry,* **37**, 369-379.

Hodges, K., Structured Interviews for Assessing Children (1993) *J. Child Psychol. Psychiatry* **34**: 49-68

Rutter, M., Tizard, J., and, Whitmore, K., (1970) *Education, health and behaviour*, Longmans, London

Verhulst, F.C., Berden, G.F.M.G., Sanders-Woudstra, J.A.R., (1985), "Mental health in Dutch children: (II) the prevalence of psychiatric disorder and relationship between measures" in *Acta Psychiatr. Scand. Suppl.* **324**, 1-45

Vikan, A., (1985) Psychiatric epidemiology in a sample of 1510 ten-tear-old children, I. *J. Child Psychol. Psychiatry*, **26**: 55-75

World Health Organisation (1993) *The ICD-10 classification of mental and behavioural disorders: diagnostic criteria for research.* World Health Organisation: Geneva

Young, J.G., O'Brien, J.D., Gutterman, E.M. & Cohen, P., (1987) Research on the clinical interview. *J. Am. Acad. Child Adol. Psychiatry* **26**, 5: 613-620

3 Sampling and survey procedures

3.1 Introduction

This chapter covers three main topics: the sampling design, the organisation of the survey and survey response.

3.2 Sample design

The sampling design for the survey was different from and many other surveys carried out by ONS in that the Postcode Address File was not used as the sampling frame. Instead the sample was drawn from Child Benefit Records held by the Child Benefit Centre (CBC). Using centralised records as a sampling frame was preferred to carrying out a postal sift of over 100,000 addresses and to sampling through schools. The postal sift would have been time consuming and expensive. We did not want to sample through schools because we wanted our initial contact to be parents who then would give signed consent to approach the child's teacher.

We were aware that 90% of child benefit records have postcodes attributed to addresses. The Child Benefit Centre had no evidence that records with postcodes were different from those without. The addresses with missing postcodes probably represent a mixture of people who did not know their postcode at the time of applying for child benefit or simply forgot to enter the details on the form. If there are other factors which differentiate between households with and without postcoded addresses, the key question is to what extent these factors are related to the mental health of children. As these factors are not known, we do not know what biases have been introduced into the survey by omitting the non-postcoded addresses.

We also excluded from the original sampling frame those cases where "action" was being invoked. Examples of such action are: the death of the child and a change of address. They are simply administrative actions as distinct from some legal process concerning the child and hence should not bias the sample in any way.

Another consequence of sampling from child benefit records rather than the Postcode Address File was having less control over the proximity of addresses. In order to exert some control over this we asked the CBC to list records by postcode (e.g. AB1 2AA, AB1 2AB .... AB1 2ZY, AB1 2ZZ) and than stratify by age and sex within postcode.

In order to keep within data protection guidelines, we had to go through several steps to get our sample. First, we supplied the Child Benefit Centre with the list of 475 postal sectors we wanted covered. We then gave them details of how to calculate the sampling fraction to apply to their records in each postal sector in order to select 30 children whose parents received child benefit. We then asked them to send out a letter on our behalf telling them about our survey and giving parents an opportunity to opt-out.

To manage this process, the sectors were grouped into three waves.

Table 3.1 shows that 14,250 letters were despatched by the Child Benefit Centre on behalf of ONS: 30 letters for each of the 475 postal sectors. Nine hundred and thirty one of the sampled addresses (6.5%) contacted ONS via a free phone number to opt out and a further 790 addresses (5.5%) were found to be ineligible. The main reason for ineligibility was that the family had moved and could not be traced. This accounted for 629 of the 790 ineligibles - 4.4% overall. Other reasons for ineligibility were that the child was deceased, in foster care, outside the age criteria, 5-15, or the family had emigrated. Therefore, just over twelve and a half thousand addresses were allocated to around 300 interviewers. *(Table 3.1)*

Table 3.1	Response to initial CBC letter			
	Wave1	Wave 2	Wave 3	All
Sampled children	4183	4394	5673	14250
Opt outs	267	276	388	931
Ineligibles	196	257	337	790
Children eligible for interview	3720	3861	4948	12529

3.3 Survey procedures

Checking CBC information

When the interviewer went to the address of the sampled child, her first task was to find out if the family still lived there and if the name was correct. Experience from the pilot survey indicated that many of the addresses from the CBC were out of date. The families had changed address and not informed the CBC. Because the survey had a national coverage, attempts were made to trace the movers, and the family reallocated to another interviewer working in the vicinity of the new address.

Interviewers also found that, in many cases, the names of both the selected child and the mother had changed owing to new relationships: remarriage, change of partner, etc. In this regard, the interviewers also checked that they had the right address.

Order of interview

The first stage of the interview was the completion of the face to face interview with the parent including a five minute self-completion element (GHQ12 and Family Functioning Scale). If the parent had difficulties with the English language a special two page self-completion questionnaire available in 40 languages was available as a replacement.

After the parent interview, permission was sought to ask questions of the sampled child. Children aged 11-15 had a face to face interview and entered details of their smoking, drinking and drug-taking experiences via a self-completion questionnaire on laptop. All children, from 5 to 15 years, were administered reading and spelling tests.

When the parent and child interviews were completed, parents were asked for written consent to contact the child's teacher. Parents were asked to nominate the teacher who they felt knew the child best. If the child had been expelled or excluded from school within the last few months, contact names for teachers were still sought.

Before the teachers' questionnaire was posted out, various steps were taken to maximise response:

- A paragraph describing the survey was inserted into a journal which goes to all teachers.
- Chief Education Officers were notified of the plans for the survey and the extent of teachers' involvement.
- A week before any postal questionnaires were sent off to teachers, the head teachers in all schools of the sampled children were notified that some of their teachers would be sent a questionnaire to fill in.
- The sample design with 475 postal sectors and the stratification of the CBC list were intended to reduce the burden on teachers so that most would not have to fill in more than two questionnaires.

3.4 Survey response rates

Information was collected on 83% of the 12,529 children eligible for interview from up to three sources resulting in 10,438 achieved interviews. *(Table 3.2)*

Among the co-operating families, almost all the parents and most of the children took part. Four out of five teachers also returned their questionnaires, based on an initial mail out and one reminder letter. *(Table 3.3)*

Table 3.2 Response to interview

	Wave1		Wave 2		Wave 3		All	
All interviews	3100	(83%)	3191	(83%)	4147	(85%)	10438	(83%)
Refusals	545	(15%)	543	(14%)	686	(13%)	1774	(15%)
Non-contacts	76	(2%)	127	(3%)	114	(2%)	317	(2%)
Base=set sample	*3721*		*3861*		*4947*		*12529*	

Table 3.3	Achieved interviews by type of informant	
	Number	%
Parent interviews	10405	(99.7%)
Child interviews/assessments	9347	(95.3%)
Teacher questionnaire	8382	(80.3%)
Base= achieved interviews	*10438*	

3.5   Interviewing procedures

Choice of parent to interview

In most interviews, over 95%, the interview with the parent was carried out with the mothers as they tended to be more available when the interviewer called. In the cases where the father was interviewed, the mother did not speak sufficient English to cope with the interview. The remainder were cases of lone fathers or fathers who were at home by themselves most of the time.

Logistics of arranging interviews

The unpredictable length of the interview meant that interviewers had to make appointments when mothers would have a clear 90-120 minutes. This was often difficult for those mothers who had several children with different 'pick-up' times from school and nursery, and mothers with full or part time jobs. In some areas, this meant that the interviewer could arrange an interview in the morning, but could not start again until children were back from school and parents, if employed, were back from work. Interviewers reported that some of the children had even busier 'social calendars' than their parents and a lot of flexibility (on the interviewer's part) was needed to complete both the parent and the child interview.

Privacy

The need for privacy in the interviews (for both parent and child) also affected the logistics of appointment making. It was obviously easier for the mother if none of her children were around (not just the selected child). This was clearly difficult if the mother worked during the day. Children's interviews, by definition, had to be done when the children were home from school, leading to the

problems of excluding the rest of the family from the living room for a considerable period of time. Some parents were initially taken aback that the interviewer needed to see the child on his/her own, though the great majority were happy with the explanations given. A technique successfully used by interviewers when parents refused to leave the room was to sit side by side with the child, reading out the questions but then asking the child to key in their own answers into the laptop computer.

Use of laptop computers

The use of laptop computers to ask sensitive questions - awkward and troublesome behaviour and smoking, drinking and drug taking - of children aged 11-15 worked successfully. However, the reporting of all types of substance use and abuse were under-reported compared with the national surveys of smoking and drinking carried out by group administration in school settings (Goddard and Higgins, 1999a; Goddard and Higgins, 1999b)

Language difficulties

In some circumstances, neither parent had a sufficient grasp of English to be interviewed, especially as some of the questions on the mental health of children, e.g., obsessions and compulsions were quite difficult to formulate in English. To overcome this difficulty, the two-page, Strengths and Difficulties Questionnaire was made available in approximately 40 languages. This was used, in a self-completion format, instead of the face-to-face parent interview.

Incentive payments

During the pilot stages of the survey, the need for incentive payments was investigated. Most teenagers agreed to be interviewed without an incentive payment. The lack of an incentive payment did not appear to affect response in the main stage of the survey, as shown by the high response rate by all children, 96% of co-operating families. One or two young people may have agreed to an interview with an incentive payment but this was not sufficiently widespread to recommend the universal use of incentive payments.

References

Goddard, E., and Higgins, V. (1999a) *Smoking, drinking and drug use among teenagers, Volume 1, England* London: The Stationary Office.

Goddard, E., and Higgins, V. (1999b) *Smoking, drinking and drug use among teenagers, Volume 2, Scotland* London: The Stationary Office.

4 Prevalence of mental disorders

4.1 Introduction

The prevalence of mental disorders among children and adolescents was based on a clinical evaluation of parent, teacher and child data collected by lay, ONS interviewers from questionnaires designed by the Department of Child and Adolescent Psychiatry, Institute of Psychiatry in London. Chapter 2 of this report describes the assessment process in some detail and the questionnaire is reproduced in Appendix E.

Four broad categories of mental disorders were identified and specific disorders were subsumed under these three headings.

Emotional disorders

Anxiety disorders
Separation anxiety
Specific phobia
Social phobia
Panic
Agoraphobia
Post Traumatic Stress Disorder (PTSD)
Obsessive-Compulsive Disorder (OCD)
Generalised Anxiety Disorder (GAD)
Other anxiety

Depression
Depressive episode
Other depressive episode

Conduct disorders

Oppositional defiant disorder
Conduct disorder (family context)
Unsocialised conduct disorder
Socialised conduct disorder
Other conduct disorder

Hyperkinetic disorder

Hyperkinesis
Other hyperkinetic disorder

Less common disorders

Pervasive developmental disorder
Psychotic disorder
Tic disorders
Eating disorders
Other psychiatric disorders

Prevalence rates for all disorders are shown in the tables as percentages to one decimal point. Therefore, rates per thousand of the population can be calculated by multiplying the percentages by ten. The percentages in the text and figures which refer to the numbers in the tables are rounded to the nearest integer. Sampling errors around these estimates are shown in Appendix C.

The figures in the tables in this chapter are weighted to take account of differential sampling, non-response by age, sex and region and adjusted to take account of missing teacher data. The weighting and adjustment strategies are fully described in Appendix A.

4.2 Prevalence of mental disorders by personal characteristics

Among children aged 5 -15 years, 5% had clinically significant conduct disorders; 4% were assessed as having emotional disorders – anxiety and depression – and 1% were rated as hyperactive. As their name suggests, the less common disorders (autistic disorders, tics and eating disorders) were attributed to half a percent of the sampled population. The overall rate of 10% includes some children who had more than one type of disorder. *(Table 4.1)*

These rates are based on the diagnostic criteria for research using the ICD-10 Classification of Mental and Behavioural Disorders with strict impairment criteria - the disorder causes distress to the child or has a considerable impact on the child's day to day life.

Sex and age

The proportion of children and adolescents with any mental disorder was greater among boys than girls: 11% compared with 8%. This disparity was evident in both younger and older children. Among 5-10 year olds, 10% of boys and 6% of girls had a mental disorder. In the older age group, the 11-15 year olds, the proportions of children with any mental disorder were 13% for boys and 10% for girls. *(Figure 4.1)*

Whereas the rates of emotional disorders were similar for boys and girls, the prevalence of conduct disorders was found to be approximately twice as common among boys than girls and for hyperkinetic disorders the ratio was even greater: 2% among boys of all ages compared with about half a percent of girls. *(Table 4.1)*

Age and sex differences of this magnitude have been found in other national surveys on the mental health of children and adolescents. (Zubrick et al., 1995)

Owing to these age and sex differences, all the subsequent tables showing the prevalence rates by child, family and household characteristics, are presented by age and sex.

Table 4.1 also shows the prevalence rates of specific mental disorders (e.g. social phobia, oppositional-defiant disorder, hyperkinesis etc.) by age and sex. These data have been presented for reference purposes. Owing to the relatively low rates of the specific disorders, all the remaining tables in this chapter focus on the broad groups of disorder.

Ethnicity

Nearly 10% of white children and 12% of black children were assessed as having a mental health problem whereas the prevalence rates among Asian children were 8% of the Pakistani and Bangladeshi and 4% of the Indian samples. *(Figure 4.2)*

Despite the large number of interviews achieved in this survey, over ten thousand, ethnic differences are difficult to interpret because of the small numbers in the sample who regarded themselves as belonging to particular ethnic groups. When the ethnic groups are categorised by age and by sex the bases are smaller still and make the differences between distributions correspondingly more

difficult to interpret. Nevertheless, Indian children, particularly girls seem to have far lower rates of mental disorder than both white or black children. *(Table 4.2)*

4.3 Prevalence of mental health disorders by family characteristics

Family type and marital status

Two questions were asked to obtain the marital status of the interviewed parent. The first asked: "Are you single, that is never married, married and living with your husband/wife, married and separated from your husband/wife, divorced or widowed?". The second question asked of everyone except those married and living with husband/wife was, "May I just check, are you living with someone else as a couple?". As neither the stability of the relationship nor the length of the period of cohabitation was assessed, it is not possible to draw conclusions about cohabitation per se.

Children of lone parents were about twice as likely to have a mental health problem than those living with married or cohabiting couples: 16% compared with 8%. This relationship was also found in the Western Australian survey of 14,100 children. (Zubrick et al., 1995)

> "Children from single parent families were more likely (odds ratio 2:1) to have a mental health morbidity than those in two-parent families"

Within the GB sample of children of lone parents, the prevalence of mental disorders did not differ markedly by whether the lone parent was single or widowed, divorced or separated. *(Figure 4.3)*

However, children living with cohabiting as distinct from married couples were more likely to have a mental health problem, in particular, conduct disorders: 8% compared with 4%. *(Table 4.3)*

There were also sex differences in the family type relationship. Nearly 1 in 5 of boys of lone parents had a mental health problem, with most of them having a conduct disorder. Among the girls in lone parent families, about 1 in 8 had a mental disorder, equally distributed among conduct and emotional disorders. *(Table 4.3)*

In an attempt to explain the relationship between family type and the mental health of children, Fombonne (1995) comments:

> "On the whole, secular changes in patterns of family life expose children and adolescents to more frequent and earlier challenges: marital discord, parental breakdown and divorce, remarriage or cohabitation, and single parent families, which have all been shown to be associated with negative outcomes in young people, with boys and girls being affected in different ways...... It is possible that secular changes in patterns of family life have led to an increase in the conditions of family functioning that lead to depression.. among adolescents"

Zubrick (1995) also explains that family type differences are not simply due to the structure of the family but represent a multiplicative interaction of factors:

> "In view of the fact that rates of child mental health morbidity can vary according to a family's social, economic and financial circumstances, family structure alone would not provide a satisfactory backdrop against which to assess rates of child mental health morbidity. Two additional factors that modify the initial finding (on family structure) were considered - parental income and quality of the parents' relationships."

This cautionary note is amply demonstrated in the GB survey which shows large differences in the socio-economic and social functioning of lone and two parent families.

	Married	Co-habiting	Lone parent
	Percentage of families with each characteristic		
Interviewed parent was economically inactive	25%	31%	46%
Household gross weekly income was less than £100	1%	3%	21%
Social sector tenants	15%	38%	56%
Interviewed parent had GHQ-12 score of 4+	16%	20%	30%
"Unhealthy" family functioning	17%	21%	24%

As social and family functioning are regarded as key risk factors for childhood psychopathology, a whole chapter in this report looks at these relationships – see Chapter 9.

Reconstituted families

The relationships between family member in the household were examined to see if any of the children were step-sons or step-daughters. This search was carried out for all children in the family not just the sampled child. Thus, a family was regarded as reconstituted if step-children were present. Overall, about 9% of the surveyed children lived in reconstituted families.

Mental disorders were more prevalent among children of reconstituted families than those without step children: 15% compared with 9%. The ratio of the prevalence rates of child mental disorders by this measure of family structure was similar across all age and sex categories: 19% compared with 12% for 11-15 year old boys and 11% compared with 5% for 5-10 year old girls. The disparity in prevalence rates between the reconstituted and other families was mainly due to the differences in the proportions of children with conduct or hyperkinetic disorders rather than emotional disorders. *(Table 4.4)*

Number of children in household

A child living in a family with one other child, i.e. two children households, represent the group least likely to have been assessed as having a mental health problem. If the number of children in the household are put in ascending order of the likelihood of having a mental health problem, the order would be 2-3-1-4-5. However, the only statistically significant differences were between those in two-children households (8%) and those who were part of four- and five-children households, 13% and 18% respectively. *(Figure 4.5)*

Whereas this trend was evident for emotional and conduct disorders, there was a different pattern for hyperactivity. The prevalence of hyperkinetic disorders was highest among lone children: nearly 5% of 5-10 year old boys. *(Table 4.5)*

All these findings lend support to the trend shown by Garralda and Bailey (1986) and Ghodsian et al.

(1980) of increased mental health morbidity among children in "larger families".

Educational qualifications of parent

Among the 10,438 parents interviewed for the survey, 94% were the child's mother. Previous research has suggested a relationship between maternal educational level and mental health of the child. This was examined in the current survey. Table 4.6 shows a clear trend - the prevalence of mental disorders among children increases with a decrease in the educational level of the interviewed parent. Looking at the two extremes of the education level distribution, 15% of children of interviewed parents with no qualifications had a mental disorder compared with 6% of those whose parent had at least a degree level qualification. (*Figure 4.6*)

Having no qualifications in contrast to having any qualifications seemed to have more impact on prevalence rates than differences between educational level. For example, 15% of 11-15 year old boys whose interviewed parent had no qualifications were assessed as having a conduct disorder compared with 5-7% of the same sample whose parents had any qualification up to degree level and 2% of those with parents with at least a degree. (*Table 4.6*)

4.4 Prevalence of mental health disorders by household characteristics

Family's employment situation

Many studies have shown that unemployed adults fare worse than employed people on several measures of psychological functioning, (Meltzer et al., 1995), Similarly, the working status of the family seemed to be a major factor in understanding the differences in prevalence rates of mental disorders among children and adolescents. About one fifth of children in families without a working parent had a mental disorder, more than twice the proportion among children with at least one working member of the family. (*Figure 4.7*).

The higher prevalence rates of mental disorders among children of non-working compared with working families were shown for all the groups of disorders – emotional, behavioural and hyperkinetic – for both boys and girls and younger and older children. Among working families, the prevalence of childhood disorders did not appear to be associated with whether one or both parents were working. (*Table 4.7*)

Household income

For most families, the majority of their income comes from paid work. Therefore, the relationship between mental disorders among children and household income to some extent reflects the association described above on the family's working situation. The prevalence of any psychiatric disorder ranged from 16% among children living in families with a gross weekly household income of under £100 to 9% among children of families in the £300-399 weekly income bracket and around 6% in those families earning £500 per week or more. (*Figure 4.8*)

This trend was evident for all three groups of disorders: emotional, behavioural and hyperkinetic. The highest prevalence rate of any mental disorder was found for boys in families with a gross income of under £100 a week, 22%, in contrast to a rate of 3% among 5-10 year old girls in families with an income of at least £500. (*Table 4.8*)

State Benefits

State benefits are paid out for a variety of reasons: one parent benefit, family credit, disability related benefits, invalid care allowance, job seekers allowance etc. The benefits shown in the analysis presented in Table 4.9 have been chosen to indicate at least some degree of disability among a member of the child's household. The prevalence of mental disorders of children in relation to some of the other state benefits (e.g. lone parent benefit or family credit) are not shown in the table as equivalent data have been presented earlier - on family type and household income.

Figure 4.9 shows very strikingly that children living in households that receive Invalid Care Allowance (ICA), Attendance Allowance (AA) and Disability Allowance (DA) were far more likely than other children to have a mental disorder. Compared with the overall prevalence rate of 10%, the corresponding percentages for children in families receiving ICA, AA and DA were 29%, 23% and 22%, and these did not vary considerably by age and sex. *(Table 4.9)*

Social class

There were marked differences in the prevalence of mental disorders among children by social class (as measured by the occupation of head of household).

Children of families in Social Class V (unskilled occupations) were approximately three times more likely to have a mental disorder than those in Social Class I (professionals): 14% compared with 5%, and about twice as likely as those in Social Class II (managerial and technical): 14% compared with 7%. *(Figure 4.10)*

At a more detailed level, 10% of 5-15 year olds in Social Class V families had conduct disorders compared with 2% of their equivalents in Social Class I. These data fit in with Maughan's review on the mental health of children in Great Britain which examined social class differences from national birth cohort studies and from local epidemiological surveys. (Maughan, 1995) She states that conduct disorders, especially those rated by teachers, show clear social class trends with such disorders more common in lower social groups. She does add a cautionary note:

> "… more specific indicators of family difficulties and disturbance have been regarded as more important risk factors for children's psychological well-being than family social position per se."

Tenure

Just as there were clear social class differences in the prevalence of children and adolescents' mental health, so there was a marked difference between owner/occupiers and renters. The prevalence of any mental disorder rose from 6% among children in owner/occupier households to 13% of those with parents in private rented accommodation to 17% of children of social sector tenants, i.e. renting from local authorities

or housing associations. The principal difference in prevalence rates was between the owner/occupiers and those living in rented accommodation rather than between types of renter. *(Figure 4.11)*

Type of accommodation

The prevalence of mental disorders among children and adolescents by type of accommodation follow the pattern shown for social class, tenure and household income. The overall rate of mental disorder was highest among those living in terraced houses and flats and maisonettes, and lowest among those in detached/semi-detached houses. *(Figure 4.12 and Table 4.12)*

4.5   Prevalence of mental disorders by areal characteristics

Region

There were no significant differences in the prevalence rates of any mental disorder or the three main groups of mental disorders between England, Scotland and Wales nor between the metropolitan and non-metropolitan areas of England. *(Figure 4.13 and Table 4.13)*

This was an unexpected finding considering the variation in prevalence rates described above in terms of social class, tenure, type of accommodation and household income. The answer may lie in the fact that sociodemographic and socio-economic differences may be lost in the aggregated data. This suggests that ACORN (A Classification of Residential Neighbourhoods), a geo-demographic classification, may be a better indicator of regional trends.

ACORN

ACORN is a geo-demographic targeting classification, combining geographical and demographic characteristics to distinguish different types of people in different areas in Great Britain. Although the ACORN classification has various levels, 6 categories, 17 groups and 54 types, for the purposes of this report, the highest level, i.e. the six broad categories have been chosen for comparative analysis. The ACORN User Guide gives the following description of each category:

A Thriving
Wealthy achievers, suburban areas; affluent greys, rural communities; prosperous pensioners, retirement areas.

B Expanding
Affluent executives, family areas; well-off workers, family areas.

C Rising
Affluent urbanites, town and city areas, prosperous professionals, metropolitan areas; better off executives, inner city areas.

D Settling
Comfortable middle agers, mature home owning areas; skilled workers, home owning areas.

E Aspiring
New home owners, mature communities; white collar workers, better-off, multi-ethnic areas.

F Striving
Older people, less prosperous areas; council estate residents, better off homes; council estate residents, high unemployment; council estate residents, greater hardship, people in multi-ethnic, low-income areas.

The highest proportion of children with any mental disorder was found among families classified as *striving*, 13%. This was about twice the rate associated with the *expanding* ACORN classification (7%) and two and a half times the proportion of those in the *thriving* category (5%). The overall trend of increased morbidity among children from *striving* to *thriving* families not unexpectedly, matches the social class, tenure and household income analysis described above. *(Figure 4.14)*

Age and sex differences in the prevalence rates of mental disorders were found in each geo-demographic category. The highest prevalence rate of any mental disorder, 19%, was found for 11-15 year old boys in the *striving* category with the lowest rate, 3%, among 5-10 year old girls in *thriving* families. *(Table 4.14)*

4.6 Odds ratios of socio-demographic correlates of mental disorders.

Logistic regression was used to produce odds ratios for the socio-demographic correlates of any disorder and the three principal subgroups – conduct disorders, emotional disorders and hyperactivity – and the two main categories of emotional disorders: anxiety and depression.

Each odds ratio shows the increase in odds that a child has a particular disorder when in a particular group compared to a reference group. The variables entered in the model were age, sex, ethnicity, family type, number of children, family employment and the ACORN classification. The latter was chosen as the socio-economic indicator as it takes account of tenure, type of accommodation and income.

The significant odds ratios for the socio-demographic correlates of the child having a mental disorder (compared with no disorder) were: age, sex, number of children in the household, family type, the family's employment situation and the ACORN classification. The odds of having any mental disorder increased by around 50% for boys compared with girls (OR=1.58) for 11-15 year olds compared with younger children (OR=1.48) and for children of lone parents compared with couples (OR=1.57).

The two characteristics with the largest significant effect on the odds of having any mental disorder were the family's employment situation and the ACORN classification. A family with no-one working compared with all adults working nearly doubled the odds of the child having a mental disorder (OR=1.94). *Thriving* compared with *striving* families had a similar odds ratio (OR=1.95).

The one other characteristic with significant odds ratios for the child having a mental disorder was the number of children in the household. Compared with the lone child family, those with four children increased the odds by about a third (OR=1.32) and those with five children by nearly two-thirds (OR=1.63). The one characteristic entered in the model that showed no significant odds ratios was ethnicity. *(Table 4.15)*

The three broad categories of disorders

The odds ratios for the socio-demographic correlates for any mental health problem of children and adolescents presented above changed when the three groups of disorders were looked at separately.

Whereas the odds of having any mental disorder for boys compared with girls was 1.58, the corresponding odds ratio was 5.56 for hyperactivity, 2.42 for conduct disorders, and was not statistically significant for emotional disorders. Similarly, the odds of having a mental disorder for 11-15 year olds compared with 5-10 year olds at 1.48, rose to 1.84 for conduct disorders, changed very little for emotional disorders at 1.45, and was not significant for hyperactivity. The largest odds ratio for five children compared with one child in the household was found for conduct disorders (OR=2.23) while the corresponding odds ratio for emotional problems was 1.43 and not statistically significant for hyperactivity.

Working versus non-working families and *thriving* as distinct from *striving* households seemed to have the greatest effect on the odds ratio of having a hyperkinetic disorder. The odds ratio for non-working compared with working families associated with a hyperkinetic disorder was 2.13 and 2.41 for *thriving* compared with *striving* families.

At a third level of analysis, odds ratios were calculated for the socio-demographic correlates of the two categories of emotional disorders: anxiety and depression. The most significant finding was the odds of having a depressive episode for 11-15 year olds compared to 5-10 year olds was 8.55. *(Table 4.16)*

Odds ratios for the co-occurrence of psychiatric disorders

Odds ratios were also calculated to estimate the extent of comorbidity between the three main groups of mental disorders and between the two categories of emotional disorders. Following the precedent set by the ECA study, odds ratios were taken to be significant when the ratio exceeded 10.00 and the lower bound of the 95% confidence interval exceeded 4.00. (Robins and Regier, 1991)

Conduct disorders were significantly comorbid with hyperkinetic disorders with an odds ratio of 38.43 (26.87 – 54.96) and any anxiety and any depressive episode frequently co-occurred having an odds ratio of 20.13 (13.18 – 39.75) Odds ratios were not calculated for the comorbidity of specific disorders both within and across ICD-10 categories as the base numbers for children with each disorder were too small.

References

CACI Information Services, (1993), *ACORN User Guide*, CACI Limited 1994. All Rights Reserved. Source: ONS and GRO(S) © Crown Copyright 1991. All Rights Reserved.

Garralda, M.E., Bailey, D., (1986) "Children with psychiatric disorders in primary care" in *Journal of Child Psychology and Psychiatry*, 27:611-24

Ghodsian, M., Fogelman, K., Tibbenham, A.,(1980) Changes in behaviour ratings of a national sample of children *British Journal of Social and Clinical Psychology* 19:247-56

Maughan, B., (1995) "Mental Health" Chapter 12 in *The Health of Children"*, London: HMSO

Robins, L. N. , Locke, B. Z., and Regier, D. An Overview of Psychiatric Disorders in America in Robins L.N and Regier, D (eds) Psychiatric Disorders in America: The Epidemiologic Catchment Area Study (1991) Free Press: New York

Standard Occupation Classification 1990 Vol. 1 (1991) Structure and definition of major, minor and unit groups. HMSO: London

Zubrick, S.R., Silburn, S.R., Garton, A., Burton, P., Dalby, R., Carlton, J., Shepherd, C., Lawrence, D. (1995) *Western Australian Child Health Survey: Developing Health and Well-being in the nineties,* Perth, Western Australia: ABS and ICHR.

Table 4.1 Prevalence of mental disorders
by age and sex

	5-10 year olds			11-15 year olds			All children		
	Boys	Girls	All	Boys	Girls	All	Boys	Girls	All
	Percentage of children with each disorder								
Emotional disorders	3.3	3.3	3.3	5.1	6.1	5.6	4.1	4.5	4.3
Anxiety disorders	3.2	3.1	3.1	3.9	5.3	4.6	3.5	4.0	3.8
Separation anxiety	1.0	1.0	1.0	0.7	0.3	0.5	0.9	0.7	0.8
Specific phobia	1.1	1.0	1.1	0.7	1.1	0.9	0.9	1.1	1.0
Social phobia	0.4	0.2	0.3	0.3	0.4	0.4	0.4	0.3	0.3
Panic	-	-	-	0.4	0.3	0.3	0.2	0.1	0.1
Agoraphobia	-	-	-	0.1	0.2	0.2	0.1	0.1	0.1
PTSD	0.0	-	0.0	0.2	0.5	0.4	0.1	0.2	0.2
OCD	0.1	0.1	0.1	0.5	0.5	0.5	0.3	0.2	0.2
GAD	0.3	0.4	0.4	0.8	1.1	0.9	0.5	0.7	0.6
Other anxiety	0.9	0.5	0.7	1.3	2.3	1.8	1.1	1.3	1.2
Depression	0.2	0.3	0.2	1.7	1.9	1.8	0.9	1.0	0.9
Depressive episode	0.2	0.2	0.2	1.2	1.4	1.3	0.6	0.7	0.7
Other depressive episode	-	0.1	0.1	0.5	0.5	0.5	0.2	0.3	0.2
Conduct disorders	6.5	2.7	4.6	8.6	3.8	6.2	7.4	3.2	5.3
Oppositional defiant disorder	4.8	2.1	3.5	2.8	1.3	2.1	3.9	1.8	2.9
Conduct disorder (family context)	-	0.1	0.0	0.1	0.4	0.2	0.0	0.2	0.1
Unsocialised conduct disorder	0.5	0.2	0.4	1.0	0.3	0.6	0.7	0.2	0.5
Socialised conduct disorder	0.6	0.0	0.3	2.8	1.1	1.9	1.5	0.5	1.0
Other conduct disorder	0.6	0.3	0.4	2.0	0.7	1.4	1.2	0.5	0.9
Hyperkinetic disorders	2.6	0.4	1.5	2.3	0.5	1.4	2.4	0.4	1.4
Hyperkinesis	2.3	0.4	1.3	1.9	0.4	1.2	2.1	0.4	1.3
Other hyperkinetic disorder	0.3	0.0	0.2	0.4	0.0	0.2	0.3	0.0	0.2
Less common disorders	0.8	0.2	0.5	0.5	0.7	0.6	0.7	0.4	0.5
Pervasive developmental disorder	0.6	0.2	0.4	0.3	0.0	0.2	0.5	0.1	0.3
Psychotic disorder	-	-	-	-	-	-	-	-	-
Tic disorders	0.1	-	0.1	0.1	0.1	0.1	0.1	0.0	0.1
Eating disorders	-	-	-	0.1	0.4	0.3	0.0	0.2	0.1
Any disorder	10.4	5.9	8.2	12.8	9.6	11.2	11.4	7.6	9.5
Base	*2909*	*2921*	*5830*	*2310*	*2299*	*4609*	*5219*	*5219*	*10438*

Figure 4.1 Prevalence of any mental disorder by age and sex

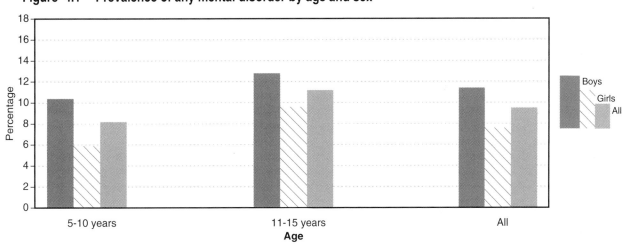

Table 4.2   Prevalence of mental disorders

by ethnicity, age and sex

All children

			Ethnic group			
	White	Black	Indian	Pakistani & Bangladeshi	Other groups	All
BOYS			*Percentage of children with each disorder*			
5-10 year olds						
Emotional disorders	3.2	1.7	5.3	2.6	7.1	3.3
Conduct disorders	6.6	6.9	3.6	6.1	4.7	6.5
Hyperkinetic disorders	2.8	-	-	-	1.6	2.6
Less common disorders	0.8	1.6	-	-	2.8	0.8
Any disorder	10.4	10.0	7.3	5.7	13.6	10.4
Base	*2667*	*70*	*61*	*39*	*72*	*2909*
11-15 year olds						
Emotional disorders	4.9	4.9	5.5	12.4	6.3	5.1
Conduct disorders	8.6	17.8	2.3	4.6	7.2	8.6
Hyperkinetic disorders	2.5	1.5	-	-	-	2.3
Less common disorders	0.6	-	-	-	-	0.5
Any disorder	12.6	22.1	5.8	15.3	13.5	12.8
Base	*2077*	*70*	*60*	*51*	*51*	*2309*
All boys						
Emotional disorders	4.0	3.3	5.4	8.2	6.8	4.1
Conduct disorders	7.5	12.3	3.0	5.2	5.7	7.4
Hyperkinetic disorders	2.6	0.7	-	-	0.9	2.4
Less common disorders	0.7	0.8	-	-	1.7	0.7
Any disorder	11.4	16.0	6.6	11.2	13.6	11.4
Base	*4745*	*140*	*121*	*89*	*123*	*5217*
GIRLS						
5-10 year olds						
Emotional disorders	3.3	4.2	-	1.7	5.0	3.2
Conduct disorders	2.8	3.1	1.9	1.9	2.6	2.7
Hyperkinetic disorders	0.5	-	-	-	-	0.4
Less common disorders	0.2	-	-	-	-	0.2
Any disorder	5.9	7.4	1.8	3.6	7.8	5.9
Base	*2638*	*73*	*60*	*61*	*86*	*2917*
11-15 year olds						
Emotional disorders	6.4	2.0	-	5.3	4.1	6.1
Conduct disorders	3.9	6.3	-	-	2.1	3.8
Hyperkinetic disorders	0.5	-	-	-	-	0.5
Less common disorders	0.7	-	-	-	-	0.7
Any disorder	10.1	8.1	-	5.6	6.4	9.7
Base	*2091*	*59*	*43*	*45*	*57*	*2295*
All						
Emotional disorders	4.7	3.2	-	3.2	4.6	4.5
Conduct disorders	3.3	4.6	1.1	1.1	2.4	3.2
Hyperkinetic disorders	0.5	-	-	-	-	0.4
Less common disorders	0.5	-	-	-	-	0.4
Any disorder	7.8	7.7	1.0	4.4	7.2	7.6
Base	*4729*	*132*	*103*	*106*	*143*	*5213*

Table 4.2	(continued) Prevalence of mental disorders
	by ethnicity, age and sex

All children

	Ethnic group					All
	White	Black	Indian	Pakistani & Bangladeshi	Other groups	
All	*Percentage of children with each disorder*					
5-10 year olds						
Emotional disorders	3.2	2.9	2.7	2.0	6.0	3.3
Conduct disorders	4.7	5.0	2.8	3.5	3.6	4.6
Hyperkinetic disorders	1.6	-	-	-	0.7	1.5
Less common disorders	0.5	0.8	-	-	1.3	0.5
Any disorder	8.2	8.6	4.6	4.4	10.5	8.1
Base	*5305*	*143*	*121*	*99*	*158*	*5826*
11-15 year olds						
Emotional disorders	5.7	3.6	3.2	9.0	5.2	5.6
Conduct disorders	6.3	12.6	1.3	2.4	4.5	6.2
Hyperkinetic disorders	1.5	0.8	-	-	-	1.4
Less common disorders	0.7	-	-	-	-	0.6
Any disorder	11.3	15.7	3.4	10.7	9.7	11.2
Base	*4168*	*129*	*103*	*96*	*107*	*4604*
All children						
Emotional disorders	4.3	3.3	2.9	5.5	5.6	4.3
Conduct disorders	5.4	8.6	2.1	3.0	3.9	5.3
Hyperkinetic disorders	1.6	0.4	-	-	0.4	1.4
Less common disorders	0.6	0.4	-	-	0.8	0.5
Any disorder	9.6	12.0	4.0	7.5	10.2	9.5
Base	*9474*	*271*	*224*	*196*	*265*	*10430*

Figure 4.2   Prevalence of any mental disorder by ethnicity

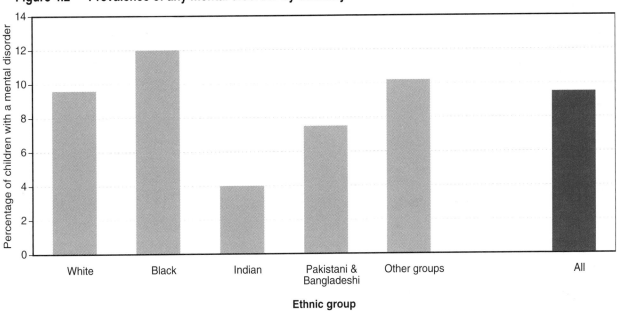

Table 4.3   Prevalence of mental disorders

by family type, age and sex

All children

				Child's family type			
	Married	Cohabiting	All couples	Lone parent - single	Lone parent - widow, divorced, separated	All lone parents	All
BOYS				*Percentage of children with each disorder*			
5-10 year olds							
Emotional disorders	2.2	5.4	2.5	6.2	6.2	6.2	3.3
Conduct disorders	4.3	8.6	4.8	12.4	13.0	12.8	6.5
Hyperkinetic disorders	2.0	1.3	1.9	6.5	4.0	4.9	2.6
Less common disorders	0.9	-	0.8	1.3	0.8	1.0	0.8
Any disorder	7.7	11.6	8.1	18.7	18.9	18.8	10.4
Base	*2046*	*242*	*2287*	*233*	*388*	*621*	*2909*
11-15 year olds							
Emotional disorders	4.4	3.9	4.4	4.3	8.2	7.5	5.1
Conduct disorders	5.7	17.0	6.6	17.6	14.5	15.1	8.6
Hyperkinetic disorders	1.9	3.9	2.0	1.0	3.6	3.1	2.3
Less common disorders	0.5	2.2	0.6	-	0.3	0.2	0.5
Any disorder	9.8	18.4	10.5	20.1	20.2	20.2	12.8
Base	*1626*	*138*	*1764*	*103*	*444*	*546*	*2310*
All boys							
Emotional disorders	3.2	4.8	3.3	5.6	7.3	6.8	4.1
Conduct disorders	4.9	11.7	5.6	14.0	13.8	13.8	7.4
Hyperkinetic disorders	1.9	2.2	2.0	4.8	3.8	4.1	2.4
Less common disorders	0.7	0.8	0.7	0.9	0.5	0.6	0.7
Any disorder	8.6	14.1	9.1	19.1	19.6	19.5	11.4
Base	*3672*	*379*	*4051*	*336*	*832*	*1168*	*5219*
GIRLS							
5-10 year olds							
Emotional disorders	3.0	2.6	3.0	4.6	4.2	4.4	3.3
Conduct disorders	1.8	3.3	2.0	8.3	3.4	5.4	2.7
Hyperkinetic disorders	0.2	0.4	0.2	2.4	0.3	1.2	0.4
Less common disorders	0.2	0.4	0.2	-	0.3	0.2	0.2
Any disorder	4.9	6.2	5.0	12.4	6.8	9.1	5.9
Base	*2002*	*269*	*2271*	*264*	*387*	*650*	*2921*
11-15 year olds							
Emotional disorders	4.8	6.4	4.9	4.8	11.3	9.9	6.1
Conduct disorders	2.7	6.0	3.0	7.8	5.9	6.3	3.8
Hyperkinetic disorders	0.6	0.7	0.6	-	-	-	0.5
Less common disorders	0.5	-	0.4	-	1.9	1.5	0.7
Any disorder	7.3	12.5	7.8	11.6	16.7	15.6	9.6
Base	*1591*	*158*	*1749*	*118*	*432*	*550*	*2299*
All girls							
Emotional disorders	3.8	4.0	3.8	4.7	7.9	6.9	4.5
Conduct disorders	2.2	4.3	2.4	8.1	4.7	5.8	3.2
Hyperkinetic disorders	0.4	0.5	0.4	1.7	0.1	0.6	0.4
Less common disorders	0.3	0.2	0.3	-	1.1	0.8	0.4
Any disorder	6.0	8.5	6.2	12.2	12.0	12.1	7.6
Base	*3593*	*427*	*4019*	*382*	*818*	*1200*	*5219*

Table 4.3   (continued) Prevalence of mental disorders

by family type, age and sex

All children

	Married	Cohabiting	**All couples**	Lone parent - single	Lone parent - widow, divorced, separated	**All lone parents**	All
					Child's family type		
ALL			*Percentage of children with each disorder*				
5-10 year olds							
Emotional disorders	2.6	3.9	2.7	5.4	5.2	5.3	3.3
Conduct disorders	3.1	5.8	3.4	10.2	8.2	9.0	4.6
Hyperkinetic disorders	1.1	0.8	1.1	4.4	2.1	3.0	1.5
Less common disorders	0.5	0.2	0.5	0.6	0.5	0.6	0.5
Any disorder	6.3	8.8	6.6	15.4	12.9	13.8	8.2
Base	*4047*	*510*	*4558*	*497*	*775*	*1272*	*5829*
11-15 year olds							
Emotional disorders	4.6	5.3	4.6	4.6	9.7	8.7	5.6
Conduct disorders	4.2	11.1	4.8	12.3	10.3	10.7	6.2
Hyperkinetic disorders	1.2	2.2	1.3	0.5	1.8	1.6	1.4
Less common disorders	0.5	1.0	0.5	-	1.1	0.8	0.6
Any disorder	8.6	15.3	9.1	15.5	18.5	17.9	11.2
Base	*3217*	*295*	*3513*	*221*	*875*	*1096*	*4609*
All children							
Emotional disorders	3.5	4.4	3.6	5.1	7.6	6.8	4.3
Conduct disorders	3.6	7.8	4.0	10.9	9.3	9.8	5.3
Hyperkinetic disorders	1.2	1.3	1.2	3.2	2.0	2.3	1.4
Less common disorders	0.5	0.5	0.5	0.4	0.8	0.7	0.5
Any disorder	7.3	11.2	7.7	15.4	15.8	15.7	9.5
Base	*7264*	*806*	*8070*	*718*	*1650*	*2368*	*10438*

Figure 4.3   Prevalence of any mental disorder by age, sex and family type

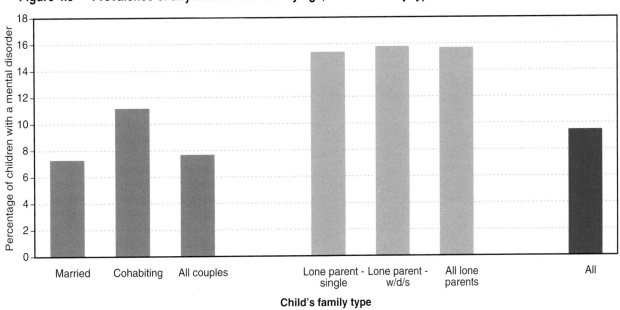

Table 4.4	Prevalence of mental disorders
	by family structure, age and sex

All Children

	Reconstituted family		
	No	Yes	All
BOYS	*Percentage of children with each disorder*		
5-10 year olds			
Emotional disorders	3.2	4.4	3.3
Conduct disorders	6.1	11.4	6.5
Hyperkinetic disorders	2.3	5.7	2.6
Less common disorders	0.8	1.3	0.8
Any disorder	9.9	16.3	10.4
Base	*2679*	*230*	*2909*
11-15 year olds			
Emotional disorders	4.7	9.0	5.1
Conduct disorders	7.9	14.7	8.6
Hyperkinetic disorders	2.3	1.9	2.3
Less common disorders	0.5	0.5	0.5
Any disorder	12.0	19.3	12.8
Base	*2083*	*227*	*2310*
All boys			
Emotional disorders	3.9	6.7	4.1
Conduct disorders	6.9	13.0	7.4
Hyperkinetic disorders	2.3	3.8	2.4
Less common disorders	0.7	0.9	0.7
Any disorder	10.8	17.8	11.4
Base	*4762*	*456*	*5219*
GIRLS			
5-10 year olds			
Emotional disorders	3.2	3.6	3.3
Conduct disorders	2.3	6.9	2.7
Hyperkinetic disorders	0.3	1.8	0.4
Less common disorders	0.2	0.4	0.2
Any disorder	5.4	11.3	5.9
Base	*2672*	*249*	*2921*
11-15 year olds			
Emotional disorders	6.1	6.1	6.1
Conduct disorders	3.1	9.6	3.8
Hyperkinetic disorders	0.4	1.0	0.5
Less common disorders	0.7	0.8	0.7
Any disorder	9.2	13.9	9.6
Base	*2059*	*240*	*2299*
All girls			
Emotional disorders	4.5	4.8	4.5
Conduct disorders	2.7	8.2	3.2
Hyperkinetic disorders	0.3	1.4	0.4
Less common disorders	0.4	0.6	0.4
Any disorder	7.1	12.6	7.6
Base	*4730*	*489*	*5219*

Table 4.4   (continued) Prevalence of mental disorders

by family structure, age and sex

All Children

	Reconstituted family		
	No	Yes	All
ALL	*Percentage of children with each disorder*		
5-10 year olds			
Emotional disorders	3.2	4.0	3.3
Conduct disorders	4.2	9.0	4.6
Hyperkinetic disorders	1.3	3.7	1.5
Less common disorders	0.5	0.8	0.5
Any disorder	7.7	13.7	8.2
Base	*5351*	*479*	*5829*
11-15 year olds			
Emotional disorders	5.4	7.5	5.6
Conduct disorders	5.5	12.1	6.2
Hyperkinetic disorders	1.4	1.4	1.4
Less common disorders	0.6	0.7	0.6
Any disorder	10.6	16.5	11.2
Base	*4142*	*467*	*4609*
All children			
Emotional disorders	4.2	5.7	4.3
Conduct disorders	4.8	10.5	5.3
Hyperkinetic disorders	1.3	2.6	1.4
Less common disorders	0.5	0.7	0.5
Any disorder	8.9	15.1	9.5
Base	*9493*	*946*	*10438*

Figure 4.4   Prevalence of any mental disorder by family structure

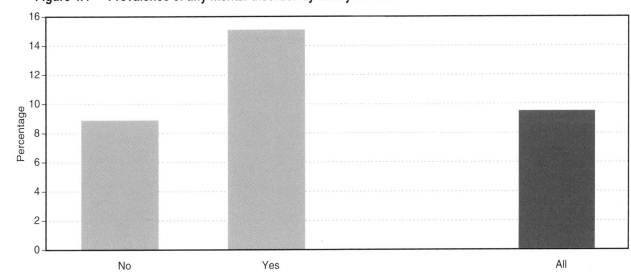

Table 4.5   Prevalence of mental disorders

by number of children in household, age and sex

All children

	Number of children in household					
	1	2	3	4	5 or more	All
BOYS	*Percentage of children with each disorder*					
5-10 year olds						
Emotional disorders	4.0	2.6	2.9	4.7	10.2	3.3
Conduct disorders	7.4	5.0	6.3	9.3	18.3	6.5
Hyperkinetic disorders	4.5	2.1	2.6	2.1	1.3	2.6
Less common disorders	0.9	0.8	0.7	1.5	-	0.8
Any disorder	13.2	8.4	9.3	14.2	24.5	10.4
Base	*448*	*1385*	*726*	*258*	*92*	*2909*
11-15 year olds						
Emotional disorders	4.3	4.7	5.3	12.0	3.8	5.1
Conduct disorders	8.0	7.9	6.8	18.2	19.5	8.6
Hyperkinetic disorders	2.1	2.7	1.8	2.5	2.0	2.3
Less common disorders	0.6	0.5	0.5	-	-	0.5
Any disorder	11.5	12.4	11.2	23.8	20.5	12.8
Base	*657*	*993*	*470*	*133*	*58*	*2310*
All						
Emotional disorders	4.2	3.5	3.8	7.2	7.7	4.1
Conduct disorders	7.7	6.2	6.5	12.3	18.7	7.4
Hyperkinetic disorders	3.1	2.3	2.3	2.2	1.6	2.4
Less common disorders	0.7	0.7	0.6	1.0	-	0.7
Any disorder	12.2	10.1	10.1	17.4	22.9	11.4
Base	*1104*	*2378*	*1196*	*390*	*151*	*5219*
GIRLS						
5-10 year olds						
Emotional disorders	3.5	2.8	3.7	3.2	5.9	3.3
Conduct disorders	2.5	2.2	2.6	5.0	6.3	2.7
Hyperkinetic disorders	0.5	0.4	0.4	-	2.8	0.4
Less common disorders	0.5	0.1	0.3	-	-	0.2
Any disorder	6.6	4.8	6.3	7.5	12.4	5.9
Base	*435*	*1383*	*741*	*277*	*85*	*2921*
11-15 year olds						
Emotional disorders	6.0	5.4	7.8	4.9	7.7	6.1
Conduct disorders	2.6	3.8	4.7	4.8	7.5	3.8
Hyperkinetic disorders	0.2	0.6	0.5	0.7	-	0.5
Less common disorders	0.6	0.6	0.9	0.7	1.7	0.7
Any disorder	9.5	8.8	11.1	9.9	13.5	9.6
Base	*653*	*958*	*463*	*160*	*64*	*2299*
All						
Emotional disorders	5.0	3.9	5.3	3.8	6.7	4.5
Conduct disorders	2.5	2.8	3.4	4.9	6.8	3.2
Hyperkinetic disorders	0.3	0.5	0.4	0.3	1.6	0.4
Less common disorders	0.5	0.3	0.5	0.3	0.7	0.4
Any disorder	8.3	6.5	8.1	8.4	12.9	7.6
Base	*1088*	*2341*	*1204*	*437*	*149*	*5219*

Table 4.5 (continued) Prevalence of mental disorders

by number of children in household, age and sex

All children

	Number of children in household					
	1	2	3	4	5 or more	All
ALL	*Percentage of children with each disorder*					
5-10 year olds						
Emotional disorders	3.8	2.7	3.3	3.9	8.1	3.3
Conduct disorders	5.0	3.6	4.5	7.1	12.5	4.6
Hyperkinetic disorders	2.5	1.2	1.5	1.0	2.0	1.5
Less common disorders	0.7	0.5	0.5	0.7	-	0.5
Any disorder	10.0	6.6	7.8	10.7	18.7	8.2
Base	*883*	*2768*	*1467*	*535*	*177*	*5829*
11-15 year olds						
Emotional disorders	5.2	5.1	6.5	8.1	5.9	5.6
Conduct disorders	5.3	5.9	5.8	10.8	13.2	6.2
Hyperkinetic disorders	1.1	1.7	1.2	1.5	1.0	1.4
Less common disorders	0.6	0.5	0.7	0.4	0.9	0.6
Any disorder	10.5	10.6	11.2	16.2	16.8	11.2
Base	*1310*	*1951*	*933*	*293*	*123*	*4609*
All children						
Emotional disorders	4.6	3.7	4.6	5.4	7.2	4.3
Conduct disorders	5.2	4.5	5.0	8.4	12.8	5.3
Hyperkinetic disorders	1.7	1.4	1.4	1.2	1.6	1.4
Less common disorders	0.6	0.5	0.6	0.6	0.4	0.5
Any disorder	10.3	8.3	9.1	12.7	17.9	9.5
Base	*2192*	*4719*	*2400*	*828*	*300*	*10438*

Figure 4.5 Prevalence of any mental disorder by number of children in household

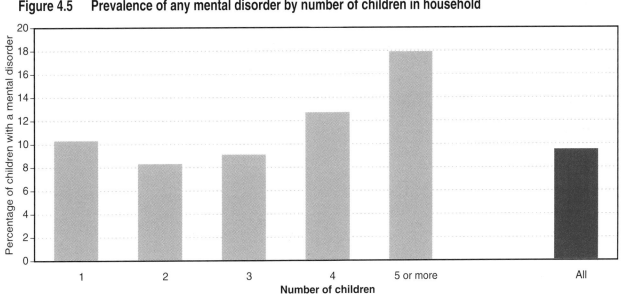

Table 4.6	Prevalence of mental disorders

by educational qualifications of parent, age and sex

All children

	Education level (interviewed parent)							
	Degree level	Teaching/ HND/ Nursing level	A-level (or equivalent)	GCSE grades A-C or equivalent	GCSE grades D-F or equivalent	Other qualification	No qualification	All
BOYS	*Percentage of children with each disorder*							
5-10 year olds								
Emotional disorders	2.0	1.7	2.6	2.8	4.0	2.6	5.9	3.3
Conduct disorders	2.8	2.9	4.6	5.0	8.4	3.1	13.1	6.5
Hyperkinetic disorders	1.9	1.5	2.1	1.5	3.5	14.1	4.2	2.6
Less common disorders	0.8	0.3	1.6	0.3	1.3	-	1.2	0.8
Any disorder	6.9	5.6	7.7	8.1	13.3	13.7	18.2	10.5
Base	*372*	*304*	*316*	*887*	*370*	*38*	*598*	*2884*
11-15 year olds								
Emotional disorders	2.2	3.7	5.8	4.6	3.6	2.6	8.0	5.1
Conduct disorders	2.2	4.8	6.6	7.4	5.9	18.4	14.7	8.6
Hyperkinetic disorders	1.0	0.5	2.5	2.1	3.2	2.9	3.5	2.3
Less common disorders	0.8	0.4	0.9	0.5	-	1.2	0.4	0.5
Any disorder	5.8	8.0	12.5	11.6	10.0	17.4	19.4	12.8
Base	*243*	*252*	*227*	*624*	*244*	*80*	*603*	*2273*
All boys								
Emotional disorders	2.0	2.6	3.9	3.6	3.9	2.6	7.0	4.1
Conduct disorders	2.6	3.7	5.4	6.0	7.4	13.5	13.9	7.5
Hyperkinetic disorders	1.5	1.0	2.2	1.7	3.4	6.5	3.9	2.5
Less common disorders	0.8	0.4	1.3	0.4	0.8	0.8	0.8	0.7
Any disorder	6.5	6.7	9.7	9.6	12.0	16.2	18.8	11.5
Base	*615*	*556*	*543*	*1511*	*614*	*118*	*1201*	*5157*
GIRLS								
5-10 year olds								
Emotional disorders	1.7	3.3	2.2	2.7	5.1	2.6	4.8	3.3
Conduct disorders	1.6	1.4	1.9	1.9	3.5	2.8	5.4	2.8
Hyperkinetic disorders	-	-	0.3	0.1	0.9	1.4	1.1	0.4
Less common disorders	0.6	0.3	-	0.2	-	-	0.2	0.2
Any disorder	3.9	4.4	4.5	4.5	7.5	5.3	10.3	6.0
Base	*351*	*300*	*322*	*886*	*348*	*76*	*597*	*2881*
11-15 year olds								
Emotional disorders	4.4	4.3	3.9	5.3	6.4	6.7	8.7	6.1
Conduct disorders	3.2	3.0	4.2	2.7	4.2	1.2	5.9	3.9
Hyperkinetic disorders	0.4	1.0	0.6	0.4	0.5	-	0.4	0.5
Less common disorders	0.9	0.9	-	0.8	-	2.1	0.7	0.7
Any disorder	7.3	8.5	7.0	8.0	10.3	10.5	13.4	9.7
Base	*255*	*232*	*193*	*639*	*252*	*94*	*592*	*2256*
All girls								
Emotional disorders	2.8	3.7	2.9	3.8	5.7	4.8	6.8	4.5
Conduct disorders	2.3	2.1	2.8	2.3	3.8	1.9	5.6	3.3
Hyperkinetic disorders	0.2	0.4	0.4	0.2	0.7	0.6	0.7	0.5
Less common disorders	0.7	0.6	-	0.4	-	1.2	0.4	0.4
Any disorder	5.3	6.2	5.4	6.0	8.7	8.2	11.9	7.6
Base	*606*	*532*	*515*	*1525*	*600*	*170*	*1189*	*5137*

Table 4.6	(continued) Prevalence of mental disorders

by educational qualifications of parent, age and sex

All children

	Education level (interviewed parent)							
	Degree level	Teaching/ HND/ Nursing level	A-level (or equivalent)	GCSE grades A-C or equivalent	GCSE grades D-F or equivalent	Other qualification	No qualification	All
ALL	*Percentage of children with each disorder*							
5-10 year olds								
Emotional disorders	1.8	2.5	2.4	2.7	4.6	2.6	5.4	3.3
Conduct disorders	2.2	2.1	3.2	3.4	6.0	2.9	9.3	4.6
Hyperkinetic disorders	1.0	0.7	1.2	0.8	2.2	5.6	2.7	1.5
Less common disorders	0.7	0.3	0.8	0.3	0.7	0.7	0.5	
Any disorder	5.4	5.0	6.1	6.3	10.5	8.1	14.2	8.2
Base	*723*	*603*	*638*	*1774*	*718*	*114*	*1196*	*5766*
11-15 year olds								
Emotional disorders	3.3	4.0	5.0	5.0	5.0	4.8	8.4	5.6
Conduct disorders	2.7	3.9	5.5	5.0	5.0	9.1	10.3	6.3
Hyperkinetic disorders	0.7	0.7	1.6	1.2	1.8	1.3	1.9	1.4
Less common disorders	0.9	0.7	0.5	0.7	1.7	0.5	0.6	
Any disorder	6.6	8.2	9.9	9.8	10.2	13.7	16.4	11.2
Base	*498*	*484*	*420*	*1263*	*496*	*174*	*1195*	*4529*
All children								
Emotional disorders	2.4	3.2	3.4	3.7	4.7	3.9	6.9	4.3
Conduct disorders	2.4	2.9	4.1	4.1	5.6	6.7	9.8	5.4
Hyperkinetic disorders	0.9	0.7	1.4	1.0	2.1	3.0	2.3	1.5
Less common disorders	0.8	0.5	0.7	0.4	0.4	1.0	0.6	0.6
Any disorder	5.9	6.5	7.6	7.8	10.4	11.5	15.3	9.6
Base	*1221*	*1087*	*1058*	*3036*	*1214*	*288*	*2390*	*10294*

Figure 4.6   Prevalence of any mental disorder by education qualifications of parent

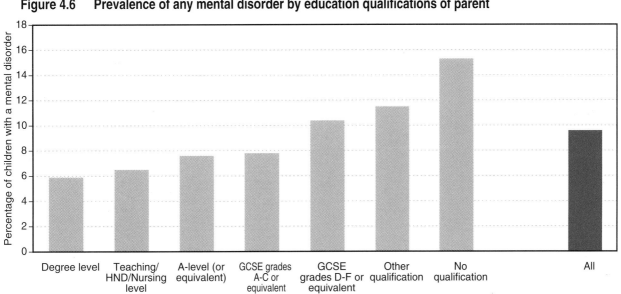

Table 4.7	Prevalence of mental disorders
	by family's employment, age and sex

All children

	Family's employment			
	Both parents working (inc. lone parents)	One parent working	Neither parents working (inc. lone parents)	All
BOYS	*Percentage of children with each disorder*			
5-10 year olds				
Emotional disorders	2.4	3.3	7.3	3.3
Conduct disorders	5.2	5.0	14.7	6.5
Hyperkinetic disorders	2.0	2.5	5.4	2.6
Less common disorders	0.5	1.3	1.7	0.8
Any disorder	8.2	9.7	21.4	10.4
Base	*1834*	*644*	*414*	*2892*
11-15 year olds				
Emotional disorders	3.8	6.5	10.3	5.1
Conduct disorders	6.5	8.5	20.0	8.6
Hyperkinetic disorders	1.9	2.4	4.4	2.3
Less common disorders	0.4	1.2	0.4	0.5
Any disorder	10.2	13.0	26.5	12.8
Base	*1612*	*360*	*303*	*2275*
All boys				
Emotional disorders	3.1	4.4	8.6	4.1
Conduct disorders	5.8	6.2	16.9	7.4
Hyperkinetic disorders	1.9	2.5	5.0	2.5
Less common disorders	0.4	1.2	1.1	0.7
Any disorder	9.1	10.9	23.5	11.5
Base	*3446*	*1004*	*717*	*5166*
GIRLS				
5-10 year olds				
Emotional disorders	2.4	3.9	6.4	3.3
Conduct disorders	2.1	1.7	7.3	2.8
Hyperkinetic disorders	0.3	0.2	1.6	0.4
Less common disorders	0.3	-	0.2	0.2
Any disorder	4.5	5.4	13.7	6.0
Base	*1859*	*619*	*407*	*2884*
11-15 year olds				
Emotional disorders	5.2	5.9	11.3	6.0
Conduct disorders	2.9	4.2	8.7	3.9
Hyperkinetic disorders	0.3	1.7	-	0.5
Less common disorders	0.5	1.2	1.4	0.7
Any disorder	8.0	10.4	18.4	9.6
Base	*1634*	*339*	*288*	*2261*
All girls				
Emotional disorders	3.7	4.6	8.4	4.5
Conduct disorders	2.5	2.6	7.9	3.2
Hyperkinetic disorders	0.3	0.7	1.0	0.5
Less common disorders	0.3	0.4	0.7	0.4
Any disorder	6.1	7.2	15.7	7.6
Base	*3493*	*958*	*695*	*5146*

Table 4.7   (continued) Prevalence of mental disorders

by family's employment, age and sex

All children

	Family's employment			
	Both parents working (inc. lone parents)	One parent working	Neither parents working (inc. lone parents)	All
ALL	*Percentage of children with each disorder*			
5-10 year olds				
Emotional disorders	2.4	3.6	6.9	3.3
Conduct disorders	3.7	3.4	11.0	4.6
Hyperkinetic disorders	1.1	1.4	3.5	1.5
Less common disorders	0.4	0.6	1.0	0.5
Any disorder	6.4	7.6	17.6	8.2
Base	*3693*	*1262*	*821*	*5776*
11-15 year olds				
Emotional disorders	4.5	6.2	10.8	5.6
Conduct disorders	4.7	6.4	14.5	6.3
Hyperkinetic disorders	1.1	2.1	2.3	1.4
Less common disorders	0.4	1.2	0.9	0.6
Any disorder	9.1	11.7	22.5	11.2
Base	*3249*	*699*	*591*	*4536*
All children				
Emotional disorders	3.4	4.5	8.5	4.3
Conduct disorders	4.1	4.5	12.5	5.3
Hyperkinetic disorders	1.1	1.6	3.0	1.5
Less common disorders	0.4	0.9	0.9	0.6
Any disorder	7.6	9.1	19.7	9.5
Base	*6939*	*1961*	*1411*	*10312*

Figure 4.7   Prevalence of any mental disorder by family's employment

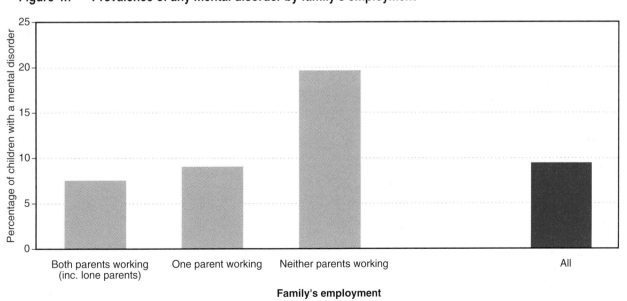

Table 4.8   Prevalence of mental disorders

by gross weekly household income, age and sex

All children (where income data available)

	Under £100	£100 - £199	£200 - £299	£300 - £399	£400 - £499	£500 - £599	£600 - £770	Over £770	All
BOYS	*Percentage of children with each disorder*								
5-10 year olds									
Emotional disorders	5.8	5.5	2.9	3.4	2.5	0.7	2.2	3.1	3.3
Conduct disorders	14.3	12.7	7.6	5.0	5.8	3.7	2.1	3.0	6.7
Hyperkinetic disorders	5.6	4.5	2.6	1.9	2.4	2.6	1.7	0.6	2.6
Less common disorders	0.6	0.6	1.7	0.6	1.5	0.3	1.2	0.2	0.8
Any disorder	21.1	16.9	11.9	9.0	8.2	5.3	6.9	6.6	10.6
Base	*173*	*496*	*416*	*354*	*269*	*278*	*320*	*436*	*2741*
11-15 year olds									
Emotional disorders	7.7	9.5	7.2	5.0	1.9	2.7	2.2	2.8	5.0
Conduct disorders	17.0	16.2	11.7	7.4	6.1	3.7	5.1	3.7	8.7
Hyperkinetic disorders	2.0	4.2	3.1	1.6	1.4	1.0	2.1	2.2	2.4
Less common disorders	-	0.9	0.5	0.4	-	-	0.4	1.2	0.5
Any disorder	22.2	22.6	16.7	11.9	7.2	6.8	7.7	7.6	12.7
Base	*107*	*377*	*328*	*261*	*221*	*220*	*278*	*358*	*2150*
All boys									
Emotional disorders	6.5	7.2	4.8	4.1	2.2	1.6	2.2	3.0	4.0
Conduct disorders	15.3	14.2	9.4	6.1	5.9	3.7	3.5	3.3	7.5
Hyperkinetic disorders	4.2	4.4	2.8	1.8	2.0	1.9	1.9	1.3	2.5
Less common disorders	0.4	0.7	1.2	0.5	0.8	0.2	0.8	0.7	0.7
Any disorder	21.5	19.4	14.0	10.3	7.8	6.0	7.3	7.1	11.5
Base	*280*	*872*	*744*	*616*	*490*	*498*	*598*	*794*	*4891*
GIRLS									
5-10 year olds									
Emotional disorders	4.5	4.0	5.1	2.1	4.1	1.8	2.3	2.1	3.2
Conduct disorders	3.1	6.2	3.5	4.8	1.8	0.4	1.0	0.5	2.8
Hyperkinetic disorders	-	1.6	0.3	0.7	-	0.4	-	-	0.5
Less common disorders	-	0.4	-	0.3	-	-	0.3	0.4	0.2
Any disorder	7.1	10.1	8.2	6.8	5.7	2.7	3.1	3.1	6.0
Base	*177*	*521*	*362*	*319*	*308*	*266*	*325*	*456*	*2735*
11-15 year olds									
Emotional disorders	8.7	11.0	7.7	6.2	2.5	4.6	3.2	3.3	6.0
Conduct disorders	3.6	7.4	4.9	3.2	2.6	2.9	0.9	2.0	3.6
Hyperkinetic disorders	-	-	0.3	1.4	0.5	0.5	-	0.3	0.4
Less common disorders	3.1	1.4	-	-	0.5	0.9	0.5	0.5	0.7
Any disorder	14.8	16.9	11.9	9.2	5.1	8.1	4.3	5.6	9.5
Base	*97*	*376*	*342*	*259*	*219*	*239*	*262*	*355*	*2150*
All girls									
Emotional disorders	6.0	6.9	6.4	4.0	3.4	3.1	2.7	2.6	4.5
Conduct disorders	3.3	6.7	4.2	4.1	2.1	1.6	0.9	1.2	3.2
Hyperkinetic disorders	-	1.0	0.3	1.0	0.2	0.5	-	0.1	0.4
Less common disorders	1.1	0.8	-	0.1	0.2	0.4	0.4	0.5	0.4
Any disorder	9.8	12.9	10.0	7.9	5.4	5.3	3.6	4.2	7.6
Base	*275*	*898*	*704*	*578*	*527*	*505*	*587*	*811*	*4885*

Table 4.8	(continued) Prevalence of mental disorders

by gross weekly household income, age and sex

All children (where income data available)

	Gross weekly household income								
	Under £100	£100 - £199	£200 - £299	£300 - £399	£400 - £499	£500 - £599	£600 - £770	Over £770	All
ALL	*Percentage of children with each disorder*								
5-10 year olds									
Emotional disorders	5.1	4.7	3.9	2.8	3.4	1.2	2.3	2.6	3.3
Conduct disorders	8.6	9.3	5.7	4.9	3.6	2.1	1.5	1.7	4.7
Hyperkinetic disorders	2.8	3.0	1.6	1.3	1.1	1.5	0.8	0.3	1.5
Less common disorders	0.3	0.5	0.9	0.4	0.7	0.2	0.7	0.3	0.5
Any disorder	14.0	13.4	10.2	8.0	6.9	4.0	5.0	4.8	8.3
Base	*350*	*1017*	*778*	*674*	*576*	*543*	*646*	*891*	*5476*
11-15 year olds									
Emotional disorders	8.2	10.3	7.4	5.6	2.2	3.7	2.7	3.0	5.5
Conduct disorders	10.6	11.8	8.2	5.3	4.4	3.3	3.1	2.8	6.2
Hyperkinetic disorders	1.0	2.1	1.7	1.5	1.0	0.7	1.1	1.2	1.4
Less common disorders	1.5	1.1	0.3	0.2	0.2	0.5	0.4	0.9	0.6
Any disorder	18.7	19.8	14.2	10.6	6.2	7.5	6.0	6.6	11.1
Base	*204*	*753*	*669*	*520*	*441*	*459*	*540*	*714*	*4300*
All children									
Emotional disorders	6.3	7.1	5.6	4.0	2.9	2.4	2.5	2.8	4.2
Conduct disorders	9.4	10.4	6.9	5.1	3.9	2.6	2.2	2.2	5.4
Hyperkinetic disorders	2.1	2.6	1.6	1.4	1.1	1.2	0.9	0.7	1.5
Less common disorders	0.7	0.8	0.6	0.3	0.5	0.3	0.6	0.6	0.6
Any disorder	15.7	16.1	12.0	9.1	6.6	5.6	5.4	5.6	9.5
Base	*555*	*1770*	*1447*	*1194*	*1017*	*1003*	*1186*	*1605*	*9776*

Figure 4.8   Prevalence of any mental disorder by gross weekly household income

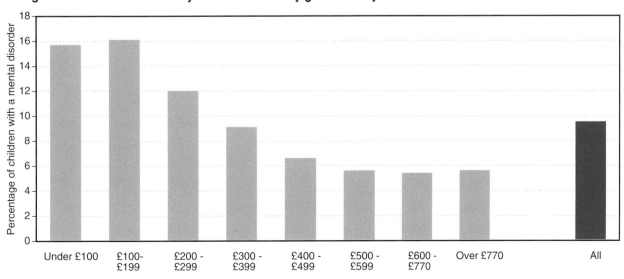

Table 4.9   Prevalence of mental disorders

by receipt of disability benefits, age and sex

| | Receipt of disability benefits | | | | | |
	Invalid care allowance	Attendance allowance	Disability allowance	Severe disablement allowance	Incapacity allowance	All
BOYS			*Percentage of children with each disorder*			
5-10 year olds						
Emotional disorders	5.6	-	11.6	-	5.9	7.5
Conduct disorders	15.3	[1]	16.0	[3]	8.3	13.1
Hyperkinetic disorders	4.9	[2]	6.5	[1]	5.1	6.4
Less common disorders	13.3	[2]	9.6	[1]	-	6.7
Any disorder	31.5	[4]	31.3	[4]	14.4	24.5
Base	68	12	103	28	64	210
11-15 year olds						
Emotional disorders	13.9	4.8	12.4	-	9.0	10.6
Conduct disorders	17.9	16.6	17.1	[2]	18.0	16.0
Hyperkinetic disorders	3.1	5.6	5.9	[2]	5.1	3.6
Less common disorders	5.0	2.3	3.0	-	-	2.4
Any disorder	33.2	18.1	26.4	[3]	22.1	24.3
Base	72	36	73	14	42	187
All boys						
Emotional disorders	9.9	3.6	11.9	-	7.1	8.9
Conduct disorders	16.6	15.4	16.4	13.8	12.1	14.5
Hyperkinetic disorders	4.0	9.0	6.3	8.9	5.1	5.1
Less common disorders	9.0	6.0	6.8	2.3	-	4.6
Any disorder	32.4	22.8	29.3	18.6	17.5	24.4
Base	140	48	176	42	107	397
GIRLS						
5-10 year olds						
Emotional disorders	17.1	[5]	9.6	[3]	7.4	11.0
Conduct disorders	11.8	[2]	5.6	-	-	5.0
Hyperkinetic disorders	3.4	-	1.2	-	-	1.1
Less common disorders	1.6	-	-	-	-	0.5
Any disorder	30.9	[7]	15.4	[3]	7.9	17.0
Base	64	18	93	19	52	189
11-15 year olds						
Emotional disorders	12.8	[2]	10.4	-	11.6	11.5
Conduct disorders	17.4	[0]	9.2	[1]	2.0	8.0
Hyperkinetic disorders	-	-	1.5	[1]	1.9	1.4
Less common disorders	-	-	-	-	-	-
Any disorder	27.2	[2]	18.3	[1]	14.1	18.4
Base	40	21	76	11	59	164
All girls						
Emotional disorders	15.4	18.1	9.9	9.9	9.6	11.2
Conduct disorders	13.9	6.6	7.2	4.0	1.1	6.4
Hyperkinetic disorders	2.1	-	1.3	3.9	1.0	1.3
Less common disorders	1.0	-	-	-	-	0.3
Any disorder	29.5	25.5	16.7	14.3	11.2	17.6
Base	103	39	169	30	111	352

Table 4.9   (continued) Prevalence of mental disorders

by receipt of disability benefits, age and sex

	Receipt of disability benefits					
	Invalid care allowance	Attendance allowance	Disability allowance	Severe disablement allowance	Incapacity allowance	All
ALL	*Percentage of children with each disorder*					
5-10 year olds						
Emotional disorders	11.1	16.6	10.6	6.3	6.6	9.2
Conduct disorders	13.6	11.9	11.0	7.9	4.6	9.3
Hyperkinetic disorders	4.2	7.6	4.0	3.0	2.8	3.9
Less common disorders	7.6	6.7	5.0	2.1	-	3.8
Any disorder	31.2	38.9	23.8	16.5	11.5	20.9
Base	*132*	*30*	*197*	*47*	*116*	*399*
11-15 year olds						
Emotional disorders	13.5	6.6	11.4	-	10.5	11.0
Conduct disorders	17.7	11.2	13.1	[3]	8.7	12.3
Hyperkinetic disorders	2.0	3.5	3.7	[3]	3.3	2.6
Less common disorders	3.2	1.5	1.5	-	-	1.3
Any disorder	31.1	15.9	22.3	[4]	17.5	21.5
Base	*112*	*56*	*148*	*25*	*102*	*350*
All children						
Emotional disorders	12.2	10.1	11.0	4.1	8.4	10.0
Conduct disorders	15.5	11.4	11.9	9.7	6.5	10.7
Hyperkinetic disorders	3.2	5.0	3.8	6.8	3.0	3.3
Less common disorders	5.6	3.3	3.5	1.4	-	2.6
Any disorder	31.2	24.0	23.1	16.8	14.3	21.2
Base	*244*	*87*	*345*	*72*	*218*	*750*

Figure 4.9   Prevalence of any mental disorder by receipt of disability benefits

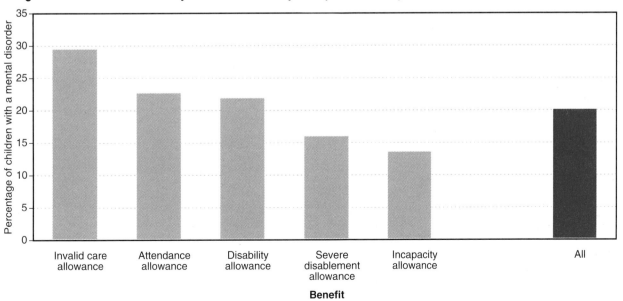

Table 4.10   Prevalence of mental disorders

by social class, age and sex

				Family's social class				
	I Professional	II Managerial and technical occupations	IIIN Skilled occupations non-manual	IIIM Skilled occupations manual	IV Partly-skilled occupations	V Unskilled occupations	Never worked	All*
BOYS				*Percentage of children with each disorder*				
5-10 year olds								
Emotional disorders	2.7	2.3	4.8	2.8	4.5	3.9	9.5	3.3
Conduct disorders	2.4	3.4	6.2	7.4	9.3	15.4	17.0	6.5
Hyperkinetic disorders	0.9	1.5	4.2	2.9	3.2	1.7	8.4	2.6
Less common disorders	1.4	0.8	1.5	0.5	0.4	1.4	1.9	0.8
Any disorder	6.7	7.0	13.7	10.4	12.6	17.7	27.7	10.4
Base	*222*	*873*	*340*	*734*	*458*	*131*	*55*	*2909*
11-15 year olds								
Emotional disorders	1.2	3.6	6.7	5.9	7.1	6.2	9.5	5.1
Conduct disorders	5.7	5.9	10.1	7.1	14.2	14.3	34.8	8.6
Hyperkinetic disorders	2.7	1.1	2.6	2.1	5.4	1.8	-	2.3
Less common disorders	2.4	0.7	-	0.2	0.1	-	-	0.5
Any disorder	8.1	9.1	14.9	12.5	18.8	17.3	33.0	12.8
Base	*166*	*750*	*262*	*572*	*329*	*122*	*23*	*2310*
All boys								
Emotional disorders	2.1	2.9	5.6	4.1	5.6	5.0	9.5	4.1
Conduct disorders	3.8	4.6	7.9	7.3	11.3	14.9	22.3	7.4
Hyperkinetic disorders	1.7	1.3	3.5	2.5	4.1	1.7	5.9	2.4
Less common disorders	1.8	0.8	0.8	0.4	0.3	0.7	1.3	0.7
Any disorder	7.3	8.0	14.2	11.3	15.2	17.5	29.3	11.4
Base	*387*	*1623*	*603*	*1306*	*786*	*252*	*79*	*5219*
GIRLS								
5-10 year olds								
Emotional disorders	1.5	2.6	4.4	3.5	3.4	5.0	6.0	3.3
Conduct disorders	1.0	1.7	3.2	2.1	4.2	5.0	9.1	2.7
Hyperkinetic disorders	-	0.1	0.6	0.5	1.0	0.8	1.1	0.4
Less common disorders	-	0.4	-	0.1	-	0.7	-	0.2
Any disorder	2.6	4.2	8.1	5.8	7.5	9.2	12.3	5.9
Base	*207*	*853*	*339*	*740*	*437*	*138*	*85*	*2921*
11-15 year olds								
Emotional disorders	1.7	5.4	5.5	6.8	8.0	8.4	11.6	6.1
Conduct disorders	1.4	2.8	5.7	3.5	4.0	5.9	15.8	3.8
Hyperkinetic disorders	-	0.8	0.4	0.4	-	1.0	-	0.5
Less common disorders	1.2	0.5	0.4	0.2	1.6	0.8	2.8	0.7
Any disorder	3.7	8.0	10.1	9.7	12.3	14.4	24.0	9.7
Base	*183*	*722*	*283*	*540*	*325*	*121*	*37*	*2299*
All girls								
Emotional disorders	1.6	3.9	4.9	4.9	5.4	6.6	7.7	4.5
Conduct disorders	1.2	2.2	4.4	2.7	4.1	5.4	11.1	3.2
Hyperkinetic disorders	-	0.4	0.5	0.4	0.6	0.9	0.8	0.4
Less common disorders	0.5	0.5	0.2	0.1	0.7	0.8	0.9	0.4
Any disorder	3.1	6.0	9.0	7.5	9.5	11.6	15.9	7.6
Base	*390*	*1575*	*622*	*1280*	*762*	*259*	*122*	*5219*

* No answers, members of the Armed Forces, full-time students are excluded from the six social class categories but included in the 'All' category.

Table 4.10   (continued) Prevalence of mental disorders

by social class, age and sex

	I Professional	II Managerial and technical occupations	IIIN Skilled occupations non-manual	IIIM Skilled occupations manual	IV Partly-skilled occupations	V Unskilled occupations	Never worked	All*
ALL			*Percentage of children with each disorder*					
5-10 year olds								
Emotional disorders	2.1	2.5	4.6	3.1	3.9	4.5	7.4	3.3
Conduct disorders	1.8	2.6	4.7	4.8	6.8	10.0	12.2	4.6
Hyperkinetic disorders	0.5	0.8	2.4	1.7	2.1	1.2	4.0	1.5
Less common disorders	0.7	0.6	0.7	0.3	0.2	1.1	0.7	0.5
Any disorder	4.7	5.6	10.9	8.1	10.1	13.3	18.4	8.2
Base	*429*	*1727*	*679*	*1474*	*894*	*268*	*141*	*5829*
11-15 year olds								
Emotional disorders	1.5	4.5	6.1	6.3	7.6	7.3	10.7	5.6
Conduct disorders	3.4	4.4	7.8	5.3	9.1	10.1	23.1	6.2
Hyperkinetic disorders	1.3	1.0	1.5	1.3	2.7	1.4	-	1.4
Less common disorders	1.8	0.6	0.2	0.2	0.8	0.4	1.7	0.6
Any disorder	5.8	8.6	12.4	11.1	15.5	15.8	27.5	11.2
Base	*348*	*1472*	*545*	*1112*	*654*	*243*	*60*	*4609*
All children								
Emotional disorders	1.8	3.4	5.3	4.5	5.5	5.8	8.4	4.3
Conduct disorders	2.5	3.4	6.1	5.0	7.8	10.1	15.5	5.3
Hyperkinetic disorders	0.8	0.9	2.0	1.5	2.4	1.3	2.8	1.4
Less common disorders	1.2	0.6	0.5	0.3	0.5	0.8	1.0	0.5
Any disorder	5.2	7.0	11.6	9.4	12.4	14.5	21.1	9.5
Base	*777*	*3199*	*1225*	*2586*	*1548*	*511*	*201*	*10438*

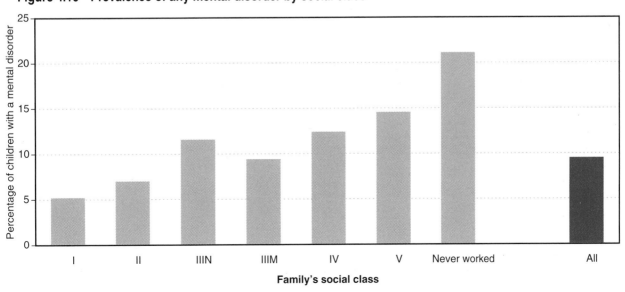

Figure 4.10   Prevalence of any mental disorder by social class

Table 4.11	Prevalence of mental disorders
	by tenure, age and sex

All children

	Tenure			
	Owners	Social sector tenants	Private renters	All
BOYS	*Percentage of children with each disorder*			
5-10 year olds				
Emotional disorders	2.2	5.8	4.6	3.3
Conduct disorders	3.3	14.3	6.9	6.5
Hyperkinetic disorders	1.8	4.0	4.5	2.6
Less common disorders	0.8	0.9	1.0	0.8
Any disorder	6.8	18.6	13.0	10.4
Base	*1927*	*783*	*198*	*2908*
11-15 year olds				
Emotional disorders	3.6	9.2	5.0	5.1
Conduct disorders	5.1	16.5	15.5	8.6
Hyperkinetic disorders	1.5	4.1	3.5	2.3
Less common disorders	0.5	0.5	1.2	0.5
Any disorder	8.5	23.1	17.2	12.8
Base	*1590*	*596*	*122*	*2308*
All boys				
Emotional disorders	2.8	7.3	4.7	4.1
Conduct disorders	4.1	15.3	10.2	7.4
Hyperkinetic disorders	1.7	4.0	4.1	2.4
Less common disorders	0.6	0.7	1.1	0.7
Any disorder	7.6	20.6	14.6	11.4
Base	*3517*	*1379*	*320*	*5216*
GIRLS				
5-10 year olds				
Emotional disorders	2.4	4.8	6.2	3.3
Conduct disorders	1.4	5.8	4.0	2.7
Hyperkinetic disorders	0.1	1.2	1.2	0.4
Less common disorders	0.2	0.3	-	0.2
Any disorder	3.9	9.9	10.4	5.9
Base	*1957*	*771*	*193*	*2921*
11-15 year olds				
Emotional disorders	4.5	9.9	8.3	6.1
Conduct disorders	2.1	8.5	5.1	3.8
Hyperkinetic disorders	0.3	0.8	0.9	0.5
Less common disorders	0.6	0.7	1.5	0.7
Any disorder	6.5	17.4	13.7	9.6
Base	*1596*	*564*	*135*	*2295*
All girls				
Emotional disorders	3.3	7.0	7.1	4.5
Conduct disorders	1.7	6.9	4.5	3.2
Hyperkinetic disorders	0.2	1.0	1.1	0.4
Less common disorders	0.4	0.5	0.6	0.4
Any disorder	5.1	13.1	11.7	7.5
Base	*3554*	*1335*	*327*	*5216*

Table 4.11   (continued) Prevalence of mental disorders

by tenure, age and sex

All children

	Tenure			
	Owners	Social sector tenants	Private renters	All
ALL	*Percentage of children with each disorder*			
5-10 year olds				
Emotional disorders	2.3	5.3	5.4	3.3
Conduct disorders	2.3	10.1	5.5	4.6
Hyperkinetic disorders	0.9	2.6	2.9	1.5
Less common disorders	0.5	0.6	0.5	0.5
Any disorder	5.3	14.3	11.7	8.2
Base	*3884*	*1554*	*390*	*5828*
11-15 year olds				
Emotional disorders	4.0	9.6	6.7	5.6
Conduct disorders	3.6	12.6	10.0	6.2
Hyperkinetic disorders	0.9	2.5	2.1	1.4
Less common disorders	0.5	0.6	1.3	0.6
Any disorder	7.5	20.3	15.3	11.2
Base	*3186*	*1160*	*257*	*4603*
All children				
Emotional disorders	3.1	7.1	5.9	4.3
Conduct disorders	2.9	11.2	7.3	5.3
Hyperkinetic disorders	0.9	2.6	2.6	1.4
Less common disorders	0.5	0.6	0.9	0.5
Any disorder	6.3	16.9	13.2	9.5
Base	*7071*	*2713*	*648*	*10432*

Figure 4.11   Prevalence of any mental disorder by tenure

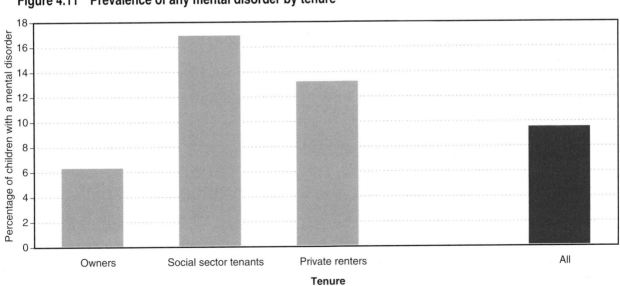

Table 4.12   Prevalence of mental disorders

by type of accommodation type, age and sex

All children

	Accommodation type					
	Detached	Semi-detached	Terraced house	Flat/ maisonette	Other	All
BOYS	*Percentage of children with each disorder*					
5-10 year olds						
Emotional disorders	2.6	2.9	3.8	6.2	-	3.3
Conduct disorders	2.6	6.1	9.6	7.0	-	6.5
Hyperkinetic disorders	1.1	2.4	3.5	4.4	-	2.6
Less common disorders	0.8	0.8	0.8	1.1	-	0.8
Any disorder	6.3	9.9	13.3	14.2	-	10.4
Base	*688*	*1083*	*946*	*187*	*4*	*2909*
11-15 year olds						
Emotional disorders	2.6	4.4	8.0	7.2	-	5.1
Conduct disorders	3.8	8.5	12.6	10.9	-	8.6
Hyperkinetic disorders	1.9	2.1	2.9	2.5	-	2.3
Less common disorders	0.8	0.6	0.3	-	-	0.5
Any disorder	7.3	11.7	18.3	16.8	-	12.8
Base	*581*	*931*	*657*	*135*	*6*	*2310*
All boys						
Emotional disorders	2.6	3.6	5.5	6.7	-	4.1
Conduct disorders	3.1	7.2	10.8	8.6	-	7.4
Hyperkinetic disorders	1.5	2.2	3.3	3.6	-	2.4
Less common disorders	0.8	0.7	0.6	0.6	-	0.7
Any disorder	6.7	10.7	15.3	15.3	-	11.4
Base	*1269*	*2014*	*1603*	*322*	*10*	*5219*
GIRLS						
5-10 year olds						
Emotional disorders	2.0	3.3	3.3	7.0	-	3.3
Conduct disorders	1.4	2.7	3.7	3.1	-	2.7
Hyperkinetic disorders	0.2	0.3	0.8	0.5	-	0.4
Less common disorders	0.3	0.1	0.3	-	-	0.2
Any disorder	3.6	5.9	6.8	9.9	-	5.9
Base	*692*	*1089*	*915*	*218*	*8*	*2921*
11-15 year olds						
Emotional disorders	4.5	5.2	8.3	7.4	[1]	6.1
Conduct disorders	1.2	5.1	4.6	3.4	-	3.8
Hyperkinetic disorders	0.6	0.5	0.3	-	-	0.5
Less common disorders	0.2	0.7	1.2	-	-	0.7
Any disorder	6.3	9.8	12.3	10.2	[1]	9.6
Base	*597*	*873*	*685*	*136*	*8*	*2299*
All girls						
Emotional disorders	3.2	4.1	5.5	7.2	[1]	4.5
Conduct disorders	1.3	3.7	4.1	3.2	-	3.2
Hyperkinetic disorders	0.4	0.4	0.6	0.3	-	0.4
Less common disorders	0.2	0.4	0.7	-	-	0.4
Any disorder	4.8	7.6	9.2	10.0	[1]	7.6
Base	*1288*	*1962*	*1600*	*353*	*16*	*5219*

Table 4.12   (continued) Prevalence of mental disorders

by type of accommodation type, age and sex

All children

	Accommodation type					
	Detached	Semi-detached	Terraced house	Flat/ maisonette	Other	All
ALL	*Percentage of children with each disorder*					
5-10 year olds						
Emotional disorders	2.3	3.1	3.6	6.7	-	3.3
Conduct disorders	2.0	4.4	6.7	4.9	-	4.6
Hyperkinetic disorders	0.6	1.3	2.2	2.3	-	1.5
Less common disorders	0.6	0.4	0.5	0.5	-	0.5
Any disorder	4.9	7.9	10.1	11.9	-	8.2
Base	*1380*	*2172*	*1861*	*405*	*12*	*5829*
11-15 year olds						
Emotional disorders	3.6	4.7	8.2	7.3	[1]	5.6
Conduct disorders	2.5	6.8	8.5	7.1	-	6.2
Hyperkinetic disorders	1.2	1.3	1.6	1.3	-	1.4
Less common disorders	0.5	0.6	0.8	-	-	0.6
Any disorder	6.8	10.8	15.2	13.5	[1]	11.2
Base	*1178*	*1804*	*1342*	*271*	*14*	*4609*
All children						
Emotional disorders	2.9	3.8	5.5	6.9	[1]	4.3
Conduct disorders	2.2	5.5	7.5	5.8	-	5.3
Hyperkinetic disorders	0.9	1.3	1.9	1.9	-	1.4
Less common disorders	0.5	0.5	0.6	0.3	-	0.5
Any disorder	5.8	9.2	12.3	12.5	[1]	9.5
Base	*2558*	*3976*	*3203*	*676*	*26*	*10438*

Figure 4.12   Prevalence of any mental disorder by type of accommodation

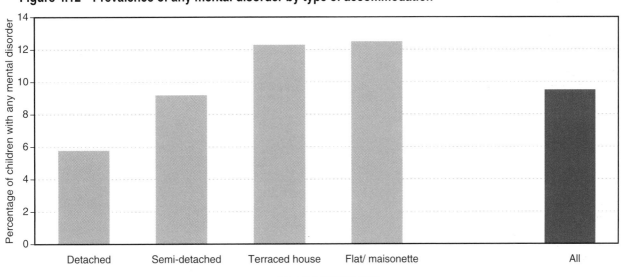

Table 4.13   Prevalence of mental disorders

by region, age and sex

All Children

	Country/Region							
	London Inner	London outer	Other Met England	Non-Met England	England	Scotland	Wales	All
BOYS	*Percentage of children with each disorder*							
5-10 year olds								
Emotional disorders	3.7	3.5	3.8	3.1	3.4	3.0	2.4	3.3
Conduct disorders	5.5	5.4	7.6	6.1	6.6	5.7	6.2	6.5
Hyperkinetic disorders	3.2	1.9	2.1	3.1	2.6	1.6	3.3	2.6
Less common disorders	-	0.6	0.8	1.1	0.9	0.3	0.6	0.8
Any disorder	9.1	10.2	11.5	10.5	10.8	8.2	7.7	10.4
Base	*128*	*180*	*903*	*1306*	*2517*	*251*	*140*	*2909*
11-15 year olds								
Emotional disorders	9.2	4.8	4.7	5.1	5.2	3.9	5.6	5.1
Conduct disorders	11.4	7.2	7.1	9.6	8.7	7.8	8.7	8.6
Hyperkinetic disorders	3.1	1.9	1.5	3.0	2.4	2.5	0.8	2.3
Less common disorders	-	1.0	0.9	0.1	0.4	1.0	0.8	0.5
Any disorder	20.4	13.9	11.2	13.4	13.1	10.1	12.1	12.8
Base	*131*	*115*	*730*	*1000*	*1977*	*210*	*124*	*2310*
All boys								
Emotional disorders	6.5	4.0	4.2	3.9	4.2	3.4	3.9	4.1
Conduct disorders	8.5	6.1	7.4	7.6	7.5	6.7	7.4	7.4
Hyperkinetic disorders	3.1	1.9	1.8	3.0	2.5	2.0	2.1	2.4
Less common disorders	-	0.8	0.8	0.7	0.7	0.6	0.7	0.7
Any disorder	14.8	11.6	11.4	11.7	11.8	9.0	9.8	11.4
Base	*259*	*295*	*1633*	*2306*	*4494*	*461*	*264*	*5219*
GIRLS								
5-10 year olds								
Emotional disorders	4.1	4.8	3.4	2.6	3.2	5.7	1.2	3.3
Conduct disorders	1.9	3.4	2.6	3.0	2.8	1.3	3.9	2.7
Hyperkinetic disorders	0.9	-	0.4	0.5	0.4	0.4	0.6	0.4
Less common disorders	-	0.6	0.2	0.1	0.2	0.4	0.6	0.2
Any disorder	6.1	8.2	6.0	5.5	5.9	7.3	5.0	5.9
Base	*143*	*176*	*904*	*1330*	*2553*	*231*	*137*	*2921*
11-15 year olds								
Emotional disorders	6.5	4.0	6.1	6.0	5.9	5.8	9.7	6.1
Conduct disorders	1.2	2.6	4.9	3.7	3.9	3.8	2.3	3.8
Hyperkinetic disorders	-	-	0.7	0.6	0.5	-	-	0.5
Less common disorders	1.1	-	0.9	0.6	0.7	0.4	0.7	0.7
Any disorder	8.0	5.8	11.1	9.3	9.6	8.8	11.9	9.6
Base	*115*	*142*	*674*	*1041*	*1971*	*201*	*126*	*2299*
All								
Emotional disorders	5.1	4.4	4.6	4.1	4.3	5.8	5.3	4.5
Conduct disorders	1.6	3.0	3.6	3.3	3.3	2.5	3.2	3.2
Hyperkinetic disorders	0.5	-	0.5	0.5	0.5	0.2	0.3	0.4
Less common disorders	0.5	0.3	0.5	0.3	0.4	0.4	0.7	0.4
Any disorder	6.9	7.1	8.1	7.2	7.5	8.0	8.3	7.6
Base	*258*	*318*	*1578*	*2370*	*4524*	*432*	*264*	*5219*

Table 4.13   Prevalence of mental disorders

by region, age and sex

All Children

	Country/Region							
	London Inner	London outer	Other Met England	Non-Met England	England	Scotland	Wales	All
ALL	*Percentage of children with each disorder*							
5-10 year olds								
Emotional disorders	3.9	4.2	3.6	2.9	3.3	4.3	1.8	3.3
Conduct disorders	3.6	4.4	5.1	4.5	4.7	3.6	5.1	4.6
Hyperkinetic disorders	2.0	1.0	1.2	1.8	1.5	1.0	2.0	1.5
Less common disorders	-	0.6	0.5	0.6	0.5	0.4	0.6	0.5
Any disorder	7.5	9.2	8.7	8.0	8.3	7.7	6.4	8.2
Base	*271*	*356*	*1807*	*2636*	*5070*	*481*	*278*	*5829*
11-15 year olds								
Emotional disorders	7.9	4.3	5.3	5.6	5.5	4.8	7.7	5.6
Conduct disorders	6.6	4.6	6.0	6.6	6.3	5.8	5.5	6.2
Hyperkinetic disorders	1.6	0.9	1.1	1.7	1.5	1.3	0.4	1.4
Less common disorders	0.5	0.5	0.9	0.4	0.6	0.7	0.7	0.6
Any disorder	14.6	9.4	11.2	11.3	11.3	9.4	12.0	11.2
Base	*246*	*257*	*1404*	*2041*	*3948*	*411*	*250*	*4609*
All children								
Emotional disorders	5.8	4.2	4.4	4.0	4.3	4.6	4.6	4.3
Conduct disorders	5.0	4.5	5.5	5.4	5.4	4.6	5.3	5.3
Hyperkinetic disorders	1.8	0.9	1.2	1.8	1.5	1.1	1.2	1.4
Less common disorders	0.2	0.5	0.7	0.5	0.5	0.5	0.7	0.5
Any disorder	10.9	9.3	9.8	9.4	9.6	8.5	9.0	9.5
Base	*517*	*613*	*3211*	*4677*	*9018*	*892*	*527*	*10438*

Figure 4.13   Prevalence of any mental disorder by country/region

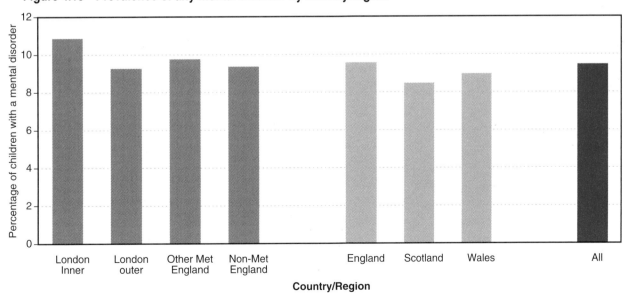

Table 4.14   Prevalence of mental disorders

by ACORN* classification, age and sex

All children

	ACORN classification						
	A - Thriving	B - Expanding	C - Rising	D - Settling	E - Aspiring	F - Striving	All
BOYS	*Percentage of children with each disorder*						
5-10 year olds							
Emotional disorders	2.3	2.9	4.7	1.7	4.0	5.0	3.3
Conduct disorders	3.7	3.3	5.4	5.7	8.3	10.0	6.4
Hyperkinetic disorders	1.1	2.7	4.0	2.7	3.2	2.6	2.5
Less common disorders	0.2	0.7	1.2	1.2	1.2	0.7	0.8
Any disorder	6.1	7.8	12.2	8.9	13.0	14.2	10.4
Base	*534*	*408*	*179*	*630*	*405*	*749*	*2904*
11-15 year olds							
Emotional disorders	3.2	3.6	1.5	5.5	5.9	7.3	5.1
Conduct disorders	3.1	6.2	8.8	6.8	11.4	13.8	8.6
Hyperkinetic disorders	1.0	1.1	2.6	2.2	3.5	3.2	2.3
Less common disorders	0.7	-	0.7	0.6	0.4	0.5	0.5
Any disorder	6.4	8.9	10.9	12.2	15.9	18.5	12.8
Base	*433*	*293*	*136*	*535*	*317*	*595*	*2309*
All boys							
Emotional disorders	2.7	3.2	3.3	3.4	4.8	6.0	4.1
Conduct disorders	3.4	4.5	6.9	6.2	9.7	11.7	7.4
Hyperkinetic disorders	1.0	2.0	3.4	2.5	3.3	2.9	2.4
Less common disorders	0.4	0.4	1.0	1.0	0.8	0.6	0.7
Any disorder	6.3	8.3	11.6	10.4	14.3	16.1	11.4
Base	*967*	*701*	*314*	*1165*	*721*	*1344*	*5213*
GIRLS							
5-10 year olds							
Emotional disorders	1.9	2.3	3.8	3.7	3.2	4.2	3.3
Conduct disorders	1.0	2.1	3.2	2.7	3.0	4.0	2.7
Hyperkinetic disorders	0.2	-	-	0.5	0.6	0.8	0.4
Less common disorders	0.4	-	-	0.1	0.5	0.1	0.2
Any disorder	3.4	4.2	6.4	6.5	6.8	7.6	5.9
Base	*512*	*417*	*182*	*697*	*358*	*749*	*2916*
11-15 year olds							
Emotional disorders	4.0	6.6	6.4	5.0	4.7	9.4	6.1
Conduct disorders	2.1	1.5	2.6	3.0	7.5	5.5	3.8
Hyperkinetic disorders	0.2	-	-	1.2	0.4	0.4	0.5
Less common disorders	0.5	0.3	1.7	0.8	1.3	0.4	0.7
Any disorder	5.9	8.7	8.4	8.3	10.5	14.4	9.7
Base	*453*	*328*	*135*	*509*	*321*	*549*	*2296*
All girls							
Emotional disorders	2.9	4.2	4.9	4.3	3.9	6.4	4.5
Conduct disorders	1.5	1.8	3.0	2.8	5.2	4.7	3.2
Hyperkinetic disorders	0.2	-	-	0.8	0.5	0.7	0.4
Less common disorders	0.4	0.1	0.7	0.4	0.9	0.2	0.4
Any disorder	4.6	6.2	7.3	7.2	8.5	10.5	7.6
Base	*966*	*745*	*317*	*1206*	*680*	*1298*	*5211*

* CACI Limited 1994. All rights reserved. Source: ONS and GRO(S) © Crown Copyright 1991. All rights Reserved.

Table 4.12   (continued) Prevalence of mental disorders

by ACORN* classification, age and sex

All children

	A - Thriving	B - Expanding	C - Rising	D - Settling	E - Aspiring	F - Striving	All
	ACORN classification						
ALL	*Percentage of children with each disorder*						
5-10 year olds							
Emotional disorders	2.1	2.6	4.3	2.8	3.6	4.6	3.3
Conduct disorders	2.4	2.7	4.3	4.1	5.8	7.0	4.6
Hyperkinetic disorders	0.6	1.3	2.0	1.5	2.0	1.7	1.5
Less common disorders	0.3	0.4	0.6	0.7	0.9	0.4	0.5
Any disorder	4.8	6.0	9.3	7.6	10.1	10.9	8.2
Base	*1046*	*825*	*361*	*1327*	*763*	*1498*	*5819*
11-15 year olds							
Emotional disorders	3.6	5.2	4.0	5.2	5.3	8.3	5.6
Conduct disorders	2.6	3.7	5.7	4.9	9.4	9.9	6.2
Hyperkinetic disorders	0.6	0.5	1.3	1.7	1.9	1.9	1.4
Less common disorders	0.6	0.2	1.2	0.7	0.8	0.4	0.6
Any disorder	6.2	8.8	9.7	10.3	13.2	16.6	11.2
Base	*887*	*621*	*271*	*1044*	*638*	*1144*	*4605*
All children							
Emotional disorders	2.8	3.7	4.1	3.9	4.4	6.2	4.3
Conduct disorders	2.5	3.1	4.9	4.5	7.5	8.2	5.3
Hyperkinetic disorders	0.6	1.0	1.7	1.6	2.0	1.8	1.4
Less common disorders	0.4	0.3	0.9	0.7	0.9	0.4	0.5
Any disorder	5.4	7.2	9.4	8.8	11.5	13.3	9.5
Base	*1933*	*1446*	*631*	*2371*	*1401*	*2642*	*10424*

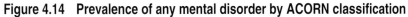

Figure 4.14   Prevalence of any mental disorder by ACORN classification

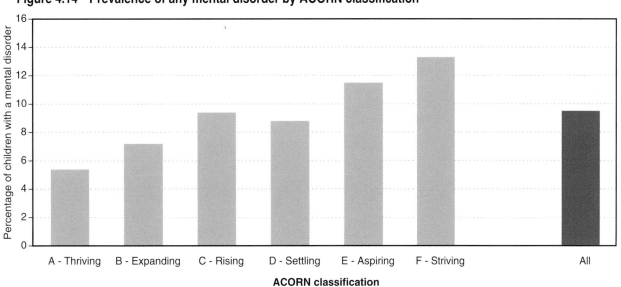

Table 4.15 Odds ratios for sociodemographic correlates of mental disorders

All children

Variable	Conduct disorders		Emotional disorders		Hyperkinetic disorders		Any disorder	
	Adjusted Odds ratio	95% C.I.	Adjusted Odds ratio	95% C.I.	Adjusted Odds ratio	95% C.I.	Adjusted Odds ratio	95% C.I.
Age								
5-10	1.00	-	1.00	-	1.00	-	1.00	-
11-15	1.45***	(1.20 - 1.75)	1.84***	(1.51-2.23)	0.96	(0.68-1.37)	1.48***	(1.29-1.70)
Sex								
Female	1.00	-	1.00	-	1.00	-	1.00	-
Male	2.42***	(1.98-2.96)	0.89	(0.74-1.08)	5.56***	(3.49-8.88)	1.58***	(1.37-1.81)
Number of children								
1	1.00	-	1.00	-	1.00	-	1.00	-
2	1.05	(0.81-1.35)	0.96	(0.74-1.25)	0.92	(0.60-1.43)	0.94	(0.78-1.12)
3	1.11	(0.82-1.48)	1.13	(0.84-1.50)	0.79	(0.47-1.33)	0.98	().80-1.21)
4	1.8***	(1.27-2.53)	1.23	(0.85-1.80)	0.65	().31-1.40)	1.32*	(1.01-1.73)
5	2.23***	(1.43-3.48)	1.43	(0.86-2.38)	0.71	(0.24-2.09)	1.63**	(1.14-2.34)
Family type								
Two parents	1.00	-	1.00	-	1.00	-	1.00	-
Lone parents	1.68***	(1.32-2.14)	1.55***	(1.20-2.00)	1.42	(0.89-2.27)	1.57***	(1.31-1.88)
ACORN Group								
Thriving	1.00	-	1.00	-	1.00	-	1.00	-
Expanding	1.27	(0.82-1.97)	1.40	(0.95-2.07)	1.61	(0.72-3.62)	1.39*	(1.04-1.86)
Rising	1.84*	(1.10-3.05)	1.48	(0.91-2.43)	3.00*	(1.22-7.36)	1.72**	(1.20-2.46)
Settling	1.68**	(1.16-2.42)	1.34	(0.95-1.90)	2.47**	(1.25-4.89)	1.58***	(1.23-2.04)
Aspiring	2.48***	(1.70-3.61)	1.33	(0.91-1.95)	2.78**	(1.35-5.73)	1.85***	(1.41-2.43)
Striving	2.45***	(1.73-3.48)	1.73**	(1.24-2.41)	2.41*	(1.22-4.79)	1.96***	(1.54-2.50)
Family's employment								
Both parents working	1.00	-	1.00	-	1.00	-	1.00	-
One parent working	1.14	(0.87-1.50)	1.44**	(1.10-1.87)	1.73*	(1.09-2.73)	1.3**	(1.07-158)
Neither working	1.9***	(1.47-2.46)	1.82***	(1.37-2.41)	2.13**	(1.29-3.15)	1.94***	(1.59-2.37)

*** p<0.001,   ** p<0.01,   * p<0.05

Table 4.16 Odds ratios for sociodemographic correlates of emotional disorders

Children with emotional disorders

Variable	Anxiety disorders		Depressive disorders		Emotional disorders	
	Adjusted Odds ratio	95% C.I.	Adjusted Odds ratio	95% C.I.	Adjusted Odds ratio	95% C.I.
Age						
5-10	1.00	-	1.00	-	1.00	-
11-15	1.56***	(1.27 - 1.93)	8.55***	(4.81-15.20)	1.84***	(1.51-2.23)
Sex						
Female	1.00	-	1.00	-	1.00	-
Male	0.85	(0.70-1.05)	0.84	(0.55-1.27)	0.89	(0.74-1.08)
Number of children						
1	1.00	-	1.00	-	1.00	-
2	0.97	(0.74-1.28)	1.26	(0.70-2.25)	0.96	(0.74-1.25)
3	1.15	(0.85-1.56)	1.58	(0.84-2.98)	1.13	(0.84-1.50)
4	1.06	(0.70-1.61)	2.64**	(1.27-5.45)	1.23	(0.85-1.80)
5	1.37	(0.79-2.36)	1.64	(0.53-5.06)	1.43	(0.86-2.38)
Family type						
Two parents	1.00	-	1.00	-	1.00	-
Lone parent	1.54**	(1.17-2.02)	1.69	(0.98-2.90)	1.55***	(1.20-2.00)
ACORN Group						
Thriving	1.00	-	1.00	-	1.00	-
Expanding	1.39	(0.93-2.09)	1.68	(0.72-3.93)	1.40	(0.95-2.07)
Rising	1.43	(0.85-2.42)	1.25	(0.38-4.06)	1.48	(0.91-2.43)
Settling	1.25	(0.87-1.80)	1.50	(0.70-3.24)	1.34	(0.95-1.90)
Aspiring	1.68**	(0.87-1.95)	1.18	(0.49-2.84)	1.33	(0.91-1.95)
Striving	2.45***	(1.18-2.38)	1.82	(0.87-3.79)	1.73**	(1.24-2.41)
Family's employment						
Both parents working	1.00	-	1.00	-	1.00	-
One parent working	1.38*	(1.04-1.83)	1.61	(0.89-2.92)	1.44**	(1.10-1.87)
Neither working	1.75***	(1.30-2.37)	2.48**	(1.40-4.41)	1.82***	(1.37-2.41)

*** p<0.001, ** p<0.01, * p<0.05

5 Characteristics of children with mental disorders

5.1 Introduction

The second part of this report focuses on children who were identified as having a mental disorder and looks at their physical health, social functioning, scholastic achievement, and lifestyle behaviours. Overall 936 children were assessed as having a mental disorder (before adjustment for missing teacher data). The numbers of children with each type of disorder were: 450 with an emotional disorder, 495 had a conduct disorder, 139 had a hyperkinetic disorder and 57 children had a less common disorder. Children who were assessed as having more than one disorder were included in each category.

This chapter compares children with each type of mental disorder with those who do not have a disorder by looking at the distribution of biographic and socio-demographic characteristics among the two groups of children. The characteristics considered were:

- sex
- age
- ethnicity
- family type
- number of children in the child's household
- educational qualifications of the interviewed parent
- employment status
- social class
- gross weekly household income
- type of accommodation
- tenure
- ACORN classification of the child's home
- country and region where the child lives

The commentary on the comparison between children with a disorder and those with no disorder is based on the data shown in Tables 5.1 to 5.5 and illustrated in Figures 5.1 to 5.5. The findings are presented in table order, rather than order of significance. Although some of the variables in the tables are interrelated, the strength of independent effects are not considered here. Chapter 4 of this report shows the odds ratios of socio-demographic and socio-economic correlates in relation to the prevalence of mental disorders.

5.2 Characteristics of children with any disorder

Compared with children who do not have a mental disorder, those with a disorder were more likely to be boys (60% compared with 49%) and 11-15 years old (52% compared with 43%).

Children with any mental disorder were:

more likely to be living:
- with a lone parent (37% compared with 21%)
- in a reconstituted family (14% compared with 9%)
- in a household where the interviewed parent had no qualifications (37% compared with 22%)
- in a lower income household, less than £200 per week (40% compared with 22%)
- in social sector housing (46% compared with 24%)
- in a family where neither parent was working (28% compared with 12%)
- in a terraced house (40% compared with 30%)
- in a household with an ACORN classification of F-striving (36% compared with 24%)

less likely to be living:
- with married parents (53% compared with 71%)
- in a household where the interviewed parent had qualifications above A-level or equivalent (14% compared with 23%)
- in social class II households (managerial and technical) (23% compared to 31%)
- in owner occupied households (45% compared with 70%)
- in a detached house (15% compared with 25%)
- in a household with an ACORN classification of A - thriving (11% compared with 19%)

In general, children with a mental disorder, compared with other children, were more likely to be male, living in a lower income household, in social sector housing and with a lone parent. They were less likely to be living with married parents or in social class I or II households.

5.3 Emotional disorders

Compared with children who do not have any mental disorder, those with an emotional disorder were more likely to be 11-15 years olds (57% compared with 43%).

Children with emotional disorders were:

more likely to be living:
- with a lone parent, divorced/widowed/separated (28% compared with 15%)
- in a household where the interviewed parent had no qualifications (37% compared with 22%)
- in a household where neither parent was working (27% compared with 12%)
- in a lower income household, less than £200 per week (38% compared with 22%)
- in social sector housing (43% compared with 24%)
- in a household with an ACORN classification of F-striving (36% compared with 24%)

less likely to be living:
- with a married couple (56% compared with 71%)
- in a household where the interviewed parent had qualifications above A-level or equivalent (14% compared with 23%)
- with two working parents (53% compared with 69%)
- in social classes II (managerial and technical) (23% compared with 31%)
- in accommodation owned by their parent(s) (48% compared with 70%)
- in a detached house (16% compared with 25%)

In summary, children with an emotional disorder in contrast to those with no mental disorder were more likely to be 11 - 15 years olds, living in social sector housing and in lower income households.

They were less likely to live in a home that is owned by their parents and for both their parents to be working.

5.4 Conduct disorders

Compared with children who do not have any mental disorder, those with a conduct disorder were more likely to be boys (70% compared with 49%) and 11-15 years old (52% compared with 43%).

Children with conduct disorders were:

more likely to be living:
- in lone parent families (42% compared with 21%)
- in a reconstituted family (18% compared with 9%)
- with interviewed parent who had no educational qualifications (42% compared with 22%)
- in a family where neither parents are working (32% compared with 12%)
- with parent(s) who had never worked (6% compared with 2%)
- in social class V household (22% compared with 14%)
- in a lower income household, less than £200 per week (45% compared with 22%)
- in social sector housing (55% compared with 24%)
- in a terraced house (43% compared with 30%)
- in a household with an ACORN classification of F-striving (39% compared with 24%)

less likely to be living:
- with married parents (47% compared with 71%)
- in a household where the interviewed parent had qualifications above A-level or equivalent (11% compared with 23%)
- in a family with both parents working (52% compared with 69%)
- in a social class I and II households (24% compared with 39%)
- in accommodation owned by their parent(s) (37% compared with 70%)
- in a detached house (10% compared with 25%)
- in a household with an ACORN classification of A-thriving (9% compared with 19%)

In general, children with a conduct disorder were more likely than children without a mental disorder to be living in social sector housing, with neither parents working, and where the interviewed parent had no educational qualifications. They were less likely to be living with married parents and in accommodation owned by their parent (s).

5.5   Hyperkinetic disorders

Compared with children who do not have any mental disorder, those with a hyperkinetic disorder were more likely to be boys (85% compared with 49%).

Children with hyperkinetic disorders were:

more likely to be living:
- in lone parent family (37% compared with 21%)
- with interviewed parent who had no educational qualifications (36% compared with 12%)
- in a reconstituted family (16% compared with 9%)
- in a family where neither parent was working (28% compared with 12%)
- in a lower income household, between £100 - £199 per week (41% compared with 22%)
- in social class IV and V households (28% compared with 19%)

- in social sector housing (46% compared with 24%)
- in a terraced house (41% compared with 30%)

less likely to be living:
- with married parents (56% compared with 71%)
- in a household where the interviewed parent had qualifications above A-level or equivalent (12% compared with 23%)
- in a family where both parents were working (51% compared with 69%)
- in a social class I or II households (23% compared with 39%)
- in a household with an ACORN classification of A - thriving (8% compared with 19%)

To summarise children with a hyperkinetic disorder were more likely than children without a mental disorder to be living in social sector housing, in a lower income household, and whose interviewed parent had no educational qualifications. They were less likely to be living in a social class I or II households and with parents who were working.

5.6   Less common disorders

Because of the small number of the children who had a less common disorder, such as autism, eating or tic disorders, a comparison could not be made between those who had any of these disorders and the sample of children with no mental disorder.

Figure 5.1   Sex distribution by type of mental disorder

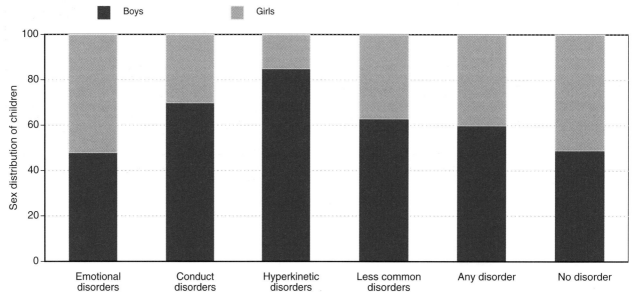

Figure 5.2 Family's employment situation by type of mental disorder

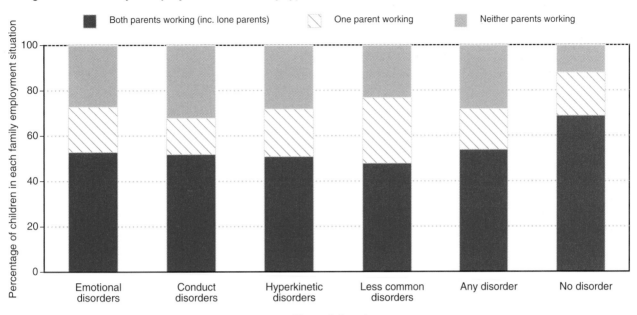

Figure 5.3 Gross weekly household income by type of mental disorder

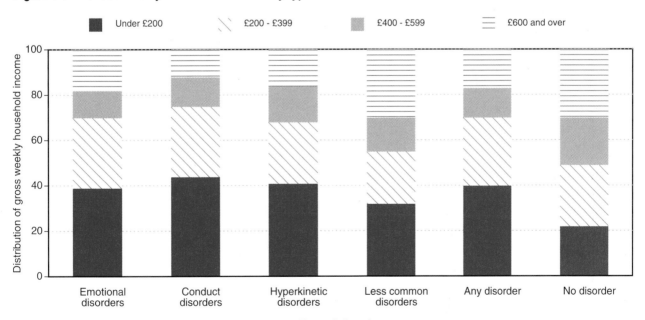

Figure 5.4   Tenure by type of mental disorder

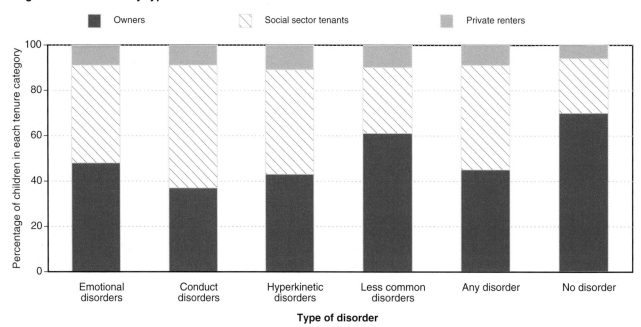

Figure 5.5   ACORN classification by type of mental disorder

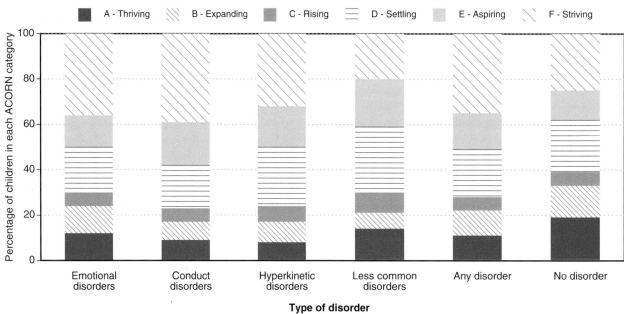

Table 5.1 Number of children with each mental disorder

by age and sex

All children

| | Type of mental disorder | | | | | | |
	Emotional disorders	Conduct disorders	Hyperkinetic disorders	Less common disorders	Any disorder•	No disorder	All
	Number of children with each disorder						
5-10 years							
Boys	96	168	68	24	285	2624	2909
Girls	95	71	12	6	164	2757	2921
All	192	239	80	30	449	5381	5829
11-15 years							
Boys	118	177	49	12	278	2032	2310
Girls	140	78	10	16	209	2089	2299
All	258	255	58	27	487	4121	4609
All children							
Boys	214	345	117	36	563	4656	5219
Girls	236	149	21	21	373	4847	5219
All	450	495	139	57	936	9502	10438

* The number of children with any mental disorder exceeds the sum of the numbers of children with each disorder because children could have been assessed as having more than one type of disorder.

Table 5.2 Child's personal characteristics

by type of mental disorder

All children

| | Type of mental disorder | | | | | | |
	Emotional disorders	Conduct disorders	Hyperkinetic disorders	Less common disorders	Any disorder	No disorder	All
	%	%	%	%	%	%	%
Sex							
Boys	48	70	85	63	60	49	50
Girls	52	30	15	37	40	51	50
Age							
5-10 years	43	48	58	52	48	57	56
11-15 years	57	52	42	48	52	43	44
Ethnicity							
White	91	92	99	94	92	91	91
Black	2	4	1	2	3	3	3
Indian	1	1	-	-	1	2	2
Pakistani & Bangladeshi	2	1	-	-	1	2	2
Other	3	2	1	4	3	3	3
Base	*450*	*495*	*139*	*57*	*936*	*9502*	*10438*

Table 5.3	Family characteristics
	by type of mental disorder

All children

	Type of mental disorder						
	Emotional disorders	Conduct disorders	Hyperkinetic disorders	Less common disorders	Any disorder	No disorder	All
	%	%	%	%	%	%	%
Family type							
Married	56	47	56	64	53	71	70
Cohabiting	8	11	7	7	9	8	8
Lone parent - single	8	14	15	6	11	6	7
Lone parent - w/d/s	28	28	22	23	26	15	16
Reconstituted family							
No	88	82	84	88	86	91	91
Yes	12	18	16	12	14	9	9
Number of children in household							
1	22	20	25	25	23	21	21
2	39	39	44	41	39	46	45
3	24	22	21	23	22	23	23
4	10	13	7	9	11	8	8
5 or more	5	7	3	2	5	3	3
Parents educational qualifications							
Degree level	7	5	7	16	7	12	12
Teaching/HND/Nursing level	8	6	5	9	7	11	11
A-level (or equivalent)	8	8	9	12	8	10	10
GCSE grades A-C or equivalent	25	23	19	23	24	30	29
GCSE grades D-F or equivalent	13	12	17	9	13	12	12
Other qualification	3	3	6	5	3	3	3
No qualification	37	42	36	25	37	22	23
Base	*450*	*495*	*139*	*57*	*936*	*9502*	*10438*

Table 5.4	Family's employment status, social class and income
	by type of mental disorder

All children

	Type of mental disorder						
	Emotional disorders	Conduct disorders	Hyperkinetic disorders	Less common disorders	Any disorder	No disorder	All
	%	%	%	%	%	%	%
Family's employment status							
Both parents working (inc. lone parents)	53	52	51	48	54	69	67
One parent working	20	16	21	29	18	19	19
Neither parents working	27	32	28	23	28	12	14
Family's social class							
Professional	3	4	4	16	4	8	7
Managerial and technical	24	20	19	35	23	31	31
Skilled non-manual	14	13	16	10	14	11	12
Skilled manual	26	23	26	12	25	25	25
Partly skilled	19	22	24	13	19	14	15
Unskilled	7	9	4	7	7	5	5
Armed forces	0	0	-	2	0	0	0
FT student	1	2	1	-	1	1	1
NA inadeq description	2	1	2	2	2	2	2
Never worked	4	6	4	4	4	2	2
Gross weekly household income							
Under £100	8	10	8	7	9	5	6
£100 - £199	30	35	33	24	31	17	18
£200 - £299	19	19	16	16	19	14	15
£300 - £399	12	12	12	7	12	12	12
£400 - £499	7	8	8	9	7	11	10
£500 - £599	6	5	8	6	6	11	10
£600 - £770	7	5	8	13	7	13	12
Over £770	11	7	8	17	10	17	16
Base	*450*	*495*	*139*	*57*	*936*	*9502*	*10438*

Table 5.5	Household and geographical characteristics
	by type of mental disorder

All children

	Type of mental disorder						
	Emotional disorders	Conduct disorders	Hyperkinetic disorders	Less common disorders	Any disorder	No disorder	All
	%	%	%	%	%	%	%
Type of accommodation							
Detached	16	10	15	23	15	25	25
Semi-detached	34	40	35	37	37	38	38
Terraced house	39	43	41	36	40	30	31
Flat/maisonette	10	7	8	4	9	6	6
Tenure							
Owners	48	37	43	61	45	70	68
Social sector tenants	43	55	46	29	46	24	26
Private renters	9	9	11	10	9	6	6
ACORN classification							
A - Thriving	12	9	8	14	11	19	19
B - Expanding	12	8	9	7	11	14	14
C - Rising	6	6	7	9	6	6	6
D - Settling	20	19	25	28	21	23	23
E - Aspiring	14	19	18	21	16	13	13
F - Striving	36	39	32	20	36	24	25
Region							
London inner	7	5	6	2	6	5	5
London outer	6	5	4	6	6	6	6
Other met England	31	32	25	39	32	31	31
Non-met England	42	46	54	39	44	45	45
Country							
England	86	88	89	85	88	86	86
Scotland	9	7	7	8	8	9	9
Wales	5	5	4	6	5	5	5
Base	*450*	*495*	*139*	*57*	*936*	*9502*	*10438*

Part 2: Children and adolescents with specific mental disorders

6 Mental disorders and physical complaints

6.1 Introduction

This chapter looks at the extent to which physical complaints co-occur with mental disorders among children and adolescents. In the survey, data were collected on several aspects of the physical health of children. However, all information came from the interview with parents.

The topics covered were:

- General health
- Presence or absence of specified physical complaints
- Life threatening illnesses
- Accidents and injuries

Specific physical complaints were chosen on the basis of their common occurrence in childhood and adolescence (e.g. asthma), findings from previous research showing a strong association with mental disorders (e.g. epilepsy), problems frequently mentioned by parents during the pilot stage of this survey (e.g. food allergies) and their inclusion in other national mental health surveys.

Previous research has shown that children with physical health problems or disabilities seem especially vulnerable to mental health problems. Rutter (1970) found in the Isle of Wight studies that children with asthma, epilepsy and neurological disorders in general were far more likely than the general population to have a mental disorder. In a national survey of disabled children in Great Britain, mental and behavioural problems were found among a large proportion of children with physical disabilities (Bone and Meltzer, 1989). They also found that nearly all the children with the most severe disabilities had a mental health disability.

In the present study, parents were also asked if they thought their child had: emotional problems, behavioural problems, hyperactivity, learning difficulties and dyslexia. The chapter concludes with a comparison of parents' perceptions and the clinical evaluation of emotional, behavioural and hyperkinetic disorders. Specific and learning difficulties in relation to mental disorders are discussed in Chapter 8.

6.2 General health

The child's general health was rated by parents on a five point scale: very good, good, fair, bad or very bad. The overall proportion of children with a fair, bad or very bad rating was 7%, the corresponding proportion among children with a mental disorder was 20% compared with 6% of those without a disorder. This pattern was found for all types of mental disorder. *(Table 6.1)*

6.3 Physical complaints

To what extent are physical complaints more commonly found in children with mental disorders, and conversely, to what extent are mental disorders more prevalent among children with specific physical complaints? These two questions are answered in this section. Physical complaints can vary in their severity, chronicity, and treatability. This survey did not cover these aspects; the parent just said "yes" if the child had the health problem or condition presented on three lists.

Asthma	Hyperactivity	Diabetes
Eczema	Behavioural problems	Obesity
Hay fever	Emotional problems	Cystic fibrosis
Glue ear or otitis media or grommets	Learning difficulties	Spina bifida
Bed wetting	Dyslexia	Kidney, urinary tract problems
Soiling pants	Cerebral palsy	Missing fingers, hands, arms, toes, feet or legs
Stomach or digestive problems or tummy pains	Migraine or severe headaches	Any stiffness or deformity of the foot, leg, fingers, arms or back
A heart problem	Chronic Fatigue Syndrome	Any muscle disease or weakness
Any blood disorder	Eye or sight problems	Any difficulty with co-ordination
Epilepsy	Speech or language problems	A condition present since birth such as club foot or cleft palate
Food allergy Some other allergy	Hearing problems	Cancer

Figure 6.1   Percentage of children with a mental disorder by type of physical complaint

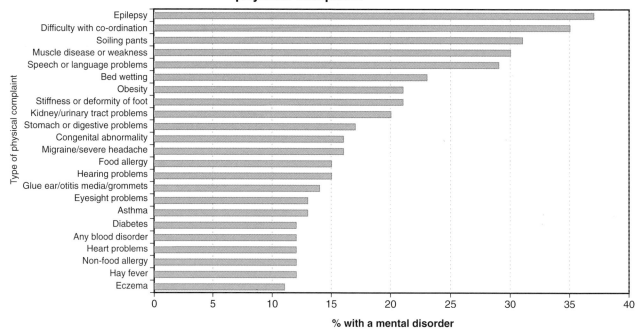

Approximately two-thirds of children with a mental disorder had one of the physical complaints listed above (i.e. excluding hyperactivity, emotional problems, behavioural problems, learning difficulties and dyslexia) compared with about half the children who were assessed as not having a mental disorder. *(Table 6.2)*

The most commonly reported physical complaints among the ten and a half thousand children and adolescents were: asthma (16%), eczema (12%) eyesight problems (11%) and hay fever (10%). Although these four complaints occurred more frequently among children with a mental disorder (compared with those with no disorder) the differences in proportions were not particularly large. The physical illness or health conditions which showed the greatest disparity in prevalence rates between children with a mental disorder and those with no disorder were: bedwetting (12% compared with 4%), speech or language problems (12% compared with 3%), co-ordination difficulties (8% compared with 2%), and soiling pants (4% compared with 1%). Among children with any disorder, stomach and digestive problems and migraine and severe headaches were most prevalent among children with emotional problems, 15% and 12% respectively, most probably reflecting the somatic symptoms associated with anxiety and depression. *(Table 6.2)*

Logistic regression analysis shows that having any physical complaint (compared with no physical health condition) increased the odds of having a mental disorder by 82% having adjusted for biographic, socio-demographic, socio-economic and geo-demographic factors. *(Table 6.3)*

Looking at the prevalence of mental disorders by particular physical complaints, children with neurological problems - epilepsy and co-ordination difficulties - were more frequently assessed as having a mental disorder. There were six physical complaints where over 22% of sufferers had a mental disorder: epilepsy (37%), difficulties with co-ordination (35%), soiling pants (31%), muscle disease or weakness (30%), speech or language problems (29%) and enuresis (23%). *(Figure 6.1, Table 6.4)*

6.4   Life threatening illness

Parents were also asked if their child was ever so ill that they thought s/he may die. Whereas 12% of the parents said "Yes" to this question, a greater proportion was found among children with mental disorders than with no disorder: 22% compared with 11%. There was little difference in the proportions of children who had experienced a life-threatening illness by type of mental disorder, ranging from 26% of those with emotional disorders to 19% of those with conduct disorders. *(Table 6.5)*

Looking at the same data from a different perspective, among children who had a life-threatening illness, about 1 in 6 were found to have a mental disorder.

6.5 Accidents and injuries

The general health section of the questionnaire asked parents to say whether their children ever had four types of accident or injury:

- Head injury with loss of consciousness
- Accident causing broken bone (excluding head injury)
- Burn requiring hospitalisation
- Accidental poisoning requiring hospital admission

Not unexpectedly, a broken bone was the most frequently mentioned accident, reported for 16% of children. Five percent of children had suffered a head injury causing loss of consciousness at some time in their lives, two percent of children had received a burn requiring hospital admission and two percent of children had been accidentally poisoned to the extent that they required hospitalisation. Children with a mental disorder were more likely than those without a disorder to have experienced each of these accidents or injuries: 20% had fractured a bone, 9% had a serious head injury, 5% had a burn requiring hospitalisation, and 5% also had been accidentally poisoned. There was no apparent association between type of accident or injury and type of mental disorder. *(Table 6.6)*

Another way of presenting these data is to look at the prevalence of mental disorders among children with accidents and injuries. Fourteen per cent of children who had any of the four types of injury had a mental disorder compared with eight percent of the sample with no injury. Children who had accidental poisoning had the highest rate of mental disorder, 25%, whereas the prevalence among children who had a broken bone at 12% was just above the national average. *(Table 6.7)*

6.6 Parents' views of their child's mental health

Because parents were asked at the start of the interview to indicate whether their child had any of the thirty four health conditions shown above, they had an opportunity to say whether they thought their child had hyperactivity, emotional problems or behavioural problems before being asked the detailed questions on which the assessments of disorders were made. Whereas parents views covered problems (of all severity), the clinical ratings assessed disorders on strict impairment criteria. Therefore, the most meaningful question is - what proportion of children described by their parents as hyperactive or having behavioural or emotional problems were clinically assessed as having mental disorders?

Parents could not be expected to differentiate between emotional, behavioural or hyperkinetic disorders but might be aware of their child's mental health problem. Among the 928 children with a clinical rating on any of the three types of disorder, about a half of their parents thought their child had a mental health problem. This is a surprising result because a clinical diagnosis was only given to children where the mental problem had a significant effect on the child's life or caused distress to others. A higher proportion might have been expected. Parents may have felt it too embarrassing to say that their child had such problems so early in the interview. The finding that about 6% of children not given a diagnosis during the clinical review were described by their parent as having a problem is not so surprising as the child may exhibit symptoms that do not meet research diagnostic criteria or have several symptoms with minimal social impairment. *(Table 6.8)*

Parents tend to use the terms, emotional problems, conduct problems and hyperactivity to cover a wide range of situations. A thousand parents (10% of those interviewed) said their child had one of the three listed problems: emotional problems (435), behavioural problems (574) and hyperactivity (355). Parents' attributions compared with the clinical diagnoses suggest that parents use the terms hyperactivity, emotional and behavioural problems in everyday language to express a difference between what they expect of their children and how they behave. This underlines the necessity of including some sort of clinical assessment in psychiatric morbidity surveys among children rather than relying solely on self-reported, general assessments by parents. (*Table 6.9*)

References

Bone, M., and Meltzer, H. (1989) *OPCS Surveys of disability in Great Britain, Report 3, The prevalence of disability among children,* London: HMSO

Rutter, M., Tizard, J. and Whitmore, K. (1970) *Education, Health and Behaviour,* London: Longmans.

Table 6.1	General health rating
	by type of mental disorder

All children

	Type of mental disorder						All
	Emotional disorders	Conduct disorders	Hyperkinetic disorders	Less common disorders	Any disorder	No disorder	
General health rating	%	%	%	%	%	%	%
Very good	43	52	46	37	49	70	69
Good	32	29	34	42	31	24	24
Fair	19	17	17	12	17	6	6
Bad	5 } 24	2 } 19	4 } 21	4 } 22	3 } 20	0 } 6	1 } 7
Very bad	0	-	-	6	0	0	0
Base	444	492	139	57	927	9380	10307

Table 6.2	Type of physical complaint

by type of mental disorder

All children

	Type of mental disorder						
	Emotional disorders	Conduct disorders	Hyperkinetic disorders	Less common disorders	Any disorder	No disorder	All
	Proportion of children with each type of physical complaint						
Asthma	23	20	25	22	20	15	16
Eczema	15	12	12	10	14	12	12
Eyesight problems	14	15	15	15	14	10	11
Hay fever	12	11	9	6	11	9	10
Stomach or digestive problems	15	8	8	9	11	6	6
Non-food allergy	8	6	7	8	7	6	6
Migraine/severe headache	12	7	4	6	8	5	5
Glue ear/otitis media/grommets	6	7	9	10	7	5	5
Bed wetting	11	12	18	18	12	4	5
Hearing problems	5	7	7	7	7	4	4
Speech or language problems	11	10	16	38	12	3	4
Food allergy	5	6	6	12	6	3	4
Difficulty with co-ordination	7	7	15	32	8	2	2
Stiffness or deformity of foot	4	4	4	4	4	2	2
Heart problems	2	1	2	-	2	1	1
Soiling pants	3	4	7	14	4	1	1
Muscle disease or weakness	4	2	5	3	3	1	1
Kidney/urinary tract problems	3	2	3	-	2	1	1
Obesity	2	2	2	4	2	1	1
Congenital abnormality	1	1	4	4	1	1	1
Epilepsy	2	2	1	11	2	1	1
Any blood disorder	1	1	1	2	1	0	1
Diabetes	1	1	1	-	1	0	1
Any physical complaint	**71**	**64**	**71**	**84**	**67**	**52**	**54**
No physical complaint	**29**	**36**	**29**	**16**	**33**	**48**	**46**
Base	*445*	*492*	*139*	*57*	*928*	*9381*	*10310*

Some physical complaints are not listed in the table above because of their rarity, i.e less than 25 cases: ME (4) Spina bifida (4) Cystic fibrosis (6) Cancer (16) Missing digits (16) Cerebral palsy (24) but are included in the any physical complaint category.

Table 6.3	Odds Ratios for physical complaints and sociodemographic correlates of mental disorders

All children

Variable	Value	Adjusted Odds ratio	95% C.I.
Physical complaint	No	1.00	-
	Yes	1.82***	(1.57-2.10)
Age	5-10	1.00	-
	11-15	1.46***	(1.27-1.68)
Sex	Female	1.00	-
	Male	1.55***	(1.35-1.79)
Number of children	1	1.00	-
	2	0.92	(0.77-1.11)
	3	0.98	(0.79-1.20)
	4	1.35*	(1.04-1.77)
	5	1.67**	(1.16-2.39)
Family type	Two parent	1.00	-
	Lone parent	1.60***	(1.33-1.92)
ACORN Group	Thriving	1.00	-
	Expanding	1.38*	(1.03-1.84)
	Rising	1.64**	(1.15-2.34)
	Settling	1.58***	(1.23-2.03)
	Aspiring	1.79***	(1.36-2.34)
	Striving	1.89***	(1.48-2.41)
Family's employment	Both parents working	1.00	-
	One parent working	1.26**	(1.04-1.53)
	Neither working	1.88***	(1.54-2.30)

*** p<0.001, ** p<0.01, * p<0.05

Table 6.4 Prevalence of mental disorders

by type of physical complaint

All children

	Emotional disorders	Conduct disorders	Hyperkinetic disorders	Less common disorders	Any disorder	Base
	Percentage of children with mental disorders for each complaint					
Epilepsy	17	18	1	10	37	67
Difficulty with co-ordination	13	17	10	8	35	235
Soiling pants	13	17	9	7	31	116
Muscle disease or weakness	18	10	8	2	30	99
Speech or language problems	12	15	7	6	29	393
Bed wetting	10	13	5	2	23	484
Stiffness or deformity of foot	10	12	3	1	21	183
Obesity	11	11	4	2	21	84
Kidney/urinary tract problems	12	10	4	-	20	96
Stomach or digestive problems	11	7	2	1	17	629
Migraine/severe headache	10	8	1	1	16	513
Congenital abnormality	6	4	8	3	16	74
Hearing problems	5	9	2	1	15	429
Food allergy	6	9	2	2	15	370
Glue ear/otitis media/grommets	5	8	2	1	14	480
Asthma	6	7	2	1	13	1604
Eyesight problems	6	7	2	1	13	1097
Hay fever	6	7	1	0	12	976
Non-food allergy	6	6	2	1	12	581
Heart problems	7	2	2	-	12	128
Any blood disorder	8	7	2	2	12	47
Diabetes	6	10	2	-	12	47
Eczema	5	6	1	0	11	1289

Table 6.5 Experience of a life threatening illness

by type of mental disorder

All children

	Type of mental disorder						
	Emotional disorders	Conduct disorders	Hyperkinetic disorders	Less common disorders	Any disorder	No disorder	All
	%	%	%	%	%	%	%
Thought child was so ill that s/he may die							
Yes: in past 12 months	2	2	1	-	2	1	1
Yes: at least 12 months ago	25	17	22	21	20	10	11
No	74	81	77	79	79	89	88
Base	*445*	*492*	*139*	*57*	*928*	*9379*	*10308*

Table 6.6	Experience of accidents and injuries
	by type of mental disorder

All children

	Type of mental disorder						
	Emotional disorders	Conduct disorders	Hyperkinetic disorders	Less common disorders	Any disorder	No disorder	All
	%	%	%	%	%	%	%
Head injury with loss of consciousness							
Yes: in past 12 months	2	1	-	2	2	1	1
Yes: at least 12 months ago	7	9	10	7	7	3	4
No	91	90	90	90	91	96	96
Accident causing broken bone							
Yes: in past 12 months	4	3	5	5	4	3	3
Yes: at least 12 months ago	17	16	14	11	16	13	13
No	79	80	81	84	80	84	84
Burn requiring hospital admission							
Yes: in past 12 months	0	0	-	-	0	0	0
Yes: at least 12 months ago	4	6	7	3	5	2	2
No	96	94	93	97	95	98	98
Accidental poisoning with hospital admission							
Yes: in past 12 months	-	0	1	-	0	0	0
Yes: at least 12 months ago	7	7	5	7	5	2	2
No	93	93	94	93	94	98	98
Base	*444*	*492*	*139*	*57*	*927*	*9380*	*10307*

Table 6.7	Prevalence of mental disorders
	by type of accident or injury

All children

	Head injury	Broken bone	Burn	Poisoning	Any injury or accident	No injury or accident	All
	Percentage of children with each disorder						
Emotional disorders	9	6	7	13	6	4	4
Conduct disorders	12	7	13	16	8	4	6
Hyperkinetic disorders	3	2	4	4	2	1	1
Less common disorders	1	1	1	2	1	1	1
Any mental disorder	**19**	**12**	**20**	**25**	**14**	**8**	**10**
Base	*456*	*1655*	*233*	*222*	*3173*	*7133*	*10306*

Table 6.8	Parental view of child's mental health
	by clinical assessment of type of mental disorder

All children

	Clinical assessment of type of mental disorder				
	Emotional disorders	Conduct disorders	Hyperkinetic disorders	Any disorder	No disorder
	Percentage of children whose parents gave each rating				
Parents' view of child's mental health					
Emotional problems	27	26	23	24	2
Behavioural problems	20	52	61	36	3
Hyperactivity	10	21	50	17	2
Any problem	**36**	**62**	**72**	**48**	**6**
Base	*445*	*492*	*139*	*928*	*9380*

Table 6.9	Clinical assessment of type of mental disorder
	by parental view of child's mental health

All children

	Parent's view of child's mental health				
	Emotional problems	Behavioural problems	Hyperactivity	Any of the 3 problems	None of the 3 problems
	Percentage of children with each type of clinical rating				
Clinical assessment of type of mental disorder					
Emotional disorders	28	15	12	16	3
Conduct disorders	34	50	32	35	2
Hyperkinetic disorders	8	16	22	11	0
Any of the 3 disorders	**51**	**58**	**43**	**46**	**5**
Base	*435*	*574*	*355*	*1000*	*9438*

7 Use of services

7.1 Introduction

Parents were asked about three types of services that their children used:

- Contact with primary health care services for any reason over the past 12 months (all children)
- Consultations with health, social or educational services (children with a mental disorder)
- Advice or help sought from family or friends (children with a mental disorder)

The questions on service use for mental health problems asked the parent to specify the area that the service provider came from, for example, specialist health care or social services. Therefore, services could not be categorised according to the four tiers of Child and Adolescent Mental Health Services (CAMHS). More detailed questions (which would have allowed for a CAMHS classification) were piloted but were dropped because parents were not always able to give the job title of the person the child had been seen by, especially if they had been in contact with more than one professional.

The chapter concludes by looking at the relationship between mental disorders and the child's contact with the police.

7.2 Use of health services for any reason

The child's contact with primary health care providers in the past 12 months was examined in relation to four types of services:

- GPs (excluding consultations for immunisation, child surveillance or development tests)
- Accident and Emergency departments
- In-patient departments
- Out-patient or day patient services

GP contacts

Overall, 36% of children (or parents on behalf of their children) had been in contact with a GP in the past 12 months. Almost a half of the children with a disorder had been in contact with a GP in the past 12 months for any reason compared with just over a third of children with no disorder. The survey did not include questions on reason for consultation. There was little difference in GP contacts by type of disorder, with proportions ranging from 45% among children with conduct disorders to 52% of those with hyperkinetic disorders. *(Table 7.1, Figure 7.1)*

Children who had a mental disorder also seemed to make more visits to their GP: 25% of those with a disorder had been in contact with their GP on three or more occasions in the past 12 months compared with 13% of those without a disorder.

Accident and Emergency departments

Just under a fifth of children (18%) had visited an Accident and Emergency department in the past 12 months and most children needed to go on one occasion only. Children with a disorder were more likely to have been taken to an Accident and Emergency department than those without a disorder (26% compared with 17%) and on more than one occasion (7% compared with 4%). This may be explained by the finding in the previous chapter that accidents and injuries were more commonly reported for children with a disorder. Children with a hyperkinetic disorder were almost twice as likely as those with no disorder to have visited an Accident and Emergency department in the last year (31% compared with 17%). *(Table 7.1, Figure 7.1)*

Inpatient stays

Inpatient stays were rare events for children aged 5-15 years. Only 5% had been in hospital in the past year. Inpatient stays were slightly more common among children with a disorder than those without (9% compared with 5%) *(Table 7.1, Figure 7.1)*

Outpatient or day patients

About 1 in 5 children had been to a hospital as an outpatient or as a day patient in the past year. These visits were in addition to the attendance at Casualty Departments. Children with a mental disorder were more likely than other children to have visited an Outpatient Department in the past year: 29% compared with 18% and children with hyperkinetic disorders and less common disorders were the most frequent visitors.
(Table 7.1, Figure 7.1)

7.3 Use of services for significant mental health problems

When parents indicated that their children had significant mental health problems, they were asked which health, social or educational service they sought help from. 71% of all children with a mental disorder had been seen by either a GP or a secondary care provider, for example, paediatrician, social worker or educational psychologist. This proportion decreased slightly, to 65% if only secondary care (excluding those who only saw their GP) was considered.

Overall, 30% of children with mental disorders had not been seen by a GP or specialist health care services. Children with emotional disorders were the least likely to have been seen by either of these health care services. This finding is not surprising because parents of children with emotional disorders may often be unaware of their child's problems; children with emotional disorders may keep their worries and anxieties to themselves. Parents also tend to take their child's emotional problems less seriously.

Contact with services varied by type of disorder: 63% of children with any emotional disorder (that is, anxiety and depression) had been in contact with services increasing to about 76% of children with behavioural problems and to 81% of those with hyperkinetic disorders. Nearly all the children and adolescents with the less common disorders (autism, tic and eating disorders) had been seen by at least one of the services. *(Figure 7.2)*

Focusing on the use of particular types of service, half the children with mental disorders had seen someone from the educational services, about a quarter had used the specialist health care services and a fifth had contact with the social services. *(Table 7.2)*

Figure 7.1 Use of services (for any reason) by mental disorder

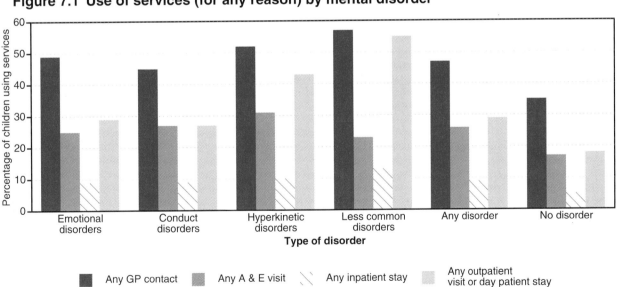

Figure 7.2 Contact with primary and secondary health services by type of mental disorder

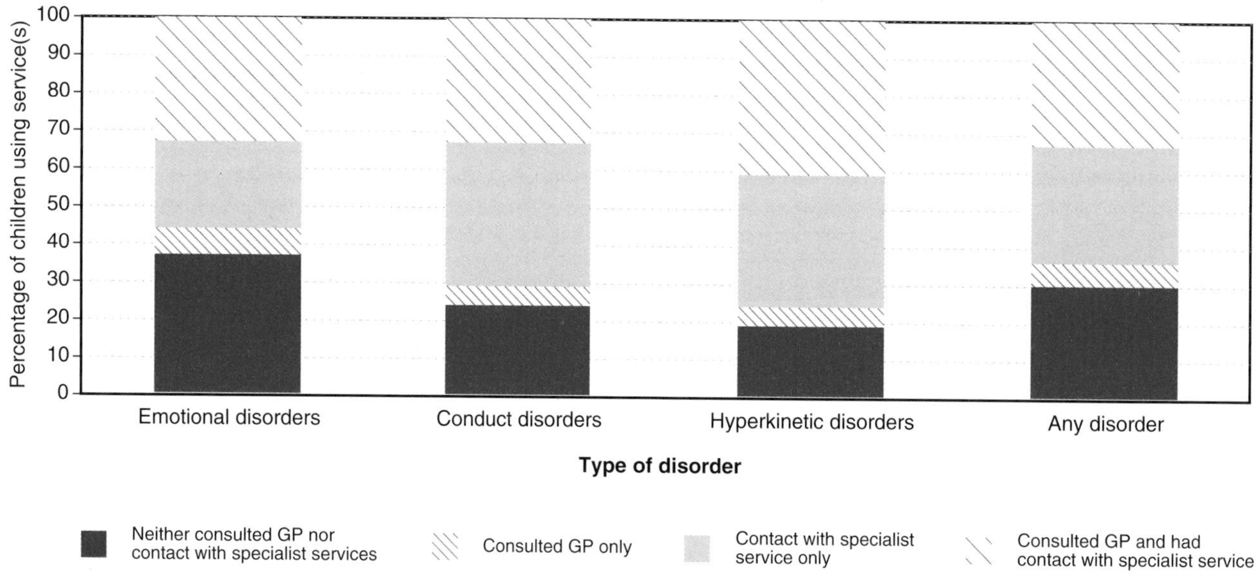

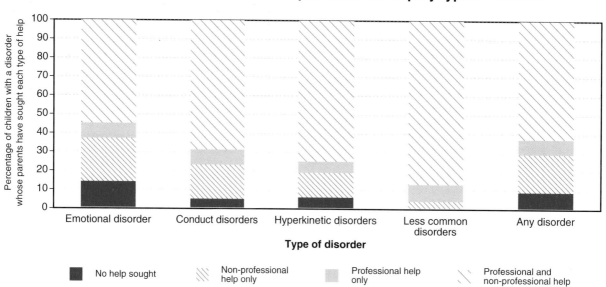

7.4   Use of professional and non-professional help

If parents are concerned about their child's well-being, they may seek the advice of friends, relatives or neighbours instead of or as well as professional help. Parents of children with a disorder were asked if they had sought non-professional help as well as professional help for their child's problem.

Approximately 9 in 10 parents had looked for some type of help or advice. The majority, 62% had sought both professional and non-professional help for their children, 20% had sought non-professional help only and 8% had sought professional help only. (*Table 7.3, figure 7.3*)

Service use varied by type of disorder. Parents of children with an emotional disorder were the

Figure 7.3 Use of professional and non-professional help by type of disorder

group most likely to have asked family or friends for advice (23%) and the least likely to have sought professional services (63%) compared with parents of children with other disorders.

Service use was also related to the number of specific mental disorders (e.g. separation anxiety, social phobia, generalised anxiety) indicating that the variety or the severity of problems may initiate the search for professional help. The proportion of parents who had sought professional help/advice increased from 66% of those with one disorder to 77% of children with two disorders and to 89% of those with three or more disorders. (*Table 7.4*)

7.5 Socio-demographic correlates of service use

In order to examine further the characteristics of children who received services, multiple logistic regression was used to produce odds ratios for the socio-demographic correlates of the use of professional services.

Each odds ratio shows the increase or decrease in odds that a parent of a child with a disorder had sought professional or non-professional advice compared with those who had not. The variables entered into the model were age, sex, number of children, family type, ACORN classification and family's employment status. ACORN was chosen as the economic indicator because it takes account of tenure, type of accommodation and income.

The significant odds ratios for the socio-demographic correlates of the parent seeking professional help (compared with not seeking professional help) were the child's sex and family's employment status. The odds of having sought professional help increased by about a half for boys compared with girls, and by around two-thirds for families with neither parent working compared with both parents working. (*Table 7.5*)

7.6 Trouble with the police

Parents were asked if their child had been in trouble with the police in the last 12 months. Overall, 2% of children had this experience. Not unexpectedly, more boys than girls and more older than younger children had been in trouble with the police. Nevertheless, the presence of a mental disorder was also a major factor. Ten per cent of children with a mental disorder had been in trouble with the police compared with just 1% of those with no disorder. One in six children with a conduct disorder had been in trouble with the police. (*Table 7.6*)

Among children who had been in trouble with the police, those with a disorder were almost three times more likely than children with no disorder to have been in this situation more than once in the past 12 months (44% compared with 12%). (*Table, not shown*)

Young people who were interviewed (11-15 year olds) and who had already admitted to troublesome behaviour were also asked (as part of the self-completion questionnaire) whether they had ever been in trouble with the police. It is important to note that the information obtained via the parents about police contact cannot be directly compared with that given by the young person, because parents may not know what their children have been up to and they were only asked if their child had been in trouble with the police in the past 12 months.

Overall, 25% of 11-15 year olds who reported awkward or troublesome behaviour said that at one point in their lives they had been in trouble with the police, which included 43% of children with a disorder and 21% of children with no disorder. Half the children with conduct disorders had been in trouble with the police compared with a third of those with emotional disorders. (*Table 7.7*)

Table 7.1	Use of health services in the past 12 months (for any reason)
	by type of mental disorder

All children

Service contacted in past 12 months	Type of mental disorder						
	Emotional disorders	Conduct disorders	Hyperkinetic disorders	Less common disorders	Any disorder	No disorder	All
	%	%	%	%	%	%	%
General practitioner							
Not at all	51	55	48	43	53	65	64
Once	10	12	14	16	11	12	12
Twice	11	11	10	9	11	10	10
Three times	6	8	7	9	7	5	5
Four or more times	22	14	21	23	18	8	9
Any GP contact	49	45	52	57	47	35	36
Base	*443*	*491*	*137*	*57*	*926*	*9375*	*10302*
A & E department							
Not at all	75	73	69	77	74	83	82
Once	18	20	21	17	18	13	14
Twice	4	5	8	4	4	3	3
Three times	2	2	-	2	2	1	1
Four or more times	1	1	1	-	1	0	1
Any A & E visit	25	27	31	23	26	17	18
Base	*445*	*492*	*139*	*57*	*928*	*9374*	*10303*
Inpatient stay							
Not at all	91	91	90	87	91	95	95
Once	8	7	8	9	7	4	4
Twice	1	1	1	-	1	1	1
Three times	0	1	1	2	1	0	0
Four or more times	1	0	-	2	0	0	0
Any inpatient stay	9	9	10	13	9	5	5
Base	*445*	*492*	*139*	*57*	*928*	*9378*	*10307*
Outpatient or day patient							
Not at all	71	73	57	45	71	82	81
Once	8	8	11	10	8	8	8
Twice	6	6	10	13	7	4	4
Three times	3	3	4	5	3	2	2
Four or more times	12	9	19	26	11	4	4
Any outpatient visit or day patient stay	29	27	43	55	29	18	19
Base	*445*	*492*	*139*	*57*	*928*	*9374*	*10303*

Table 7.2　Use of services for significant mental health problems

by type of mental disorder

All children with a disorder

Service used	Type of mental disorder				
	Emotional disorders	Conduct disorders	Hyperkinetic disorders	Less common disorders	Any disorders
	%	%	%	%	%
Primary health care services (e.g. GP or Health Visitor)	40	38	46	67	40
Specialist health care services (e.g. Paediatrician or child guidance clinic)	21	26	38	60	27
Social services (e.g. Social worker)	16	27	23	25	20
Educational services (e.g. Class teacher, educational psychologist, school counsellor)	43	55	67	72	50
Alternative therapist	6	5	4	25	6
Other specialist service	7	4	4	12	6
Any of the above services	63	76	81	96	71
Consulted GP and had contact with a specialist service	33	33	41	58	34
Contact with specialist services only	23	38	35	29	31
Consulted GP only	7	5	5	9	6
Neither consulted GP nor had contact with specialist services	**37**	**24**	**19**	**4**	**30**
Base	*397*	*403*	*134*	*56*	*793*

Table 7.3   Use of professional and non-professional help by type of mental disorder

All children with a mental disorder

Type of help sought	Type of mental disorder				
	Emotional disorders	Conduct disorders	Hyperkinetic disorders	Less common disorders	Any disorder
	%	%	%	%	%
No help sought	14	5	6	-	9
Professional help only	8	8	6	9	8
Non-professional help only	23	18	13	4	20
Professional and non-professional help	55	68	75	87	62
	Percentage of children whose parents sought each type of help				
Any professional help	*63*	*76*	*81*	*96*	*70*
Any non-professional help	*78*	*86*	*88*	*91*	*83*
Any help	*86*	*95*	*94*	*100*	*91*
Base	*397*	*403*	*134*	*56*	*793*

Table 7.4   Use of professional and non-professional help
by number of mental disorders

All children with a disorder

	Number of disorders			
	One disorder	Two disorders	Three or more disorders	Any disorder
	Percentage of children whose parents sought each type of help			
Sought professional help for significant mental health problems	66	77	88	71
Sought non-professional help for significant mental health problems	81	84	93	83
Sought any help for significant mental health problems	90	91	98	91
Base	*522*	*209*	*61*	*793*

Table 7.5   Odds Ratios for the socio-demographic correlates of service use

		Any psychiatric disorder	
Variable	Value	Adjusted Odds ratio	95% C.I.
Sex	Female	1.00	-
	Male	1.49*	(1.09 - 2.04)
Family's employment	Both parents working	1.00	-
	One parent working	0.90	(0.59 - 1.39)
	Neither working	1.63*	(1.05 - 2.53)

Others variables entered into the model that were not found to be significant were; age, number of children, family type and ACORN classification.

*** p<0.001, **p<0.01, *p<0.05

Table 7.6 In trouble with the police in the past 12 months
by type of mental disorder, age and sex

All children

	Type of mental disorder						
	Emotional disorders	Conduct disorders	Hyperkinetic disorders	Less common disorders	Any disorder	No disorder	All
Has child been in trouble with the police in the past 12 months?							
5-10 year olds							
Yes	1	4	2	-	3	0	0
No	100	96	98	100	97	100	100
Base	*192*	*239*	*80*	*30*	*449*	*5323*	*5772*
11-15 year olds							
Yes	9	27	26	[26]	17	2	4
No	91	74	74	[1]	83	98	96
Base	*253*	*253*	*58*	*27*	*480*	*4053*	*4533*
All boys							
Yes	8	18	14	-	13	2	3
No	93	82	86	100	87	98	97
Base	*213*	*343*	*117*	*36*	*559*	*4603*	*5162*
All girls							
Yes	3	10	[20]	[20]	6	1	1
No	97	90	[1]	[1]	94	100	99
Base	*232*	*149*	*21*	*21*	*369*	*4773*	*5143*
All children							
Yes	5	16	12	2	10	1	2
No	95	84	88	98	90	99	98
Base	*445*	*492*	*139*	*57*	*928*	*9376*	*10305*

Table 7.7 Ever been in trouble with the police
by type of mental disorder (11-15 years only)

All children aged 11-15 years who completed a self-completion questionnaire and had already admitted to carrying out less serious troublesome behaviour.

	Type of mental disorder						
	Emotional disorders	Conduct disorders	Hyperkinetic disorders	Less common disorders	Any disorder	No disorder	All
Whether child has ever been in trouble with the police							
Yes	34	49	40	[5]	43	21	25
No	66	51	60	[7]	57	79	75
Base	*149*	*169*	*39*	*12*	*284*	*1145*	*1430*

8 Scholastic achievement and education

8.1 Introduction

The aim of this chapter is to look at the relationship between the mental disorders among children and scholastic achievement, special educational needs (SEN) and absenteeism from school.

8.2 Special educational needs

Teachers were asked whether the child had any officially recognised special needs, and if so, to rate the level of special needs according to the five recognised stages:

- Stage 1 - Class teacher or form/year tutor has overall responsibility
- Stage 2 - SEN co-ordinator takes the lead in co-ordinating provision and drawing up individual educational plans
- Stage 3 - External specialist support enlisted
- Stage 4 - Statutory assessment by Local Education Authority (LEA)
- Stage 5 - SEN statement issued by LEA

Whereas, about 1 in 5 children had officially recognised special educational needs, those with a disorder were three times more likely than other children to have special needs: 49% compared with 15%. The proportion of children with special educational needs also varied greatly by type of disorder. Children with a hyperkinetic disorder were twice as likely as those with an emotional disorder to have special educational needs 71% compared with 37%. (*Table 8.1, Figure 8.1*)

Among all the children with special educational needs 17% were at stage 5, the level at which a statement is issued about the child by their Local Education Authority (LEA). Among the children who have a mental disorder and with special educational needs, 28% were at Stage 5. Among the children who do not have a mental disorder but do have special educational needs, 13% were at Stage 5. The distribution of children with special needs across the five stages did not vary by the three main types of disorder, but for the small number of children with a less common disorder, about three quarters were at Stage 5. (*Table 8.2*)

In Table 8.3 the data are presented so that the prevalence of mental disorders among children at different stages of special educational needs can be compared with children with no special educational needs. The prevalence rate of mental disorders ranged from 6% among children who did not have special educational needs to 40% among children who were at stage 5 of the special needs scale. (*Table 8.3, Figure 8.2*)

Figure 8.1 Officially recognised SEN by type of mental disorder

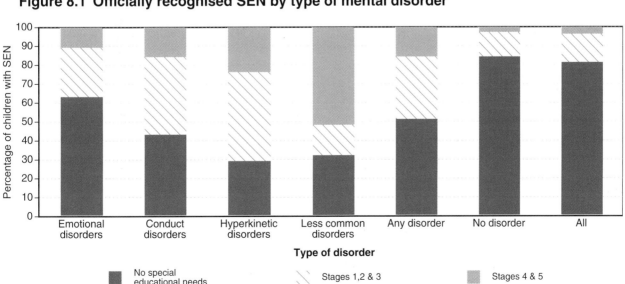

Figure 8.2 Prevalence of mental disorders by level of SEN

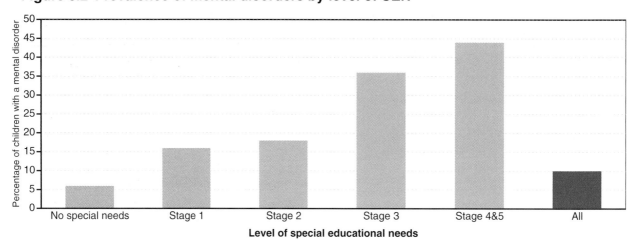

It is clear from the findings described above that children who had a mental disorder were more likely, than those without a disorder to have had officially-recognised, special educational needs. Logistic regression was used to look at the strength of the independent association between mental disorders and special educational needs taking account of socio-biographic, socio-demographic, socio-economic and geo-demographic factors.

The significant correlates of having special educational needs were: presence of a mental disorder, child's sex, child's age, number of children in family and family's employment situation. Among these five factors the presence of a mental disorder had the greatest influence on the odds of having special educational needs. Children with a mental disorder were around five times more likely (than those with no disorder) to have had special educational needs (OR=4.61) and the odds ratio for boys compared with girls was 2.04. (*Table 8.4*)

8.3   Specific learning difficulties

All children (aged 5-15 year olds) were invited to participate in a component of the survey, which aimed to explore the relationship between specific learning difficulties (SpLDs) and mental health. Children were individually assessed on their general cognitive, reading and spelling abilities by ONS interviewers who had received training in psychometric test administration. Those who completed the test of general

cognitive ability and at least the reading test were included in the analysis.

Assessment materials

General cognitive ability
The second edition of the British Picture Vocabulary Scale (BPVS-II, Dunn, Dunn, Whetton & Burley, 1997) was used to generate a standard score for receptive vocabulary; that is, the words a child recognises when spoken. The BPVS-II has been considered to be a good measure of global cognitive ability (IQ) for research studies (Dunn et al, 1997, p.4). In this study, using the BPVS-II reduced the risk of over-including children in the SpLD category who have recently arrived in the UK and may have a lack of knowledge of English.

Reading ability
Single word reading ability was assessed using the Word Reading Scale of the British Ability Scales, Second Edition (BAS-II, Elliott, Smith & McCulloch, 1996). The printed card of single words was presented to children using the standard instructions and a raw score for total correctly read words obtained. Regional variations in pronunciation were accepted within the constraints specified in the BAS-II Test Manual. Raw scores were transformed into ability scores using the Item Response Theory model developed for the BAS-II (BAS-II Technical Manual) and age-corrected standard scores generated from the BAS-II tables.

Spelling ability

Children were also invited to try the spelling items from the BAS-II and record their answers in pencil on a standard BAS-II Spelling Sheet. Researchers coded responses as correct or incorrect using BLAISE software developed for the study which subsequently presented easier or harder items depending on the accuracy of the response using decision rules specified for the BAS-II. This method minimised the number of items that were too easy or too hard that each individual had to try. Raw scores were transformed into age-based standard scores via ability scores using the method described above.

Criteria for inclusion in specific learning difficulty category

Specific learning difficulty (SpLD) was conceptualised as the failure to achieve expected academic progress in reading and spelling despite conventional instruction, adequate intelligence and sociocultural opportunity (Snowling, 1987). This was operationally defined in the current study in terms of ability-achievement discrepancy analysis (Shepard, 1980).

Regression equations were generated to predict reading and spelling ability scores from BPVS-II scores based on the entire sample, corrected to two decimal places. The resulting regression equations are shown below.

Regression equations for predicted reading and spelling ability

Predicted reading ability = 37.701 + 0.6522 x BPVS Standard Score

Predicted spelling ability = 49.832 + 0.5205 x BPVS Standard Score

The difference between predicted and actual reading and spelling score for each participant was calculated, and individuals were included in the SpLD category if their discrepancy score fell within the most extreme 5% of the sample for each year group, following the methodology developed by Yule, Lansdown & Urbanowicz (1982). In most cases where both reading and spelling scores were available, the most extreme 5% was identified on the basis of membership of the most extreme 7.5% for reading and spelling; in cases where only reading scores were available, individuals were included in the SpLD category if they were in the most extreme 5%.

Given that the rate of specific learning difficulties (SpLD) was set at 5%, children with a mental disorder were three times more likely than those with no disorder to have SpLD: 12% compared with 4%. There was little difference in the proportions of children with SpLD by type of disorder. *(Table 8.5)*

Another way of examining these data is to look at the prevalence of mental disorders among children with specific learning difficulties. Among children with SpLD, 22% had any mental disorder. In terms of the broad groups of disorders 13% had conduct disorders, 9% emotional disorders and 5% had a hyperkinetic disorder. *(Table 8.6)*

8.4 Absenteeism from school

Teachers were asked how many days the child had been absent during the last term. Overall, 67% of all children had been absent from school for a day or more during the previous term. Forty five per cent had been away from school for up to a week and 21% had been away for more than a week. *(Table 8.7)*

Children with a disorder were slightly more likely to have been absent from school during the previous term: 74% compared with 66%. However, a clearer distinction between the two groups can be seen when looking at the number of days that the child has been absent in the last term. Children with a disorder were about twice as likely as other children to have been absent from school for 11 days or more: 19% compared with 8%.

There was some variation between the proportions of children who had been absent from school by type of disorder: 25% of children with emotional disorders had been absent from school for 11 days or more compared with 21% of children with conduct disorders and 14% with hyperkinetic disorders.

8.5 Truancy

All three types of respondent (young person, parent and teacher) were asked about truanting. However, because of differences in question wording, type of administration and routing it is not possible to directly compare the information which was collected from the three sources.

The question directed at parents was: *(In the past 12 months) Has s/he often played truant ('bunked off') from school?* This was only asked of parents of children who were more troublesome than average. According to parents, 4% of the children had 'definitely' and 2% had 'perhaps' often played truant in the past year. Children who had a disorder were six times more likely, than those without a disorder, to have 'definitely' played truant in the past year: 12% compared with 2%. According to parents 1 in 5 children with conduct disorders may have or did play truant in the past twelve months. *(Table 8.8)*

The wording of the truancy question for the 11-15 year olds was the same as that asked of parents. However, owing to the sensitive nature of the topic, the question was included in the self-completion questionnaire. Five per cent of the young people reported that they had 'definitely' and 7% had 'perhaps' played truant in the past year. Whereas parents may have been unsure whether their children were playing truant, the young people themselves must have known. Therefore, those in the 'perhaps' category were probably in the 'definitely' category but were concerned about admitting it. Adding the two groups together young people with a disorder were four times more likely than other children to have played truant: 33% compared with 9%. Children with conduct disorders most frequently reported truanting behaviour, at 44%. *(Table 8.9)*

The question on truancy presented to teachers was different to those addressed to parents and children, because teachers did not have a face-to-face interview but were sent a postal questionnaire. The questionnaire included the statement: *'plays truant'* and the teacher had to respond by ticking one of three boxes labelled, not true, somewhat true or certainly true. According to the teachers 3% of children played truant. This percentage represents 15% of children assessed as having a mental disorder and just 2% of those with no disorder. Following the pattern of the parent and young person data, children with conduct disorders had the highest reported rate of truancy, 19%. *(Table 8.10)*

References

Dunn, L.M., Dunn, L.M., Whetton, C. & Burley, J. (1997). *The British Picture Vocabulary Scale Second Edition Testbook.* Windsor: NFER

Elliott, C., Smith, P. & McCulloch, K. (1996). *British Ability Scales - Second Edition: Administration and Scoring Manual.* Windsor: NFER.

Shepard, L. (1980). An evaluation of the regression discrepancy method for identifying children with learning disabilities. *Journal of Special Education,* **14** (1). 79 - 91.

Snowling, M. (1987). *Dyslexia - a Cognitive Developmental Perspective.* Oxford: Blackwell.

Yule, W., Lansdown, R. & Urbanowicz, M. (1982). Predicting educational attainment from WISC-R in a primary school sample. *British Journal of Clinical Psychology.* **21**. 43 - 46.

Table 8.1   Officially recognised special educational needs (SEN)
by type of mental disorder

All children (where teacher data available)

	Type of mental disorder						
	Emotional disorders	Conduct disorders	Hyperkinetic disorders	Less common disorders	Any disorder	No disorder	All
No special needs	63	43	29	32	51	84	81
Officially recognised special needs at:							
Stage 1	10	14	13	5	11	6	7
Stage 2	9	11	11	2	10	5	5
Stage 3	7 }37	15 }57	24 }71	9 }68	12 }49	2 }15	3 }19
Stage 4	2	3	4	-	2	0	0
Stage 5	9	13	19	52	14	2	3
Base	*339*	*399*	*120*	*47*	*736*	*7282*	*8018*

Stage 1 - Class teacher or form/year tutor has overall responsibility
Stage 2 - SENCO takes the lead in co-ordinating provision and drawing up IEP
Stage 3 - External specialist support enlisted
Stage 4 - Statutory assessment by LEA
Stage 5 - Statement issued by LEA

Table 8.2   Level of officially recognised special educational needs (SEN)
by type of mental disorder

Children with special educational needs

	Type of mental disorder						
	Emotional disorders	Conduct disorders	Hyperkinetic disorders	Less common disorders	Any disorder	No disorder	All
	%	%	%	%	%	%	%
Officially recognised special needs at:							
Stage 1	28	25	18	7	22	39	35
Stage 2	25	20	15	3	20	32	29
Stage 3	18	27	34	13	25	15	18
Stage 4	6	5	6	-	5	0	1
Stage 5	24	23	27	77	28	13	17
Base	*127*	*225*	*85*	*32*	*361*	*1133*	*1494*

Stage 1 - Class teacher or form/year tutor has overall responsibility
Stage 2 - SENCO takes the lead in co-ordinating provision and drawing up IEP
Stage 3 - External specialist support enlisted
Stage 4 - Statutory assessment by LEA
Stage 5 - Statement issued by LEA

Table 8.3 Prevalence of mental disorder
by level of officially recognised SEN

All children (where teacher data available)

	No special needs	Stage 1	Stage 2	Stage 3	Stage 4	Stage 5	All
			Percentage of children with a mental disorder				
Emotional disorders	3	7	7	8	[8]	12	4
Conduct disorders	3	12	12	26	[11]	24	6
Hyperkinetic disorders	1	3	3	12	[5]	10	2
Any disorder	**6**	**16**	**18**	**36**	**[17]**	**43**	**10**
Base	*6524*	*528*	*433*	*264*	*20*	*249*	*8018*

Table 8.4 Odds ratios for mental disorder and socio-demographic correlates of SEN

Variable	Value	Adjusted OR	95% CI
Any mental disorder	Present	1.00	
	Not present	4.61***	(3.90 - 5.44)
Age	11-15 years	1.00	
	5-10 years	1.46***	(1.28 -1.65)
Sex	Female	1.00	
	Male	2.04***	(1.80 - 2.31)
Number of children	1	1.00	
	2	1.00	(0.85 - 1.19)
	3	1.13	(0.94 - 1.37)
	4	1.30*	(1.01 - 1.66)
	5 or more	1.77**	(1.24 - 2.52)
Family's employment	Both parents working	1.00	
	One parent working	1.32***	(1.13 - 1.55)
	Neither working	1.71***	(1.40 - 2.08)

Other variables entered into the model that were not significant were ethnicity, family type and ACORN classification.

"*** p<0.001, **p<0.01, *p<0.05

Table 8.5   Specific learning difficulties by type of mental disorder

All children (who completed the tests)

	Emotional disorders	Conduct disorders	Hyperkinetic disorders	Less common disorders	Any disorder	No disorder	All
Specific learning difficulties (SpLD)							
Not present	89	87	83	85	88	96	95
Present	11	13	17	15	12	4	5
Base	*385*	*424*	*113*	*40*	*791*	*8543*	*9334*

Table 8.6   Prevalence of mental disorders by specific learning difficulties (SpLDs)

All children (who completed the tests)

	Not present	Present	All*
	Percentage of children with a mental disorder		
Emotional disorders	4	9	4
Conduct disorders	5	13	5
Hyperkinetic disorders	1	5	1
Any disorder	**8**	**22**	**9**
Base	*8865*	*468*	*9334*

*   Percentages are different to the prevalence rates shown in chapter 4 owing to the reduced number of children who undertook the SpLD assessments.

Table 8.7   Absenteeism from school by type of mental disorder

All children (where teacher data were available)

	Emotional disorders	Conduct disorders	Hyperkinetic disorders	Less common disorders	Any disorder	No disorder	All
	%	%	%	%	%	%	%
No days absent	**22**	**23**	**29**	**40**	**26**	**34**	**33**
1 - 5 days	35	38	43	30	37	46	45
6 - 10 days	18	18	15	24	17	13	13
11 - 15 days	9 } 25	9 } 21	5 } 14	3 } 6	7 } 19	4 } 8	4 } 8
16 days and over	16	12	9	3	12	4	4
Any days absent	**78**	**77**	**71**	**60**	**74**	**66**	**67**
Base	*244*	*294*	*82*	*34*	*539*	*5726*	*6265*

Table 8.8	Truancy (parent interview)
	by type of mental disorder

All children (who were more troublesome than average)

	Type of mental disorder						All
	Emotional disorders	Conduct disorders	Hyperkinetic disorders	Less common disorders	Any disorder	No disorder	
	%	%	%	%	%	%	%
No	83	80	87	91	83	97	94
Perhaps	6	5	4	3	5	2	2
Definitely	11	14	8	6	12	2	4
Base	*216*	*425*	*117*	*34*	*607*	*1970*	*2576*

Table 8.9	Truancy (young person interview)
	by type of mental disorder

All 11-15 year olds who completed the self-completion questionnaire

	Type of mental disorder						All
	Emotional disorders	Conduct disorders	Hyperkinetic disorders	Less common disorders	Any disorder	No disorder	
	%	%	%	%	%	%	%
No	68	57	60	69	65	90	88
Perhaps	11	16	8	15	13	6	7
Definitely	21	28	31	16	22	3	5
Base	*239*	*223*	*50*	*20*	*431*	*3891*	*4321*

Table 8.10	Truancy (teacher questionnaire)
	by type of mental disorder

All children (where teacher data were available)

	Type of mental disorder						All
	Emotional disorders	Conduct disorders	Hyperkinetic disorders	Less common disorders	Any disorder	No disorder	
	%	%	%	%	%	%	%
Not true	85	81	89	91	85	98	97
Somewhat true	7	8	8	-	7	1	2
Certainly true	7	11	3	9	8	0	1
Base	*345*	*408*	*123*	*47*	*752*	*7569*	*8321*

9 Social functioning of the family

9.1 Introduction

This chapter is concerned with the relationship between the mental health of the child and the social functioning of the child's family. The term, social functioning, is used in a very broad sense to refer to several aspects of parental attitudes and behaviour and for the purposes of the survey includes:

- Mental health of interviewed parent
- Family functioning
- Reward strategies and punishment regimes
- Stressful life events
- Impact of child's health on the family

9.2 Mental health of parent

The parent who was interviewed about the child's mental health, in most cases the mother, was also asked about her own mental health by means of the GHQ-12 (General Health Questionnaire, Goldberg and Williams, 1988). The GHQ-12 is a self administered screening test of twelve questions designed to detect non-psychotic psychiatric disorders in community settings.

1. Have you recently been able to concentrate on whatever you're doing?
2. Have you recently lost much sleep over worry?
3. Have you recently felt that you are playing a useful part in things?
4. Have you recently felt capable about making decisions about things?
5. Have you recently felt constantly under strain?
6. Have you recently felt you couldn't overcome your difficulties?
7. Have you recently been able to enjoy your day to day activities?
8. Have you recently been able to face up to your problems?
9. Have you recently been feeling unhappy or depressed?
10. Have you recently been losing confidence in yourself?
11. Have you recently been thinking of yourself as a worthless person?
12. Have you recently been feeling happy, all things considered?

Each item is scored with a 1 according to whether it applied more than usual (for a negative item) or less than usual (for a positive item). A score in the range of 0 (no problem) to 12 (severe problem) was calculated for each person. In the present survey the threshold score was set at 3, i.e., all those with a score of 3 or more were deemed to have screened positive for a neurotic disorder.

Of the 10,252 parents who completed the GHQ12, a quarter screened positive. This proportion is typical of that found in other community surveys. The distribution of GHQ12 scores was markedly different among parents of children with a mental disorder from those with no disorder: 47% of children assessed as having a mental disorder had a parent who scored 3 or more on the GHQ12, approximately twice the proportion of the sample of children with no disorder, 23%. The corresponding proportions for a GHQ12 score of 6 or more were 29% and 10%.

Among the sample of children with a mental disorder, the proportions having a parent with a GHQ12 score of 3 or more did not vary considerably by type of disorder, ranging from 42% of those with a hyperkinetic disorder to 50% with an emotional disorder. (*Table 9.1*)

The proportion of children with parents who screened positive on the GHQ12 increased with the severity of the child's mental health problem, as measured by the number of diagnosed, specific mental disorders. The proportion of children with GHQ12 screen-positive parents rose from 23% of the no-disorder group to 44% of children with one disorder to 50% of those with two disorders and to 68% of children with three disorders. (*Table 9.2*)

The association between the child's and the interviewed parent's mental health status can be seen most clearly in *Figure 9.1*. It shows that the proportion of children with mental disorders increased steadily by the ungrouped GHQ12 score with a minimum prevalence rate of any mental disorder of 5% among children whose parents scored zero to a maximum of 37% among children with parents who scored 11. In summary, children with parents who screened positive on the GHQ12

Figure 9.1 Children with a mental disorder by parent's GHQ-12 score

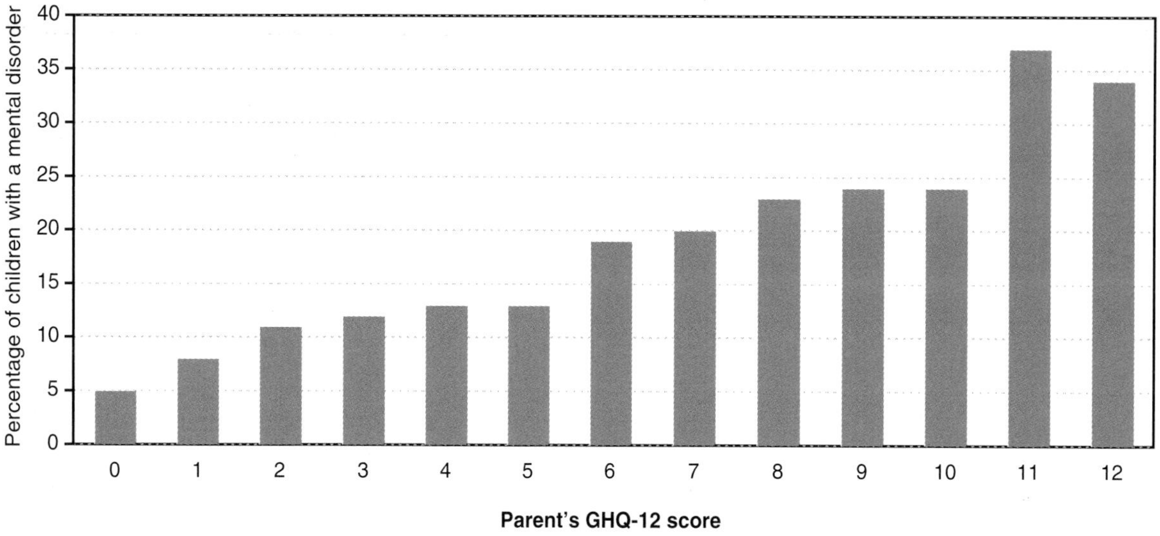

were three times more likely to have a mental disorder than those whose parents had sub-threshold scores - 18% compared with 6%. Data on the relationship between the parent GHQ12 scores and types of disorder are shown in *Tables 9.3 and 9.4.*

9.3   Family functioning

The instrument used to estimate family functioning was the General Functioning Scale of the MacMaster Family Activity Device (FAD-GFS). It comprises 12 statements that parents rate on a four point scale: strongly agree, agree, disagree and strongly disagree. The scale has been shown to have good reliability, internal consistency and validity in distinguishing between non-clinical families and families attending a psychiatric service. (Miller et al., 1985, Byles et al., 1988, Fristad., 1989)

1. Planning family activities is difficult because we misunderstand each other.
2. In times of crisis we can turn to each other for support.
3. We can not talk to each other about the sadness we feel.
4. Individuals are accepted for what they are.
5. We avoid discussing our fears and concerns.
6. We can express feelings to each other.
7. There is lots of bad feeling in the family.
8. We feel accepted for what we are.
9. Making decisions is a problem for our family.
10. We are able to make decisions on how to solve problems.
11. We don't get along well together.
12. We confide in each other.

A scoring system is used to calculated "healthy" or "unhealthy" family functioning. Overall, 19% of children lived in families assessed as having unhealthy family functioning. The Western Australian Child Health Survey also used the FAD and reported that over 12% per cent of the 1500 families surveyed were considered to have a high level of family discord.(Silburn et al., 1996) It is difficult to compare this figure with the GB survey as their method of calculating high discord was not presented. In the present survey, children with a mental disorder were twice as likely to live in families rated as unhealthy than children with no disorder: 35% compared with 17%. Among children assessed as having a conduct disorder, 43% were part of a family with an unhealthy FAD-GFS rating. (*Table 9.5*)

These findings add to the accumulated evidence from a number of sources which suggest that disordered family functioning is implicated in a wide range of psychiatric problems in children. (Tamplin et al., 1998). More specifically, they found marked differences between the mean FAD scores of control families and those with depressed adolescents.

Among the small number of children in the survey, 65 in total, who turned out to have had three or more specific mental disorders, the proportion with an unhealthy family functioning rating was 55%. (*Table 9.6*)

Another way of analysing the data on family functioning is to look at the prevalence of mental disorders among children by the level of family functioning. Given that the overall prevalence of mental disorders among children and adolescents was 10%, the rate among children in healthy functioning families was 7% compared with 18% among unhealthy, functioning families. Among the 255 children in families with the worst family functioning score, about a third had a mental disorder. (*Table 9.7*)

9.4 Reward strategies and punishment regimes

How parents reward their children for good behaviour and punish them for bad behaviour was investigated by asking parents to rate the frequency of their use of three reward strategies and six punishment regimes.

Reward strategies
1. Giving encouragement or praise.
2. Giving treats such as extra pocket money, staying up late or a special outing.
3. Giving child favourite things.

Punishment regimes
1. Sending child to his/her room.
2. Grounding or keeping him/her in.
3. Shouting or yelling at him/her.
4. Smacking him/her with your hand.
5. Hitting him/her with a strap or something else.
6. Shaking him/her.

Parents had a choice of saying whether they carried out each activity, never, seldom, sometimes or frequently. Among all children, 82% were frequently encouraged or praised, 34% were frequently treated and 30% were given favourite things. There were no great differences in the distribution of reward strategies by whether or not the children had a mental disorder. However, there was a very slight increase in the proportion of children who frequently got treats or received favourite things among children with a disorder compared to those with no disorder: 40% compared with 33% for treats and 35% compared to 30% for given favourite things. (*Table 9.8*)

The six punishment regimes listed above can be split into two groups: those involving no physical punishment (sending to room, grounding, and shouting) and those with a physical element (smacking with hand, hitting with strap, and

shaking). Looking at the differences in the frequency of punishment by the presence or type of disorder can only be done for the non-physical punishments as very few parents do or admit to sometimes or frequently smacking, hitting or shaking their children. In terms of the non-physical punishments, children with mental disorders were far more likely to be frequently punished than children with no mental disorder: 18% compared with 8% were sent to their rooms; 17% compared with 5% were grounded, and 42% compared with 26% were shouted at. Not unexpectedly, the major contribution to these differences derive from the higher rates of frequent punishment among children with conduct or hyperkinetic disorders, i.e., disorders that have a behavioural impact, in contrast to emotional problems. (*Table 9.9*)

Looking at the prevalence of mental disorders by punishment regimes is a complimentary way of looking at the association between these two characteristics. *Table 9.10* shows the higher rates of mental disorder among children more frequently punished: 20% of those frequently sent to their room; 27% of frequently grounded children; 15% of children shouted at frequently; and 38% of children frequently smacked. Conduct disorders made a major contribution to these prevalence rates. For example, 21% of frequently grounded children and 34% of frequently smacked child had a conduct disorder. (*Tables 9.10, 9.11*)

9.5 Stressful life events

All parents were asked if the child experienced ten stressful life events. The items in the list were chosen because they are thought to be highly (psychologically) threatening for the child. Goodyer (1990) has suggested that moderately or highly undesirable recent life events exert potential causal effects on the onset of emotional and behavioural symptoms in school aged children.

1. Since child was born, parent had a separation due to marital difficulties or broken off a steady relationship.
2. Since child was born, parent (or partner) had a major financial crisis such as losing the equivalent to at least three months income.
3. Since child was born, parent (or partner) had a problem with the police involving a court appearance.

4. At some stage in the child's life, s/he had a serious illness which required a stay in hospital.
5. At any stage in the child's life, s/he had been in a serious accident or badly hurt in an accident.
6. At any stage in the child's life, a parent, brother or sister died.
7. At any stage in the child's life, a close friend died.
8. At any stage in the child's life, a grandparent died.
9. At any stage in the child's life, a pet died.
10. In the past year, child has broken off a steady relationship with a boy or girl friend. (*applies if aged 13 or above*)

Children with a mental disorder were more likely than those with no disorder to have experienced eight of the ten events. For example, 50% of children with a mental disorder had at one time seen the separation of their parents, compared with 29% of the sample with no disorder. The corresponding figures for a parent having problems with the police were 15% and 5% and for a parent or sibling dying - 6% compared with 3%. The two events which showed little difference in the frequency of their occurrence by presence or absence of disorder were the death of a grandparent at around 13% and the death of a pet at 27%. There was no clear relationship between type of disorder and type of event. Nevertheless, the disorder with the greatest proportion of children who had a serious illness, 39%, was hyperkinetic disorder and children with emotional disorders included the largest percentage of those who had broken off a relationship with a boy or girl friend, 24%. (*Table 9.12*)

Many children experienced more than one stressful event in the course of their lives. Among all the children in the sample, about a third had never had a stressful life event, a third had experienced one event and around a third had to cope with two or more stressful events. Although children with a mental disorder were more likely than other children to have had one stressful life event: 82% compared with 70%, they were far more likely to have experienced three or more events: 31% compared with 13%. The proportion of children who had experienced several stressful life events was very similar for those with emotional, behavioural and hyperkinetic disorders. (*Table 9.13*)

The prevalence of mental disorder by type of event is difficult to interpret because of the relatively large proportion of children who had more than one stressful life event. Nevertheless, the data indicate that the two factors associated with the highest prevalence rates were: split with boyfriend or girlfriend (24%) and parent or partner in trouble with the police (22%). (*Table 9.14*)

The number of stressful life events does seem to have a cumulative effect on psychiatric morbidity with prevalence rates ranging from 7% among children with one event to 16% of those who had three events to 34% of children who had experienced five or more stressful life events. (*Table 9.15*)

9.6 Social functioning correlates of mental disorders

Logistic regression analysis was used to look at the increased odds of having any mental disorder (compared to no disorder) in terms of the independent association with the four factors described above - parent's GHQ12, punishment regime, family functioning and number of stressful life events. Six socio- and geo-demographic characteristics were also inserted into the model: sex, age, number of children, family structure, family employment and the ACORN measure.

A screen-positive, parental GHQ12 score increased the odds of the child having a mental disorder by 2.23. Frequent punishment increased the odds by 1.97, unhealthy family functioning by 1.82 and at least one stressful life event by 1.35. (*Table 9.16*)

9.7 Impact of child's mental disorder on the family

The last section of this chapter focuses solely on children who had been assessed as having a mental disorder and were described by their parent as having a significant health problem: 792 children. The children with a mental disorder not covered in this impact section are those where the diagnosis came primarily from the child or teacher. The parents of these children either did not mention the child's problem, or did not think it had a major significance in their lives, and thus, were routed past the impact questions.

The impact of the child's mental problems can be grouped under three headings:

- Impact of child's problems on family relationships
- Impact of child's problems on the social life of the family and stigma
- Impact of child's problems on parents' health

The questions on impact in the survey were based on the Child and Adolescent Burden Assessment. (Patrick et al., 1994)

Family relationships

Among children with a mental disorder who were living in households with two parents or a parent and partner, about 1 in 3 of their parents said the child's problem made their relationship more strained, around 1 in 6 said it made their relationship stronger and, for the remaining children, 1 in 2, it made no difference. Because we are only looking at children with mental disorders, identified by parents, within a particular family structure, the base numbers are relatively small. This means the data will be interpreted to indicate patterns rather than statistically significant differences. Conduct disorders do seem to cause a greater strain on parent and partner relationships than emotional disorders: parents of 49% of children with conduct disorders reported that the child's problem made their relationship more strained, the corresponding proportion for parents of children with emotional disorders was 27%.

Parents with no partner in the household were asked if the child's mental disorder was a contributory factor to a previous relationship breaking up. Overall, 20% of parents replied that it was a factor, which included 26% of parents of children with conduct disorders and 16% with emotional disorders.

The third family structure scenario examined was the impact of the child's problem on the parent's (and the partner's) relationship with their other children. The responses for parent and partner were similar in that 25%-30% reported the child's problem made their relationships with other children more difficult.

Finally, a quarter of parents said their children's problems caused difficulties with other family members. This proportion included a third of parents of children with conduct and hyperkinetic disorders and a fifth of parents who had children with emotional disorders. *(Table 9.17)*

Social life and stigma

About 15 % of children with any mental disorder had parents who reported their own social difficulties caused by their child's problem: difficulties with their friendships, major disruptions to their social and leisure activities, and, to a great extent, preventing them from doing things socially with the child. These difficulties seemed more likely to be experienced by parents of children with conduct or hyperkinetic than with emotional disorders. This difference by type of disorder was more distinct when looking at the parents' responses to the stigma questions - whether child's difficulties caused embarrassment and whether parent felt disapproved of or avoided because of the child's problems. Overall, the proportion of children with mental disorders whose parents expressed these views was around 30%, yet for the embarrassment question the proportion for children with conduct disorders was 46%. *(Table 9.18)*

Effect on parents' health

The mental health problems of the child had a considerable impact on the health of the interviewed parent. Eighty seven per cent of parents said their child's problems made them worried and 58% felt that their child's problems caused them to be depressed. About two thirds of parents said their child's mental health problem made them tired and a quarter said it made them physically ill. Children with emotional disorders seemed less likely to have an impact on their parents' health than those with conduct or hyperkinetic disorders. *(Table 9.19)*

Parents reacted to their worry, depression, tiredness or physical illness in different ways: 31% sought help from a doctor (of which two thirds received medication), 9% drank more alcohol and 30% increased their smoking. *(Table 9.20)*

References

Byles, J., Byrne, C., Boyle, M.H., Offord, D.R. (1988) Ontario Child Health Study: Reliability and validity of the General Functioning Scale of the MacMaster Family Assessment Device. *Family Process*, **30**(1), 116-123

Fristad, M.A. (1989) A comparison of the MacMaster and circumplex family assessment instruments. *Journal of Marital and Family* Therapy, **15**, 259-269.

Goodyer, I.M., Wright, C., and Altham. P.M.E., (1990) The Friendships and Recent Life Events of Anxious and Depressed School-Age-Children. *British Journal of Psychiatry*, **156**, (**May**), 689-698

Miller, I.W., Epstein, N.B., Bishop, D.S. and Keitner, G.I. (1985) The MacMaster Family Assessment Device: reliability and Validity. *Journal of Marital and Family* Therapy, **11**, 345-356

Patrick, M.K.S., Angold, A., Burns, B.J., and Costello, E.J., *The Child and Adolescent Burden Assessment (CABA) Parent Interview, Version 4.1*, Developmental Epidemiology Program, Duke University.

Silburn, S.R., Zubrick, S.R., Garton, A., Gurrin, L., Burton, P., Dalby, R., Carlton, J., Shepherd, C., Lawrence, D. (1996) *Western Australian Child Health survey: Family and Community Health*, Western Australia: Australian Bureau of Statistics and the TVW Telethon Institute for Child Health Research.

Tamplin, A., Goodyer, I.M. and Herbert, J. (1998) Family functioning and parent general health in families of adolescents with major depressive disorders. *Journal of Affective Disorders*, **48**, 1-13.

Table 9.1 Distribution of parent's GHQ-12 scores

by type of mental disorder

All children

| | Type of mental disorder | | | | | | |
	Emotional disorders	Conduct disorders	Hyperkinetic disorders	Less common disorders	Any disorder	No disorder	All
	%	%	%	%	%	%	%
Parent's GHQ-12							
0-2	50	51	58	52	53	77	75
3-5	16	20	18	19	18	13	13
6-8	17	14	16	17	15	6	7
9-12	17	15	8	13	14	4	5
3 or more	**50**	**49**	**42**	**48**	**47**	**23**	**25**
Base	*444*	*491*	*139*	*56*	*925*	*9297*	*10252*

Table 9.2 Distribution of parent's GHQ-12 scores

by number of mental disorders

All children

| | Number of mental disorders | | | | |
	0	1	2	3+	All
	%	%	%	%	%
Parent's GHQ-12					
0-2	77	56	50	32	75
3-5	13	17	18	24	13
6-8	6	14	18	18	7
9-12	4	13	14	26	5
3 or more	**23**	**44**	**50**	**68**	**25**
Base	*9326*	*640*	*220*	*65*	*10252*

Table 9.3 Prevalence of mental disorders

by parent's GHQ-12 score

All children

| | Parent's GHQ score | | | | | | | | | | | | | |
	0	1	2	3	4	5	6	7	8	9	10	11	12	All
	Percentage of children with each disorder													
Emotional disorders	2	4	5	5	5	6	9	10	12	13	14	19	18	4
Conduct disorders	3	4	7	7	9	9	11	8	13	16	12	21	19	6
Hyperkinetic disorders	1	2	2	2	3	1	4	2	3	1	2	5	1	1
Less common disorders	0	1	0	1	1	1	-	2	2	-	2	2	2	1
Any mental disorder	**5**	**8**	**11**	**12**	**13**	**13**	**19**	**20**	**23**	**24**	**24**	**37**	**34**	**10**
Base	*5221*	*1567*	*886*	*595*	*438*	*339*	*278*	*239*	*206*	*148*	*126*	*123*	*87*	*10252*

Table 9.4   Prevalence of mental disorders
by parent's GHQ-12 score (grouped)

All children

| | Parent's GHQ score | | | | | | |
	0-2	3-5	6-8	9-12	Below threshold	At or above threshold	All
	Percentage of children with each disorder						
Emotional disorders	3	5	10	16	3	9	4
Conduct disorders	3	8	11	17	3	10	6
Hyperkinetic disorders	1	2	3	2	1	2	1
Less common disorders	0	1	1	2	0	1	1
Any mental disorder	**6**	**13**	**20**	**30**	**6**	**18**	**10**
Base	*7673*	*1372*	*723*	*483*	*7673*	*2578*	*10252*

Table 9.5   Distribution of family functioning scores
by type of mental disorder

All children

| | Type of mental disorder | | | | | | |
	Emotional disorders	Conduct disorders	Hyperkinetic disorders	Less common disorders	Any disorder	No disorder	All
	%	%	%	%	%	%	%
Family functioning score							
Up to 1.50	27	17	21	30	23	37	36
1.51 - 2.00	39	40	42	42	41	46	46
Healthy family functioning	**66**	**57**	**64**	**73**	**65**	**83**	**81**
2.01 - 2.50	26	31	30	18	27	15	16
2.51 or higher	8	12	7	9	8	2	2
Unhealthy family functioning	**34**	**43**	**36**	**27**	**35**	**17**	**19**
Base	*438*	*485*	*139*	*56*	*915*	*9297*	*10212*

Table 9.6 Distribution of family functioning scores
by number of mental disorders

All children

	Number of mental disorders				
	0	1	2	3+	All
	%	%	%	%	%
Family functioning score					
Up to 1.50	37	25	20	20	36
1.51 - 2.00	46	42	42	27	46
Healthy family functioning	**83**	**68**	**62**	**47**	**81**
2.01 - 2.50	15	25	30	30	16
2.51 or higher	2	7	8	23	2
Unhealthy family functioning	**17**	**32**	**38**	**53**	**19**
Base	*9297*	*632*	*217*	*65*	*10212*

Table 9.7 Prrevalence of mental disorders
by family functioning score

All children

	Healthy family functioning			Unhealthy family functioning			
	1.00-1.50	1.51-2.00	All healthy	2.01-2.50	2.51-4.00	All unhealthy	All
	Percentage of children with each disorder						
Emotional disorders	3	4	4	7	15	8	4
Conduct disorders	2	4	3	10	25	12	6
Hyperkinetic disorders	1	1	1	2	4	3	1
Less common disorders	1	1	1	1	2	1	1
Any mental disorder	**6**	**8**	**7**	**16**	**32**	**18**	**10**
Base	*3621*	*4665*	*8286*	*1671*	*255*	*1926*	*10212*

Table 9.8	Reward strategies
	by type of mental disorder

All children

	Type of mental disorder						All
	Emotional disorders	Conduct disorders	Hyperkinetic disorders	Less common disorders	Any disorder	No disorder	
	%	%	%	%	%	%	%
Reward strategies							
Encouragement or praise							
Never	0	1	1	-	0	0	0
Seldom	1	2	2	2	1	1	1
Sometimes	19	23	18	16	21	16	17
Frequently	79	74	78	82	78	82	82
Treats (pocket money or staying up late)							
Never	6	4	1	8	4	4	4
Seldom	6	8	11	6	7	8	8
Sometimes	46	48	49	47	48	55	54
Frequently	43	40	39	40	40	33	34
Giving child favourite things							
Never	5	6	1	8	6	4	4
Seldom	9	11	14	4	10	10	10
Sometimes	48	48	48	55	49	56	56
Frequently	37	34	38	34	35	30	30
Base	*445*	*492*	*139*	*57*	*928*	*9376*	*10305*

Table 9.9 Punishment regimes

by type of mental disorder

All children

	Type of mental disorder						
	Emotional disorders	Conduct disorders	Hyperkinetic disorders	Less common disorders	Any disorder	No disorder	All
	%	%	%	%	%	%	%
Punishment regimes							
Sending child to his/her room							
Never	26	21	23	29	23	26	26
Seldom	27	20	18	35	25	35	34
Sometimes	35	34	34	29	34	31	31
Frequently	12	25	26	7	18	8	9
"Grounding" or keeping him/her in							
Never	28	16	19	38	23	34	33
Seldom	24	20	22	22	22	27	26
Sometimes	27	34	31	21	30	24	24
Frequently	13	24	18	8	17	5	6
Too young to go out alone	8	7	10	11	8	10	10
Shouting or yelling at him/her							
Never	8	3	5	7	5	6	6
Seldom	15	8	7	18	12	19	18
Sometimes	43	37	33	46	41	50	49
Frequently	34	53	55	29	42	26	28
Smacking him/her with your hand							
Never	58	41	37	63	49	56	55
Seldom	32	41	48	24	37	35	35
Sometimes	8	15	12	12	12	9	9
Frequently	1	3	2	-	2	0	0
Hitting him/her with strap							
Never	99	96	96	97	97	99	98
Seldom	1	3	3	2	2	1	1
Sometimes	0	1	1	2	1	0	0
Frequently	-	-	-	-	-	0	0
Shaking him/her							
Never	96	94	93	98	96	98	98
Seldom	3	5	6	-	4	2	2
Sometimes	1	1	1	2	1	0	0
Frequently	-	-	-	-	-	0	0
Base	*445*	*492*	*139*	*56*	*928*	*9374*	*10302*

Table 9.10   Prevalence of mental disorders

by type of non-physical, parental punishment

All children

	Frequency of sending child to his room				
	Never	Seldom	Sometimes	Frequently	All
	Percentage of children with each disorder				
Emotional disorders	4	3	5	6	4
Conduct disorders	4	3	6	16	6
Hyperkinetic disorders	1	1	2	4	1
Less common disorders	1	1	1	1	1
Any mental disorder	**8**	**6**	**11**	**20**	**10**
Base	*2669*	*3530*	*3215*	*884*	*10299*

	Frequency of grounding child or keeping him/her in				
	Never	Seldom	Sometimes	Frequently	All*
	Percentage of children with each disorder				
Emotional disorders	4	4	5	9	4
Conduct disorders	2	4	8	21	6
Hyperkinetic disorders	1	1	2	4	1
Less common disorders	1	1	1	1	1
Any mental disorder	**6**	**8**	**12**	**27**	**10**
Base	*3444*	*2722*	*2489*	*612*	*10300*

* Includes 1033 children too young to go out alone

	Frequency of shouting or yelling at child				
	Never	Seldom	Sometimes	Frequently	All
	Percentage of children with each disorder				
Emotional disorders	6	4	4	5	4
Conduct disorders	2	2	4	10	6
Hyperkinetic disorders	1	1	1	3	1
Less common disorders	1	1	1	1	1
Any mental disorder	**8**	**6**	**8**	**15**	**10**
Base	*565*	*1879*	*5030*	*2829*	*10303*

Table 9.11   Prevalence of mental disorders

by type of physical, parental punishment

All children

	Frequency of smacking child with hand				
	Never	Seldom	Sometimes	Frequently	All
	Percentage of children with each disorder				
Emotional disorders	5	4	4	10	4
Conduct disorders	4	7	9	34	6
Hyperkinetic disorders	1	2	2	7	1
Less common disorders	1	0	1	-	1
Any mental disorder	**8**	**11**	**13**	**37**	**10**
Base	*5690*	*3594*	*966*	*51*	*10302*

	Frequency of hitting child with a strap or something else				
	Never	Seldom	Sometimes	Frequently	All
	Percentage of children with each disorder				
Emotional disorders	4	4	[1]	-	4
Conduct disorders	6	13	[4]	-	6
Hyperkinetic disorders	1	3	[1]	-	1
Less common disorders	1	1	[1]	-	1
Any mental disorder	**10**	**16**	**[6]**	**-**	**10**
Base	*10140*	*123*	*29*	*8*	*10301*

	Frequency of shaking child				
	Never	Seldom	Sometimes	Frequently	All
	Percentage of children with each disorder				
Emotional disorders	4	7	[3]	-	4
Conduct disorders	6	16	[3]	-	6
Hyperkinetic disorders	1	5	[1]	-	1
Less common disorders	1	-	[1]	-	1
Any mental disorder	**10**	**19**	**[6]**	**-**	**10**
Base	*10081*	*187*	*27*	*7*	*10302*

Table 9.12	Stressful life events
	by type of mental disorder

All children

	Type of mental disorder						
	Emotional disorders	Conduct disorders	Hyperkinetic disorders	Less common disorders	Any disorder	No disorder	All
	Proportion of children who have experienced each stressful life event						
Stressful life event							
Since child was born parent had a separation due to marital difficulties or broken off steady relationship	49	58	47	39	50	29	31
Since child was born parent (or partner) had a major financial crisis such as losing the equivalent of three months income	28	25	20	25	24	15	16
Since child was born parent (or partner) had a problem with the police involving a court appearance	15	18	13	5	15	5	6
At some stage in the child's life s/he had a serious illness which required a stay in hospital	33	28	39	30	30	20	20
At any stage in child's life, child had been in a serious accident or badly hurt in an accident	10	9	8	8	9	5	5
At any stage in child's life, a parent, brother or sister died	5	7	8	4	6	3	3
At any stage in child's life, a close friend died	12	9	9	12	10	5	6
At any stage in child's life, a grand-parent died	16	12	17	9	14	13	13
At any stage in child's life, a pet died	32	22	27	13	27	27	27
In the past year child has broken off a steady relationship with a boy or girl friend (asked if aged 13 or above)	24	17	14	[5]	18	8	10
Base = all children	445	492	139	57	928	9376	10305
Base = children aged 13 or above	174	163	31	19	313	2347	2661

Table 9.13 Number of stressful life events
by type of mental disorder

All children

| | Type of mental disorder | | | | | | |
	Emotional disorders	Conduct disorders	Hyperkinetic disorders	Less common disorders	Any disorder	No disorder	All
	%	%	%	%	%	%	%
Number of stressful life events							
0	15	17	16	28	18	30	29
1	26	27	27	25	27	35	34
2	21	24	28	22	24	22	22
3	19	15	14	18	16	9	10
4	11	13	12	4	11	3	4
5+	7	4	4	4	4	1	1
At least one event	**85**	**83**	**84**	**72**	**82**	**70**	**71**
Base = all children	*445*	*492*	*139*	*57*	*928*	*9380*	*10309*

Table 9.14 Prevalence of mental disorders
by type of stressful life events

All children

	Marital difficulties	Financial crisis	Trouble with police*	Serious illness	Serious accident
	Percentage of children with each disorder				
Emotional disorders	7	8	10	7	8
Conduct disorders	10	9	16	7	9
Hyperkinetic disorders	2	2	3	3	2
Less common disorders	1	1	1	1	1
Any mental disorder	**16**	**15**	**22**	**14**	**16**
Base	*3151*	*1599*	*646*	*2108*	*548*

* Parent or partner's trouble with the police

	Death of parent/sibling	Death of close friend	Death of grandparent	Death of pet	Split up with boy/girl friend
	Percentage of children with each disorder				
Emotional disorders	6	10	6	5	16
Conduct disorders	11	9	4	4	11
Hyperkinetic disorders	3	2	2	1	2
Less common disorders	1	1	0	0	2
Any mental disorder	**17**	**17**	**11**	**10**	**24**
Base	*338*	*579*	*1315*	*2735*	*257*

Table 9.15 Prevalence of mental disorders by number of stressful life events

All children

	0	1	2	3	4	5+	All
	Percentage of children with each disorder						
Emotional disorders	2	3	4	9	12	24	4
Conduct disorders	3	4	6	8	18	18	6
Hyperkinetic disorders	1	1	2	2	4	4	1
Less common disorders	1	0	1	1	1	2	1
Any mental disorder	**6**	**7**	**11**	**16**	**27**	**34**	**10**
Base	*2992*	*3550*	*2264*	*979*	*396*	*128*	*10309*

Table 9.16 Odds Ratios for social functioning and socio-demographic correlates of mental disorders

Variable	Value	Adjusted OR	95% CI
Parent's GHQ-12 score	0-2	1.00	....
	3+	2.23***	(1.93-2.59)
Punishment regime	Infrequent	1.00	....
	Frequent	1.97***	(1.70-2.39)
Family functioning	Healthy	1.00	....
	Unhealthy	1.82***	(1.56 - 2.13)
Stressful life events	None	1.00	....
	At least one	1.35**	(1.12-1.63)
Age of child	5 - 10 years	1.00	....
	11-15 years	1.52***	(1.32-1.76)
Sex of child	Girl	1.00	....
	Boy	1.50***	(1.30-1.73)
Family type	Two parent family	1.00	....
	One parent family	1.33**	(1.10-1.60)
Family employment	All working	1.00	....
	One parent working	1.26*	(1.03-1.54)
	All not working	1.75***	(1.42-2.15)
ACORN classification	Thriving	1.00	....
	Expanding	1.37*	(1.02-1.84)
	Rising	1.58*	(1.11-2.26)
	Settling	1.50**	(1.16-1.94)
	Aspiring	1.71***	(1.30-2.25)
	Striving	1.67***	(1.30-2.15)

Other variables entered which were not significant were: number of children
*** p<0.001, ** p<0.01, * p<0.05

Table 9.17	Impact of child's problems on family relationships
	by type of mental disorder

	Type of mental disorder				
	Emotional disorders	Conduct disorders	Hyperkinetic disorders	Less common disorders	Any disorder
Impact of child's problems (as described by parent) on family relationships	%	%	%	%	%
Child's problems made relationship with partner......					
more strained	27	49	41	18	34
no different	54	37	43	52	49
stronger	18	14	16	30	17
Base = parent with partner	*249*	*233*	*85*	*39*	*491*
Child's problems put a strain on a previous relationship and was part of the reason the relationship broke up......					
to a great extent	9	12	8	-	9
to some extent	7	14	12	[2]	11
not at all	75	64	71	[11]	70
problem started before split	8	10	8	[2]	10
Base = parent with no partner in household	*147*	*171*	*50*	*15*	*300*
Child's problems made relationship with other children......					
more difficult	23	34	31	24	25
no different	60	54	57	55	59
stronger	11	7	2	12	9
no other children	6	6	9	10	7
Base = all parents	*395*	*402*	*134*	*54*	*789*
Child's problems made partner's relationship with his/her other children......					
more difficult	25	39	34	24	30
no different	51	44	48	57	50
stronger	14	4	3	8	9
no other children	10	12	14	11	11
Base = all parents	*372*	*378*	*122*	*49*	*736*
Child's problems caused difficulties with other family members					
Yes	19	35	35	34	26
No	81	65	65	66	74
Base = all parents	*397*	*401*	*134*	*56*	*791*

Table 9.18	Impact of child's problems on social life and stigma
	by type of mental disorder

Children with disorder whose parents reported at least one significant mental health problem of child

	Type of mental disorder				
	Emotional disorders	Conduct disorders	Hyperkinetic disorders	Less common disorders	Any disorder
Impact of child's problems (as described by parent) on social life and stigma	%	%	%	%	%
Child's problems caused difficulties with parent's own relationships with friends					
Yes	14	21	17	29	15
No	86	79	83	71	85
Child's problems disrupted parents leisure and social activities...					
to a great extent	14	18	18	27	14
to some extent	30	35	33	39	32
not at all	56	48	49	34	54
Child's difficulties have kept parent from doing things socially with child....					
to a great extent	12	21	28	25	16
to some extent	25	32	31	39	29
not at all	63	47	41	36	55
Child's difficulties have caused embarrassment to parent					
Yes	19	46	42	40	31
No	81	54	58	60	69
Parent has felt disapproved of or avoided because of child's difficulties					
Yes	23	36	41	44	29
No	77	64	59	56	71
Base = all parents	*397*	*402*	*134*	*56*	*792*

Table 9.19 Impact of child's problems on parent's health

by type of mental disorder

Children with disorder whose parents reported at least one significant mental health problem of child

Impact of child's problems (as described by parent) on parent's health	Type of mental disorder				
	Emotional disorders	Conduct disorders	Hyperkinetic disorders	Less common disorders	Any disorder
	%	%	%	%	%
Child's problems caused parent to be worried......					
to a great extent	37	44	41	57	38
to some extent	48	48	50	34	49
not at all	15	8	9	9	12
Child's problems caused parent to be depressed......					
to a great extent	19	24	20	22	19
to some extent	35	43	42	40	39
not at all	46	33	38	39	42
Child's problems caused parent to be tired......					
to a great extent	24	33	35	39	27
to some extent	38	44	44	45	41
not at all	39	23	20	16	31
Child's problems caused parent to be physically ill......					
to a great extent	11	12	11	11	10
to some extent	16	20	9	20	16
not at all	74	68	80	69	74
Base = all parents	*397*	*402*	*134*	*56*	*792*

Table 9.20	Impact of child's problems on parent's health behaviour
	by type of mental disorder

Children with disorder whose parents reported at least one significant mental health problem of child

	Type of mental disorder				
	Emotional disorders	Conduct disorders	Hyperkinetic disorders	Less common disorders	Any disorder
Parent's behaviour if child's problems had caused worry, depression, tiredness or physical illness to some or a great extent	%	%	%	%	%
Went to see a doctor					
Yes	32	35	30	37	31
No	68	65	70	63	69
Base = Parents whose child caused them health problems	*361*	*385*	*128*	*54*	*736*
Prescribed medicine by doctor					
Yes	70	64	60	[10]	63
No	30	36	40	[10]	37
Base = Parents who went to see doctor owing to health problems caused by child's problem	*114*	*135*	*38*	*20*	*227*
Drank more alcohol					
Yes	9	9	8	15	9
No	91	91	92	85	91
Base = Parents whose child caused them health problems	*361*	*385*	*128*	*54*	*736*
Smoked more cigarettes					
Yes	29	37	28	16	30
No	71	63	72	84	70
Base = Parents whose child caused them health problems	*361*	*385*	*128*	*54*	*736*

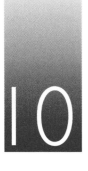

10 Children's social functioning and lifestyle behaviours

10.1 Introduction

Whereas the previous chapter looked at the relationship between mental disorders among children and measures of family functioning, this final chapter focuses on the social life of children in terms of their friendships, help-seeking behaviour and lifestyle. The term, lifestyle behaviour, is used to cover smoking, drinking and drug use.

10.2 Friendships

A child's social life usually revolves around their friends so to find out more about their friendships 11-15 year olds were asked the following questions:

- Do you have any friends?
- How much time do you spend together (with your friends)?
- How often do friends come to your home?
- How often do you go to your friend's home?
- Can you confide in any of your friends such as sharing a secret or telling them private things?
- Do you have a 'best' friend or special friend?
- Over the past 12 months have you belonged to any teams, clubs or other groups with an adult in charge?

Looking at the responses to the individual questions permits a more detailed examination of the relationship between mental disorders and friendship behaviour. In reviewing previous studies Goodyer et al. (1990) have commented that good peer relationships are probably necessary for healthy mental development. Absence of close relationships may increase the risk of psychiatric disorder.

The first question in the friendship section asked young people if they had any friends. Not surprisingly, virtually all young people reported that they had friends. However, a quarter of these children said that they did not have a 'best' or special friend. There was very little difference in the proportions of children without friends or 'best' friends by presence of or type of disorder. The only notable difference was that children with

hyperkinetic disorders were slightly more likely, than those with emotional disorders not to have a 'best' friend: 28% compared with 16%. *(Table 10.1)*

Young people spent a lot of their spare time with friends. Among all young people, who had friends, only 12% spent little or none of their spare time with their friends. Again, there was very little difference in the amount of time that children spent with their friends by presence of a mental disorder or by type of disorder. *(Table 10.1)*

The next two questions in the friendship section asked young people how often friends came to their house and how often they went to their friend's homes. Just over a quarter (28%) of all young people only had friends round to their home for just a little or none of the time. Children with a mental disorder were more likely, than those with no disorder, to have friends round infrequently: 35% compared with 27%. There was some difference by the three broad types of disorder: 15% of children with hyperkinetic disorders did not have any friends round, compared with 9% with conduct disorders, 7% with emotional disorders and 4% of children with no disorder. *(Table 10.1)*

Young people's behaviour in going round to their friend's homes followed a similar pattern to their friends coming round to their homes. Just under a quarter (24%) of children did not visit or only spent a little time at their friends. Children with a mental disorder were less likely than other children to spend time at their friends' houses: with 31% compared with 23% spending only a little or none of their spare time at their friends. There was little difference in the amount of time spent in their friends' homes by type of mental disorder. *(Table 10.1)*

Young people were also asked if they felt able to confide in any of their friends such as sharing secrets or telling them private things. Only a small proportion of children (6%) felt unable to confide in friends. Children with a mental disorder were more likely, than those with no disorder, to report that they did not feel able to confide in friends: 8% compared with 5%. This proportion varied slightly by type of disorder, ranging from 6% of those with an emotional disorder, to 8% with hyperkinetic disorder and 10% with conduct disorders. *(Table 10.1)*

The final question in the friendship section was about membership of teams, clubs or other groups (with an adult in charge) over the past 12 months. Just over a quarter (27%) of children had not been a member of a club, team or group over the past 12 months. However, this applied to over a third (36%) of children with a mental disorder. *(Table 10.1)*

An overall friendship score was computed by allocating a score of one to the more positive responses and zero to the negative answers to the friendship questions. Thus children with no friends scored zero and those who; (a) had a best friend (b) spent some or all of their spare time with friends (c) frequently had friends visiting them in their home (d) went round to their friends home some or all of the time (e) confided in their friends and (f) were club members, scored six.

Across the whole population of 11-15 year olds, just 6% had a severe lack of friendship (a score of 0 - 2). However, this proportion was greater among those with mental disorders than those with no disorder: 9% compared with 5%. The group containing the largest proportion with severe lack of friendship, 12%, were children assessed as being hyperkinetic. *(Table 10.2, Figure 10.1)*

10.3   Help-seeking behaviour

All 11-15 year olds were asked if they had ever felt so unhappy or worried that they asked someone for help. Overall, a quarter of them had sought help because they had felt so unhappy or worried in the past. Children with a disorder were almost twice as likely, as those without a disorder, to have been in this situation (41% compared with 23%). About half the children with an emotional disorder had sought help, and a third of those with hyperkinetic and conduct disorders. *(Figure 10.2)*

This group of young people, who had sought help in the past, were then asked who they had turned to for help when they needed it; this could have been more than one person. Mothers were the most frequently mentioned (58%). A special friend was the next most popular, 52%, and the child's father was the third most common response (28%).

Overall, a small proportion of children had asked for help from professional advisors, such as school nurses, doctors, social workers or had used a telephone helpline. However these services were used by a far greater proportion of children with a mental disorder than those with no disorder: 27% compared with 4%. *(Table 10.3)*

The majority of children who had sought help (56%) wanted a chance to talk things over, 15% required practical advice and 29% were seeking both practical advice and a chance to talk things over. *(Table 10.4)*

Figure 10.1   Distribution of friendship scores by type of mental disorder

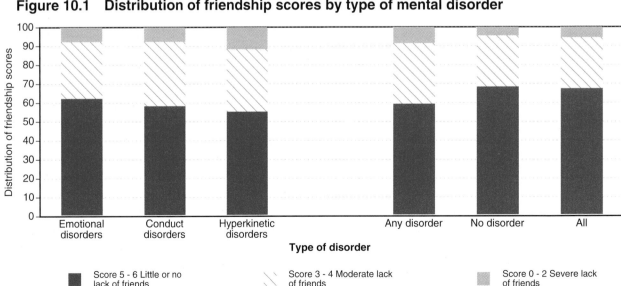

Figure 10.2 Help seeking behaviour by type of mental disorder

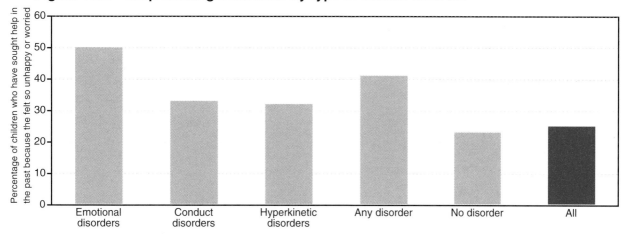

The young people who had not sought help were asked to imagine who they would turn to for assistance if they ever needed it. Again, it was the child's mother who was the most popular choice, proposed by 79% of children. The child's father and a special friend were the next two most commonly reported (46%). Twenty four per cent of children mentioned brother or sister. *(Table 10.5)*

When asked what type of help they would expect to receive, 14% hoped to get practical advice, 37% wanted the opportunity to talk things over and 49% thought they would get both practical advice and a chance to talk things over. *(Table 10.6)*

10.4 Smoking, drinking and drug use

Questions on smoking, drinking and drug use were included in the survey so that the relationship between mental disorders and life style behaviours could be examined. The questions asked in the mental health survey were taken from the national surveys of smoking, drinking and drug use among young teenagers in England and Scotland, carried out by ONS (Goddard and Higgins, 1999). Although the question wording was similar in both surveys, the mode of administration was different. In the surveys dedicated to estimating the prevalence of smoking, alcohol consumption and drug use, young people were given a paper questionnaire to complete in a group setting in school. Samples of saliva were taken from fifty percent of the children, for cotinine analysis, to monitor the accuracy of the results on smoking. For the current survey, 11-15 year olds were asked to complete a questionnaire on a lap-top computer at home.

A comparison of the data from both sources, presented in Tables 10.7, 10.8 and 10.9, suggest that children interviewed at home systematically under-report their smoking, drinking and drug use compared to the rates from the school survey.

Therefore, the only analysis presented in this report is the prevalence of mental disorders by the lifestyle behaviours of children and not the prevalence of smoking, drinking and drug use by type of mental disorder. Therefore, any differences in the rates of mental disorder by smoking, drinking or drug use are probably an underestimate of the true difference between users and non-users.

Smoking

Children were categorised into five groups according to their smoking behaviour: regular smokers, occasional smokers, those who used to smoke, children who had tried it once and those who had never smoked. Whereas the overall prevalence rate of mental disorders among 11-15 year olds was 11%, the mental health profile of regular smokers (>6 cigarettes a day) was different from all other groups: 41% of 11-15 year olds who regularly smoked were assessed as having a mental disorder (28% had a conduct disorder, 20% had an emotional disorder and 4% were rated as having a hyperkinetic disorder). The group with the second highest prevalence of mental disorders were those who used to smoke; a rate of 16%. The prevalence among children who had never smoked was 7%. *(Table 10.10)*

Drinking

Children were placed into seven groups in terms of their alcohol consumption: more than once a week, about once a week, about once a fortnight, about once a month, a few times a year, never drinks alcohol now and never had an alcoholic drink. As found for smoking, the most frequent users, those who drank alcohol more than once a week, had by far the highest proportion of children with a mental disorder, 24%. This represents three times the proportion of children with a mental disorder among the group who had never drunk any alcohol. *(Table 10.11)*

Use of cannabis

Cannabis was the most frequently used drug by 11-15 year olds: 234 children admitted to trying it. The number of children who reported using other drugs was far too small to accurately estimate their prevalence of mental disorders. Cannabis users were divided into two group - those using the drug at least once a month, 42% of all users, and the remainder who used cannabis less frequently. About one half of the frequent users had a mental disorder - 32% conduct disorders; 25% emotional disorders - compared with one fifth of the less than once a month users and one tenth of those who had never used cannabis. *(Table 10.12)*

References

Goddard, E. & Higgins, V. (1999) *Smoking, drinking and drug use among young teenagers in 1998 (Volume I : England).* London: The Stationery Office.

Goodyer, I.M., Wright, C. & Altham, P. M. E. (1990) The friendships and recent life events of anxious and depressed school-age-children. *British Journal of Psychiatry,* **156** (MAY), 689-698.

Table 10.1 Friendship behaviour

by type of mental disorder

All 11-15 year olds who completed a personal interview

	Type of mental disorder						
	Emotional disorders	Conduct disorders	Hyperkinetic disorders	Less common disorders	Any disorder	No disorder	All
	%	%	%	%	%	%	%
Do you have any friends?							
Yes	99	100	98	[20]	99	100	100
No	1	0	2	-	1	0	0
Base	*239*	*225*	*51*	*20*	*434*	*3897*	*4331*
Do you have a 'best' friend or a special friend?							
Yes	84	76	72	[14]	79	76	76
No	16	24	28	[5]	21	24	24
Base	*236*	*224*	*50*	*20*	*429*	*3892*	*4321*
How much time do you spend together...							
all of your spare time	32	41	33	[7]	34	21	23
some of your spare time	54	46	50	[7]	52	67	65
a little time	13 } 14	11 } 12	14 } 16	[5]	13 } 14	11 } 12	11 } 12
or not at all?	1	1	2	-	1	1	1
Base	*237*	*224*	*50*	*20*	*430*	*3890*	*4319*
How often do friends come to your house...							
all or most of the time	26	24	19	[7]	23	15	16
some of the time	43	39	39	[6]	42	58	56
a little time	22 } 31	30 } 37	27 } 42	[5]	27 } 35	23 } 27	24 } 28
or not at all?	9	7	15	[1]	8	4	4
Base	*237*	*224*	*50*	*20*	*430*	*3891*	*4321*
How often do you go to your friend's home...							
all or most of the time	24	26	18	[7]	23	16	16
some of the time	46	44	50	[5]	46	61	60
a little time	26 } 30	25 } 30	25 } 31	[5]	26 } 31	21 } 23	21 } 24
or not at all?	4	5	6	[2]	5	2	3
Base	*237*	*224*	*50*	*20*	*430*	*3892*	*4332*
Can you confide in any of you friends such as sharing a secret or telling them private things?							
Definitely	48	51	46	[8]	49	54	54
Sometimes	46	39	46	[8]	43	40	41
Not at all	6	10	8	[3]	8	5	6
Base	*237*	*224*	*49*	*20*	*429*	*3889*	*4318*
Over the past 12 months have you belonged to any teams, clubs or other groups with an adult in charge?							
Yes	68	61	70	[10]	64	74	73
No	32	39	30	[9]	36	26	27
Base	*239*	*225*	*50*	*20*	*433*	*3894*	*4326*

Table 10.2 Friendship score

by type of mental disorder

All 11-15 year olds who completed a personal interview

	Type of mental disorder						All
	Emotional disorders	Conduct disorders	Hyperkinetic disorders	Less common disorders	Any disorder	No disorder	
Friendship score *	%	%	%	%	%	%	%
0	1	1	2	-	1	0	0
1	1	1	2	[1]	1	1	1
2	6	6	8	[3]	7	4	4
3	8	14	19	[1]	12	10	10
4	22	20	14	[4]	20	17	17
5	30	33	27	[7]	31	31	31
6	31	24	29	[3]	27	37	36
Score 0 - 2 Severe	8	9	12	[4]	9	5	6
Score 3 - 4 Moderate	30	34	33	[5]	32	27	27
Score 5 - 6 Little or no lack	62	58	55	[10]	59	68	67
Base	*239*	*225*	*50*	*20*	*433*	*3893*	*4325*

* Score 1 for each of: Child spends some or all of spare time with friends;Friends visit child's home some or all of the time; Child visits friend's home some or all of the time; Child can definitely or sometimes confide with friend; Has a best or special friend; Belongs to team, club or group with adult in charge.

Table 10.3 People asked for help

by type of mental disorder

All 11-15 year olds who had been so worried or unhappy that they had asked for help

	Type of mental disorder						All
	Emotional disorders	Conduct disorders	Hyperkinetic disorders	Less common disorders	Any disorder	No disorder	
	Percentage of children seeking each type of help						
Mother	48	48	[9]	[6]	51	59	58
Special friend	54	48	[5]	[4]	52	52	52
Father	20	20	[1]	[3]	22	29	28
School teacher	21	25	[4]	[3]	22	19	20
Brother or sister	17	15	[1]	[4]	18	17	17
Telephone helpline	7	4	[-]	[1]	5	2	2
Doctor	7	9	[1]	[-]	7	1	2
School nurse	6	-	[-]	[-]	4	1	2
Social worker	8	3	[-]	[-]	5	0	1
None of these	8	4	[2]	[-]	6	7	6
Base	*119*	*74*	*16*	*11*	*175*	*884*	*1059*

Table 10.4 Type of help sought

by type of mental disorder

All 11-15 year olds who completed a personal interview and had sought help because they had felt unhappy or worried

| | Type of mental disorder | | | | | | |
	Emotional disorders	Conduct disorders	Hyperkinetic disorders	Less common disorders	Any disorder	No disorder	All disorder
Type of help	%	%	%	%	%	%	%
Practical advice	11	16	[2]	[1]	12	16	15
Talk things over	55	56	[9]	[6]	56	56	56
Both practical advice and to talk things over	35	28	[3]	[4]	32	29	29
Base	*116*	*72*	*14*	*11*	*172*	*855*	*1026*

Table 10.5 Potential helpers

by type of mental disorder

All 11-15 year olds who had not sought help in the past

| | Type of mental disorder | | | | | | |
	Emotional disorders	Conduct disorders	Hyperkinetic disorders	Less common disorders	Any disorder	No disorder	All
	Percentage of children who would seek each type of help						
Mother	72	67	59	[6]	68	80	79
Father	33	33	39	[3]	36	47	46
Special friend	44	35	36	[1]	40	47	46
Brother or sister	25	15	3	[4]	19	25	24
School teacher	14	17	15	-	16	12	12
Telephone helpline	2	1	-	-	1	2	2
School nurse	1	1	3	-	1	2	2
Doctor	2	1	-	-	2	2	2
Social worker	4	4	5	-	4	1	1
None of these	12	15	22	-	14	6	7
Base	*120*	*149*	*34*	*8*	*256*	*3005*	*3260*

Table 10.6 Type of potential help
by type of mental disorder

All 11-15 year olds who had not sought help

	Type of mental disorder						All
	Emotional disorders	Conduct disorders	Hyperkinetic disorders	Less common disorders	Any disorder disorder	No disorder	
Type of help expected	%	%	%	%	%	%	%
Practical advice	13	16	[7]	[1]	15	14	14
Talk things over	44	50	[10]	[4]	47	36	37
Both practical advice and to talk things over	43	34	[10]	[2]	38	49	49
Base	*110*	*139*	*27*	*7*	*232*	*2874*	*3106*

Table 10.7 Smoking behaviour
by age, survey source and sex

Smoking behaviour

	11	11	12	12	13	13	14	14	15	15	All	All
	School	H'hold	School	H'hold	School	H'hold	School	H'hold	School	H'hold	School	H'hold
	%	%	%	%	%	%	%	%	%	%	%	%
Boys												
Regular smoker	1	-	3	1	5	3	15	8	19	13	9	5
Occasional smoker	3	1	7	1	8	2	8	4	11	6	8	3
Used to smoke	3	1	5	3	12	4	11	7	15	10	9	5
Tried smoking	16	11	18	19	21	26	23	29	21	30	20	23
Never smoked	78	88	67	77	54	66	42	53	34	40	54	65
Base	*300*	*448*	*349*	*434*	*302*	*440*	*612*	*413*	*754*	*424*	*2317*	*2159*
Girls												
Regular smoker	1	-	3	1	9	3	19	10	29	18	12	6
Occasional smoker	3	0	6	1	9	5	13	5	11	7	8	4
Used to smoke	2	1	7	4	13	7	13	10	16	8	10	6
Tried smoking	12	9	18	17	21	20	17	28	18	24	18	19
Never smoked	82	90	66	77	48	66	37	46	26	44	51	65
Base	*303*	*441*	*375*	*442*	*390*	*441*	*670*	*416*	*673*	*420*	*2411*	*2160*
All												
Regular smoker	1	-	3	1	7	3	17	9	24	16	11	6
Occasional smoker	3	1	6	1	9	3	11	4	11	6	8	3
Used to smoke	2	1	6	3	13	6	12	9	15	9	10	5
Tried smoking	14	10	18	18	21	23	20	29	20	27	19	21
Never smoked	80	89	67	77	50	66	40	50	30	42	53	65
Base	*603*	*887*	*724*	*876*	*692*	*882*	*1282*	*831*	*1427*	*842*	*4728*	*4318*

School = Data collected at school (Goddard and Higgins, 1999) "
H'hold = Data collected from this survey at home

Table 10.8	Drinking behaviour

by age, survey source and sex

Drinking

	11	11	12	12	13	13	14	14	15	15	All	All
	School	H'hold	School	H'hold	School	H'hold	School	H'hold	School	H'hold	School	H'hold
	%	%	%	%	%	%	%	%	%	%	%	%
Boys												
Almost every day	1	1	2	-	0	1	2	1	4	1	2	1
About twice a week	2	1	2	1	5	2	9	5	18	9	8	3
About once a week	2	2	2	2	5	3	10	8	20	14	8	6
About once a fortnight	2	3	6	3	8	4	11	9	11	14	8	6
About once a month	3	3	4	4	7	8	12	16	14	15	8	9
Only a few times a year	17	13	22	22	32	29	30	27	19	30	24	24
Never drinks now	6	1	4	3	6	2	4	2	4	1	5	2
Never had a drink	68	77	58	65	38	52	22	34	11	16	38	49
Base	*287*	*447*	*335*	*436*	*294*	*439*	*601*	*414*	*741*	*424*	*2258*	*2160*
Girls												
Almost every day	0	0	0	-	1	-	2	-	1	1	0	0
About twice a week	0	0	1	-	3	1	10	1	14	9	6	2
About once a week	1	-	3	2	7	2	10	6	18	14	8	4
About once a fortnight	1	1	3	1	3	5	12	8	17	14	7	5
About once a month	3	1	4	5	11	8	12	11	15	15	9	8
Only a few times a year	10	15	25	20	30	31	28	38	19	30	23	27
Never drinks now	5	1	6	2	3	2	3	1	2	1	4	1
Never had a drink	80	82	57	69	42	51	23	35	14	16	42	52
Base	*291*	*440*	*368*	*442*	*380*	*442*	*655*	*416*	*665*	*421*	*2359*	*2161*
All												
Almost every day	0	1	1	-	1	1	2	1	3	1	2	0
About twice a week	1	1	2	1	4	2	10	3	16	8	7	3
About once a week	1	1	3	2	6	3	10	7	19	11	8	5
About once a fortnight	2	2	4	2	5	4	12	9	13	13	7	6
About once a month	3	2	4	5	10	8	12	13	14	16	9	8
Only a few times a year	13	14	24	21	31	30	29	32	19	31	23	26
Never drinks now	6	1	5	2	4	2	4	1	3	1	4	2
Never had a drink	74	80	57	67	40	51	22	34	12	20	40	51
Base	*580*	*887*	*704*	*876*	*676*	*882*	*1254*	*832*	*1405*	*843*	*4619*	*4320*

School = Data collected at school (Goddard and Higgins, 1999)
H'hold = Data collected from this survey at home

Table 10.9	Drug taking
	by survey source

All children aged 11-15 years old

	School	H'hold
	Percentage of children using each type of drug	
Ever used...		
Cannabis	**12**	5
Inhalants (Glue)	**2**	1
Ecstasy	**1**	0
Amphetamines	**3**	1
LSD	**1**	0
Tranquilisers	**0**	0
Cocaine	**1**	0
Heroin	**0**	0
Base	*4649*	*4313*

School = Data collected at school (Goddard and Higgins, 1999)
H'hold = Data collected from this survey at home

Table 10.10	Prevalence of mental disorders
	by smoking behaviour

Children aged 11-15 years old

	Regular smoker	Occasional smoker	Used to smoke	Tried smoking once	Never smoked	All children
	Percentage of children with each mental disorder					
Emotional disorders	20	6	8	6	4	6
Conduct disorders	28	6	9	8	3	6
Hyperkinetic disorders	4	1	3	2	1	1
Less common disorders	2	-	1	0	0	1
Any mental disorder	**41**	**10**	**16**	**13**	**7**	**11**
Base	*236*	*129*	*235*	*911*	*2808*	*4319*

Table 10.11 Prevalence of mental disorders

by drinking behaviour

Children aged 11-15 years old

	More than once a week	About once a week	About once a fortnight	About once a month	Only a few times a year	Never now drinks alcohol	Never had an alcohol drink	All children
	Percentage of children with each mental disorder							
Emotional disorders	14	8	7	7	5	6	5	6
Conduct disorders	15	8	6	8	7	7	4	6
Hyperkinetic disorders	2	2	1	1	1	0	1	1
Less common disorders	1	-	2	1	0	-	0	1
Any mental disorder	**24**	**14**	**15**	**14**	**10**	**13**	**8**	**11**
Base	*133*	*205*	*251*	*368*	*1101*	*67*	*2193*	*4319*

Table 10.12 Prevalence of mental disorders

by use of cannabis

Children aged 11-15 years old

	At least once a month	Less than onece a month	Has never used cannabis	All children
	Percentage of children with each mental disorder			
Emotional disorders	25	8	5	6
Conduct disorders	32	12	4	6
Hyperkinetic disorders	3	7	1	1
Less common disorders	2	1	0	1
Any mental disorder	**49**	**21**	**10**	**11**
Base	*98*	*136*	*4080*	*4314*

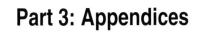

Part 3: Appendices

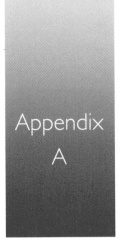

Sampling, weighting and adjustment procedures

A1   Sampling procedures

The sampling frame

The Child Benefit Register (CBR), held by the Department of Social Security, was used as the sampling frame for the survey. Of the 7,134,968 records on the file, 6,536,570 had a postcoded address (91.6%). Whereas, the Child Benefit Register had entries for 25,810 postal sectors, at the time of the sampling phase of the survey, mid 1998, in reality, there were around 9,000 valid sectors in Great Britain. Many of the non-valid sectors were clearly mistakes on the CBR caused by the transcription or imputation of a wrong letter or a number - these sectors had only one or two children in them. However, Table A1.1 shows that there were some very large sectors in the non-valid category. Further investigation found that many of these large sectors represented discontinued postcodes. *(Table A1.1)*

Table A1.1 Size of non-current sectors on the CBR file

Sector size	Frequency	Cumulative %
1	5597	31.9
2	4423	57.2
3	2194	69.7
4	1394	77.7
5	909	82.9
6-10	1757	92.9
11-20	440	95.4
21-30	112	96.0
31-50	136	96.8
51-100	127	97.5
101-200	90	98.0
201-500	103	98.6
501-1000	138	99.4
1001+	102	100.0
Total	**17522**	

The sampling design for the survey involved a two-stage process: the selection of 475 sectors with 30 children selected per sector. Because it was not possible to group small sectors prior to the selection nor vary the number of children to be selected from each sector, all sectors with fewer than 100 children were excluded from the sampling frame.

In order to reduce bias, we included all sectors, subject to the minimum size constraint and, for non-current sectors, subject to a minimum of 100 discontinued postcodes. (ONS is able to reallocate discontinued postcodes to their new versions).

This produced a population of 7905 current sectors and 360 non-current sectors. These sectors included 6,422,402 (98.3%) of the children in addresses with postcodes so the overall coverage of the CBR by the ONS-created, sampling frame was 90.0%.

After dropping the 24 sectors selected for the pilot survey, introducing another small potential bias, a Regional Health Authority (RHA) code was imputed for the 360 non-current sectors.

Stratification and selection of sectors

The frame was stratified by RHA and within that by socio-economic group (SEG) and then the sectors were selected with probability proportional to the number of children: 400 sectors were selected in England, 25 in Wales and 50 in Scotland. 5 sectors were wanted in the Scottish Highlands and Islands, i.e., those north of the Caledonian Canal plus the Islands.

Table A1.2 Allocation of the 475 sectors to (health) regions				
Region	Children	%	Sectors selected	Sectors expected
1	354,145	5.5	26	26.19
2	439,280	6.8	32	32.49
3	541,872	8.4	39	40.08
4	234,953	3.7	17	17.38
5	381,551	5.9	27	28.22
6	423,259	6.6	30	31.30
7	416,493	6.5	30	30.80
8	326,463	5.1	24	24.15
9	348,041	5.4	25	25.74
10	306,677	4.8	22	22.68
11	373,213	5.8	27	27.60
12	636,191	9.9	46	47.05
13	287,489	4.5	21	21.26
14	481,529	7.5	35	35.61
15	317,883	4.9	25	23.51
16	530,992	8.3	45	39.27
17	22,371	0.3	5	1.65
Total	6,422,402	100	475	475.00

The numbers of sectors per region were fixed in advance and were not strictly proportional to size. In particular, the Scottish Highlands and Islands would have warranted only 1-2 selections. The number of sectors chosen per country/region were preselected for practical and financial reasons with the view that the survey data would be weighted to take account of any imbalance in the distribution of sectors by geographical area. *(Table A1.2)*

A2 Weighting procedures

Weighting occurred in three steps. First, weights were applied to adjust for differential probability of postal sector selection by country. Second, sample weights were applied to take account of the variations in response by region. Third, all respondents were weighted up or down to represent the age-sex structure of the total national population of children and adolescents, aged 5-15, living in private households.

(a) Weighting to correct for over-sampling in Scotland and Wales

As described in Section A1 above, more sectors were selected in Scotland and Wales

Table A2.1 Sample weights by country	
England	1.0264
Wales	0.9404
Scotland-other	0.8727
Scotland H&I	0.3309

than would have emerged from a random sampling design for practical and financial reasons. The compensatory weights to take account of this are shown in Table A2.1.

(b) Weighting to take account of variation in response by region

Previous research in psychiatric epidemiology indicate higher prevalence rates of mental disorders among those living in cities than in rural communities (Blazer et al., 1987; Dohrenwend and Dohrenwend 1974; Giggs and Cooper, 1987; Lewis and Booth, 1994; Neff et al., 1987; Vazquez-Barquero et al., 1982) and experience from national surveys, irrespective of topic, show quite clearly, poorer co-operation from sampled respondents in urban than rural sectors. (Beerton, 1999; Brehm, 1993; House and Wolf, 1978; Goyder et al., 1992; Groves and Couper, 1998; Lievesley, 1988; Market Research Society, 1981; Smith, 1983; Steeh, 1981) These two research findings influenced the decision to take account of the different response rates by region when weighting the survey data. As expected the sample in Inner London produced the lowest response (72%) whereas the participation rate in Wales was 91%. *(Table A2.2)*

Table A2.2 Sample weights by region			
Region*	Response rate (%)	Number	Weight
Inner London	71.60	433	1.1634
Outer London	79.10	569	1.0531
Metropolitan England	83.80	3149	0.994
Non-metropolitan England	84.50	4621	0.9858
Wales	91.10	611	0.9144
Glasgow Met	78.50	487	1.0611
Other Scotland	82.70	568	1.0073
ALL	**83.30**	**10438**	

*Regions were based on groupings of the Government Office Classification of Region (Version 2).

(c) Weighting to correct for non-response bias by age and sex

The next step in the weighting process involved calculating weights to correct for non-response bias associated with age and sex. The age-sex distribution of the sample was calculated for boys and girls separately, with age grouped into one-year intervals. This was then compared with the age-sex distribution of the population (excluding children in institutions) from population projections from the 1991 Census to produce the age-sex weights shown in Table A2.3.

(d) Calculation of final weight factor

The product of the three weights for postal sector selection, response by region, and age-sex distribution was calculated. After this weight was applied to the original data, the weighted sample bases differed very slightly from the original. A final correction factor was therefore applied to return the weighted sample size to its original size.

A3 Adjustment procedures for teacher non-response

Description of the issue

The assessments of mental disorders among children and adolescents by psychiatrists were based on the data obtained from the parent,

the child (aged 11-15), and the teacher. In most cases, data were available from both the parent and child where appropriate, but for a substantial number of cases (20%), the teacher did not provide any information.

We can assume that, given a complete set of data from both home and school, the psychiatrists would on average, make the right assessment. Therefore, if they were able to use both home and school information to assess all children in the population and we were able to average the results of this census over a large number of repeats under identical circumstances, they would arrive at the prevalence level in the population. Therefore if this complete information were available for all sampled children in the survey, the estimated prevalence level would be unbiased for the actual prevalence level, differing only through sampling error and response error.

On the other hand, if repeated censuses were taken but collecting only the home information, another average prevalence would be measured. The question is: would the prevalence level measured with the school and home information taken together be the same as with just the home information? If the measures were the same, then we would not need to carry out adjustments for the missing teacher data. If the measures were different, some adjustment factor would need to be incorporated into the reported data.

Table A2.3 Distribution of children by age and sex

Age	Boys			Girls		
	Unweighted survey database	ONS pop estimates for 1998	*Weight Factor*	Unweighted survey database	ONS pop estimates for 1998	*Weight Factor*
	%	%		%	%	
5	9.2	9.03	*0.98*	9.0	9.06	*1.01*
6	9.7	9.38	*0.97*	9.2	9.41	*1.02*
7	9.2	9.50	*1.03*	10.6	9.50	*0.90*
8	8.7	9.27	*1.07*	9.5	9.28	*0.98*
9	9.7	9.22	*0.95*	9.7	9.23	*0.95*
10	9.6	9.36	*0.98*	9.3	9.33	*1.00*
11	9.7	9.08	*0.94*	8.4	9.08	*1.08*
12	9.6	9.01	*0.94*	8.7	8.97	*1.03*
13	8.3	8.93	*1.08*	8.8	8.94	*1.02*
14	7.9	8.60	*1.09*	8.7	8.58	*0.99*
15	8.4	8.67	*1.03*	8.2	8.62	*1.05*
Base	5212	4178366		5226	3968829	

Estimating and measuring the difference in the two measures

The evidence for the need to carry out this readjustment comes from looking at the ratio of parent-based to clinical-based diagnoses in no teacher information (t=0) and with teacher information (t=1) groups. If the ratio is the same, it suggests that having the teacher report doesn't make a significant contribution. If the ratio is higher for the t=1 group, it suggests that clinical diagnoses underestimate prevalence in the absence of teacher reports.

The prevalence rates for the three types of disorder and for any disorder are shown below for t=0 and t=1 conditions, followed by the clinical-parent ratios. *(Tables A3.1 and A3.2)*

These findings fit in with clinical experience, namely, that teacher reports contribute little if anything to the diagnosis of emotional disorders but make a substantial difference to the diagnosis of conduct and hyperkinetic disorders, though for rather different reasons. As far as conduct disorder is concerned, the key issue is that there are a lot of children who are oppositional, aggressive and antisocial at school but not at home. Psychiatrists rarely get to know about these children unless they have a teacher report. As far as hyperkinetic disorders are concerned, there are many children where the parental evidence is inconclusive and where the teacher report tips the balance.(Goodman, 1999)

Therefore, the adjustment factors applied to the prevalence rates of mental disorders (excluding emotional disorders), incorporated in all the tables in Chapter 4,

Table A3.2 Clinical-parent ratios by absence/presence of teacher data

	No teacher data t=0	With teacher data t=1
Emotional disorders	1.16	1.17
Conduct disorders	1.11	1.88
Hyperkinetic disorders	1.00	1.88
Any disorder	1.22	1.58

were calculated on the raw number according to the following rules.

(a) Calculate revised number of children with each clinically-assessed type of mental disorder with no teacher data:

$$N(clin)_{revised} = \frac{N(clin)_{t=1}}{N(parent)_{t=1}} \times N(parent)_{t=0}$$

$N(clin)_{t=1}$ = No. of children with disorder from a clinical assessment with teacher data
$N(parent)_{t=1}$ = No. of children with disorder from a parent only assessment with teacher data
$N(parent)_{t=0}$ = No. of children with disorder from a parent only assessment with no teacher data

(b) Calculate adjustment factor

$$Adjustment\ factor = \frac{N(clin)_{revised} + N(clin)_{t=1}}{N(clin)_{t=0} + N(clin)_{t=1}}$$

Table A3.3 Final adjustment factors

Disorder	Adjustment factor
Emotional disorders	1.00
Conduct disorders	1.12
Hyperkinetic disorders	1.09
Any disorder	**1.06**

Table A3.1 Prevalence of mental disorders by type of assessment with and without teacher data.

	Clinical diagnoses			Parental assessments		
	t=0	t=1	All	t=0	t=1	All
Emotional disorders	5.1	4.1	4.3	4.4	3.5	3.7
Conduct disorders	4.1	4.9	4.7	3.7	2.6	2.8
Hyperkinetic disorders	0.7	1.5	1.3	0.7	0.8	0.8
Any disorder	8.8	9.0	9.0	7.2	5.7	6.0

References

Beeton, R. (1999) The effect of interviewer and area characteristics on survey response rates: an exploratory analysis. *Survey Methodology Bulletin*, **45**, 7-15

Blazer, D., Bradford, A.C., George, L.K. Alcohol abuse and dependence in the rural South. *Archives of General Psychiatry*, **42:** 651-656.

Brehm, J. (1993) *The Phantom respondents: Opinion Surveys and Political Representation.* Ann Arbor: University of Mitchigan Press

Dohrenwend, B.P. and Dohrenwend, B.S. (1974) Psychiatric disorders in urban settings, in *American Handbook of Psychiatry* (ed. G Caplan) Vol II, 2nd edition, Basic Books, New York.

Giggs, J.A. and Cooper, J.F. (1987) Ecological structure and the distribution of schizophrenia and affective psychoses in Nottingham, *British Journal of Psychiatry,* **151**:627-633

Goodman, R. (1999) Personal communication.

Goyder, J., Lock, J., and McNair, T. (1992) Urbanization Effects on Survey Nonresponse: A Test Across ansd Within Cities. *Quality and Quantity*, 26, 39-48.

Groves, R.M., and Cooper, M.P. (1998) *Nonresponse in Household Interview Surveys,* John Wiley and Sons: New York.

House, J.S., and Wolf, S. (1978) Effects of Urban residence on Interpersonal Trust and Helping Behaviour. *Journal of Personality and Social* Psychology, **36, 9**, 1029-1043

Lewis, G. and Booth, M. (1994) Are cities bad for your mental health? *Psychological Medicine* **24**: 913-915

Lievesley, D. (1988) Unit nonresponse in interview surveys, Unpublished working paper, London: Social and Community Planning Research

Market Research Society (1981) Report of the Second Working Party on Respondent Co-operation : 1977-1980, *Journal of the Market Research Society,* **23**, 3-25

Neff, J. and Husaini, B.A. (1987) Urbanicity, Race, and *Psychological Distress. Journal of Community Psychology* **15**: 520-536.

Smith, T.W., (1983) The Hidden 25 Percent: An Analysis of Nonresponse on the 1980 General Social Survey, *Public Opinion Quarterly,* **47**, 386-404

Steeh, C.G. (1981) Trends in Nonresponse Rates, 1952-1979. *Public Opinion Quarterly*, **45**, 40-57

Vazquez-Banquero, J.L., Munoz, P.E., Madoz Jauregui, V. (1982) The influence of the process of urbanicity on the prevalence of neurosis: a community survey. *Acta Psychiatrica Scandinavica* **65**:161-170

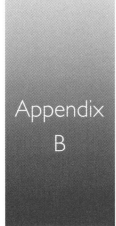

Statistical terms and their interpretation

Confidence interval

The percentages quoted in the text of this report represent summary information about a variable (e.g., presence of a mental disorder) based on the sample of people interviewed in this study. However, extrapolation from these sample statistics is required in order to make inferences about the distribution of that particular variable in the population. This is done by calculating confidence intervals around the statistic in question. These confidence intervals indicate the range within which the "true" (or population) percentage is likely to lie. Where 95% confidence intervals are calculated, this simply indicates that one is "95% confident" that the population percentage lies within this range. (More accurately, it indicates that if repeated samples were drawn from the population, the true percentage would lie within this range in 95% of the samples).

Confidence intervals are calculated on the basis of the sampling error (q.v.). The upper 95% confidence intervals are calculated by adding the sampling error multiplied by 1.96 to the sample percentage or mean. The lower confidence interval is derived by subtracting the same value. 99% confidence intervals can also be calculated by replacing the value 1.96 by the value 2.58.

Sampling errors

The sampling error is a measure of the degree to which a percentage (or other summary statistic) would vary if repeatedly calculated in a series of samples. For example, if the prevalence rate of a mental disorder was calculated for a random sample of children and adolescents drawn from the population at large, then another sample was drawn and the rate calculated again its value would be unlikely to be identical to the first. If this process was continued, the rate would continue to vary from sample to sample. Thus, the sampling error provides a measure of this variability, and is used in the calculation of confidence intervals and statistical significance tests. In this survey simple random sampling did not take place; rather, a multi-stage stratified sampling design was used. To take account of the design of this survey, sampling errors were calculated using STATA. However, this does not affect the interpretation of the sampling errors or their use in the calculation of confidence intervals.

Multiple logistic regression (MLR) and Odds Ratios (OR)

Logistic regression analysis has been used in the analysis of the survey data to provide a measure of the effect of, for example, various sociodemographic variables on mental disorders among children. Unlike the crosstabulations presented elsewhere in the report, MLR estimates the effect of any sociodemographic variable while controlling for the confounding effect of other variables in the analysis.

Logistic regression produces an estimate of the probability of an event occurring when an individual is in a particular sociodemographic category compared to a reference category. This effect is measured in terms of odds. For example, Table 4.15 shows that being in the family type "lone parent" increases the odds of having an emotional disorder compared to the reference category of "two parent family".

The amount by which the odds of this disorder actually increases is shown by the Adjusted Odds Ratio (OR). In this case, the OR is 1.55 indicating that being a child in a lone parent household increases the odds of having an emotional disorder by about one half, controlling for the possible confounding effects of the other variables in the statistical model, i.e. age, sex, number of children, family employment and the ACORN classification. To determine whether this increase is due to chance rather than to the effect of the variable, one must consult the associated 95% confidence interval.

Confidence intervals around an Odds Ratio

The confidence intervals around odds ratios can be interpreted in the manner described earlier in this section. For example, Table 4.15, shows an odds ratio of 5.56 for the association between sex and hyperkinetic disorders, with a confidence interval from 3.49 to 8.88, indicating that the 'true' (i.e., population) OR is likely to lie between these two values. If the confidence interval does not include 1.00 then the OR is likely to be significant - that is, the association between the variable and the odds of a particular disorder is unlikely to be due to chance. If the interval includes 1.00, then it is possible that the 'true' OR is actually 1.00, that is no increase in odds can be attributed to the variable.

Odds ratios and how to use them multiplicatively

The odds ratios presented in the tables show the adjusted odds due solely to membership of one particular category - for example, being a boy rather than a girl. However, odds for more than one category can be combined by multiplying them together. This provides an estimate of the increased odds of a disorder or symptom due to being a member of more than one category at once - for example, being a boy and aged 11-15. For example, in Table 4.15 being a boy rather than a girl increases the odds of any mental disorder (OR=1.48), while being aged 11-15 (compared with 5-10 year olds) also independently increases the odds (OR=1.58). The increased odds for 11-15 year old boys compared with 5-10 year old girls is therefore the product of the two independent odds ratios, 2.34.

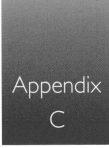

Appendix C

Sampling errors

This survey involved a multi-stage sampling design with both clustering and stratification. Clustering can lead to a substantial increase in standard error if the households or individuals within the primary sampling units (postal sectors) are relatively homogenous but the primary sampling units differ from one another. Stratification tends to reduce standard error and is of most advantage where the stratification factor is related to the characteristics of interest on the survey.

The effect of a complex sampling design on the precision of survey estimates is usually quantified by means of the design factor (deft). For any survey estimate , the deft is calculated as the ratio of the standard error allowing for the full complexity of the survey design to the standard error assuming a simple random sample. The standard error based on a simple random sample multiplied by the deft gives the standard error of a complex design.

$$se(p) = deft \times se(p)_{sys}$$

where:

$$se(p)_{sys} = \sqrt{\frac{p(1-p)}{N}}$$

The formula to measure whether the differences between the percentages is likely to be due entirely to sampling error for a complex design is:

$$se(p_1\text{-}p_2) = \sqrt{deft^2_1 \frac{p1(100\text{-}p1)}{n_1} + deft^2_2 \frac{p_2(100\text{-}p_2)}{n_2}}$$

where p1 and p2 are observed percentages for the two subsamples and n1 and n2 are the subsample sizes. The 95% confidence interval for the difference between two percentages is then given by;

$$(p_1\text{-}p_2) +/- 1.96 \times se(p_1\text{-}p_2)$$

If this confidence interval includes zero then the observed difference is considered to be a result of chance variation in the sample. If the interval does not include zero then it is unlikely (less than 5% probability) that the observed differences could have occurred by chance. The standard errors of survey measures which are not presented in the following tables for sample subgroups may be estimated by applying an appropriate value of deft to the sampling error. The choice of an appropriate value of deft will vary according to whether the basic survey measure is included in the tables. Since most deft values are relatively small (1.1 or less) the absolute effect of adjusting sampling errors to take account of the survey's complex design will be small. In most cases it will result in an increase of less than 10% over the standard error assuming simple random sampling. Whether it is considered necessary to use deft or to use the basic estimates of standard errors assuming a simple random sample is a matter of judgement and depends chiefly on how the survey results will be used.

Table C1	Standard errors and 95% confidence intervals for prevalence rates of mental disorders by sex, age and ethnicity

Base	Characteristic	%(p) (adj)	Sample size	True standard error of p	Deft	95% confidence Interval
All children	Emotional disorders	4.31	10438	0.21	1.08	3.89 - 4.73
	Conduct disorders	5.31	10438	0.23	1.09	4.81 - 5.81
	Hyperkinetic disorders	1.45	10438	0.11	0.96	1.22 - 1.68
	Any mental disorder	9.50	10438	0.30	1.07	8.88 - 10.13
Boys	Emotional disorders	4.11	5213	0.28	1.02	3.56 - 4.66
	Conduct disorders	7.41	5213	0.36	1.05	6.62 - 8.20
	Hyperkinetic disorders	2.45	5213	0.20	0.97	2.03 - 2.88
	Any mental disorder	11.44	5213	0.45	1.05	10.50 - 12.37
Girls	Emotional disorders	4.51	5225	0.30	1.04	3.92 - 5.10
	Conduct disorders	3.20	5225	0.24	1.04	2.68 - 3.73
	Hyperkinetic disorders	0.45	5225	0.09	1.02	0.25 - 0.64
	Any mental disorder	7.57	5225	0.37	1.04	6.80 - 8.34
5-10 year olds	Emotional disorders	3.29	5913	0.24	1.03	2.82 - 3.76
	Conduct disorders	4.59	5913	0.25	0.97	4.04 - 5.14
	Hyperkinetic disorders	1.50	5913	0.14	0.92	1.21 - 1.80
	Any mental disorder	8.16	5913	0.33	0.95	7.48 - 8.85
11-15 year olds	Emotional disorders	5.60	4525	0.41	1.20	4.80 - 6.40
	Conduct disorders	6.20	4525	0.38	1.12	5.37 - 7.04
	Hyperkinetic disorders	1.38	4525	0.17	1.02	0.98 - 1.74
	Any mental disorder	11.20	4525	0.55	1.20	10.06 - 12.35
White	Emotional disorders	4.31	9529	0.22	1.06	3.88 - 4.74
	Conduct disorders	5.38	9529	0.24	1.10	4.85 - 5.90
	Hyperkinetic disorders	1.57	9529	0.12	0.98	1.31 - 1.83
	Any mental disorder	9.58	9529	0.31	1.06	8.94 - 10.23
Black	Emotional disorders	3.25	247	1.07	0.95	1.15 - 5.35
	Conduct disorders	8.56	247	1.73	1.02	4.76 - 12.35
	Hyperkinetic disorders	0.38	247	0.35	0.93	-0.37 - 1.13
	Any mental disorder	11.99	247	2.02	1.00	7.79 - 16.19
Indian	Emotional disorders	2.90	215	1.20	1.05	0.55 - 5.25
	Conduct disorders	2.11	215	0.89	0.96	0.15 - 4.06
	Hyperkinetic disorders	0.00	215	0.00	0.00	0.00 - 0.00
	Any mental disorder	4.02	215	1.31	1.00	1.30 - 6.74
Pakistani and Bangladeshi	Emotional disorders	5.47	189	1.98	1.19	1.59 - 9.35
	Conduct disorders	2.99	189	1.32	1.12	0.09 - 5.89
	Hyperkinetic disorders	0.00	189	0.00	-	0.00 - 0.00
	Any mental disorder	7.52	189	2.41	1.29	2.51 - 12.52
Other	Emotional disorders	5.63	251	1.51	1.04	2.67 - 8.59
	Conduct disorders	3.94	251	1.27	1.09	1.15 - 6.73
	Hyperkinetic disorders	0.44	251	0.39	0.98	-0.40 - 1.27
	Any mental disorder	10.17	251	1.99	1.07	6.03 - 14.30

| | Table C2 | Standard errors and 95% confidence intervals for prevalence rates of mental disorders by family and household characteristics | | | | |

Base	Characteristic	%(p) (adj)	Sample size	True standard error of p	Deft	95% confidence Interval
Two parent families	Emotional disorders	3.57	8092	0.22	1.07	3.14 - 4.00
	Conduct disorders	3.99	8092	0.22	1.07	3.50 - 4.47
	Hyperkinetic disorders	1.19	8092	0.11	0.95	0.95 - 1.42
	Any mental disorder	7.67	8092	0.29	1.01	7.07 - 8.28
Lone parent families	Emotional disorders	6.87	2346	0.54	1.03	5.81 - 7.93
	Conduct disorders	9.81	2346	0.58	0.99	8.54 - 11.08
	Hyperkinetic disorders	2.34	2346	0.31	1.03	1.68 - 3.01
	Any mental disorder	15.77	2346	0.74	1.01	14.24 - 17.31
Both parent working (inc. lone parents)	Emotional disorders	3.40	6941	0.23	1.06	2.95 - 3.85
	Conduct disorders	4.14	6941	0.23	1.02	3.64 - 4.65
	Hyperkinetic disorders	1.11	6941	0.12	0.99	0.86 - 1.37
	Any mental disorder	7.62	6941	0.33	1.06	6.94 - 8.31
One parent working	Emotional disorders	4.52	1974	0.50	1.07	3.54 - 5.50
	Conduct disorders	4.46	1974	0.47	1.07	3.43 - 5.49
	Hyperkinetic disorders	1.62	1974	0.27	0.99	1.05 - 2.20
	Any mental disorder	9.05	1974	0.68	1.08	7.64 - 10.47
No parent working	Emotional disorders	8.52	1404	0.77	1.03	7.01 - 10.03
	Conduct disorders	12.50	1404	0.81	0.96	10.72 - 14.28
	Hyperkinetic disorders	3.00	1404	0.46	1.05	2.01 - 3.98
	Any mental disorder	19.66	1404	1.04	1.00	17.50 - 21.82
Owner occupiers	Emotional disorders	3.07	7072	0.20	0.97	2.68 - 3.46
	Conduct disorders	2.89	7072	0.21	1.11	2.43 - 3.35
	Hyperkinetic disorders	0.92	7072	0.12	1.11	0.66 - 1.17
	Any mental disorder	6.33	7072	0.27	0.96	5.77 - 6.89
Social sector tenants	Emotional disorders	7.12	2709	0.51	1.03	6.12 - 8.12
	Conduct disorders	11.16	2709	0.60	1.04	9.84 - 12.47
	Hyperkinetic disorders	2.56	2709	0.29	1.00	1.94 - 3.18
	Any mental disorder	16.88	2709	0.69	0.98	15.44 - 18.31
Private renters	Emotional disorders	5.92	651	0.93	1.00	4.10 - 7.74
	Conduct disorders	7.28	651	1.00	1.03	5.08 - 9.48
	Hyperkinetic disorders	2.58	651	0.61	1.02	1.28 - 3.89
	Any mental disorder	13.18	651	1.36	1.05	10.35 - 16.00

| Table C3 | Standard errors and 95% confidence intervals for prevalence rates of mental disorders by area characteristics | | | | | |

Base	Characteristic	%(p) (adj)	Sample size	True standard error of p	Deft	95% confidence Interval
ACORN: Cat.A Thriving	Emotional disorders	2.78	1928	0.36	0.96	2.07 - 3.49
	Conduct disorders	2.48	1928	0.35	1.05	1.71 - 3.24
	Hyperkinetic disorders	0.63	1928	0.16	0.92	0.29 - 0.97
	Any mental disorder	5.44	1928	0.50	0.99	4.40 - 6.48
ACORN: Cat.B Expanding	Emotional disorders	3.72	1453	0.47	0.95	2.80 - 4.64
	Conduct disorders	3.14	1453	0.44	1.02	2.17 - 4.10
	Hyperkinetic disorders	0.97	1453	0.22	0.89	0.50 - 1.44
	Any mental disorder	7.21	1453	0.64	0.97	5.88 - 8.54
ACORN: Cat.C Rising	Emotional disorders	4.14	599	0.70	0.86	2.77 - 5.51
	Conduct disorders	4.91	599	0.91	1.09	2.91 - 6.90
	Hyperkinetic disorders	1.70	599	0.51	1.01	0.61 - 2.79
	Any mental disorder	9.44	599	1.15	0.99	7.06 - 11.83
ACORN: Cat.D Settling	Emotional disorders	3.86	2381	0.45	1.14	2.98 - 4.74
	Conduct disorders	4.48	2381	0.42	1.05	3.56 - 5.40
	Hyperkinetic disorders	1.61	2381	0.26	1.05	1.06 - 2.17
	Any mental disorder	8.78	2381	0.61	1.08	7.51 - 10.04
ACORN: Cat.E Aspiring	Emotional disorders	4.36	1406	0.54	0.99	3.30 - 5.42
	Conduct disorders	7.48	1406	0.62	0.93	6.12 - 8.84
	Hyperkinetic disorders	1.95	1406	0.34	0.96	1.22 - 2.68
	Any mental disorder	11.50	1406	0.77	0.93	9.90 - 13.10
ACORN: Cat.F Striving	Emotional disorders	6.20	2657	0.48	1.03	5.26 - 7.14
	Conduct disorders	8.24	2657	0.54	1.07	7.06 - 9.43
	Hyperkinetic disorders	1.79	2657	0.25	1.01	1.25 - 2.32
	Any mental disorder	13.35	2657	0.68	1.06	11.93 - 14.76
England	Emotional disorders	4.27	8772	0.24	1.11	3.80 - 4.74
	Conduct disorders	5.38	8772	0.25	1.10	4.83 - 5.92
	Hyperkinetic disorders	1.49	8772	0.12	0.97	1.24 - 1.75
	Any mental disorder	9.62	8772	0.33	1.08	8.94 - 10.31
Scotland	Emotional disorders	4.55	1055	0.48	0.75	3.61 - 5.49
	Conduct disorders	4.64	1055	0.60	0.98	3.32 - 5.95
	Hyperkinetic disorders	1.13	1055	0.30	0.96	0.49 - 1.77
	Any mental disorder	8.52	1055	0.76	0.91	6.94 - 10.10
Wales	Emotional disorders	4.60	611	0.74	0.87	3.15 - 6.05
	Conduct disorders	5.28	611	0.88	1.03	3.34 - 7.21
	Hyperkinetic disorders	1.23	611	0.48	1.12	0.21 - 2.26
	Any mental disorder	9.03	611	1.23	1.09	6.48 - 11.59

| Table C4 | Standard errors and 95% confidence intervals for key characteristics of children within the three broad categories of mental disorders: emotional disorders |

Base	Characteristic	%(p) (adj)	Sample size	True standard error of p	Deft	95% confidence Interval
Children with emotional disorders	Seen GP in past year	49.38	441	2.35	0.99	44.77 - 53.99
	Not seen GP in past year	50.62	441	2.35	0.99	46.01 - 55.23
	Outpatient in past year	28.56	441	2.12	0.98	24.40 - 32.72
	Not outpatient in past year	71.44	441	2.12	0.98	67.28 - 75.60
	A&E visit in past year	25.43	441	2.47	1.19	20.59 - 30.27
	No A&E visit in past year	74.57	441	2.47	1.19	69.73 - 79.41
	Parental GHQ12 score 0-2	50.18	440	2.42	1.01	45.44 - 54.92
	Parental GHQ12 score 3-12	49.82	440	2.42	1.01	45.08 - 54.56
	No stressful life events	15.30	441	1.65	0.96	12.07 - 18.53
	1+ stressful life events	84.70	441	1.65	0.96	81.47 - 87.93
	Healthy family functioning	65.73	434	2.36	1.03	61.10 - 70.36
	Unhealthy family functioning	34.27	434	2.36	1.03	29.64 - 38.90
	Severe lack of friendship (score 0-2)	7.80	233	1.87	1.06	4.13 - 11.47
	Moderate lack of friendship (score 3-4)	30.49	233	3.25	1.08	24.12 - 36.86
	Little/no lack of friendship (score 5-6)	61.71	233	3.42	1.07	55.01 - 68.41
	Smoker	22.51	233	2.74	1.00	17.14 - 27.88
	Non-smoker	77.49	233	2.74	1.00	72.12 - 82.86
	Regular drinker (once a week or more)	14.81	233	2.21	0.95	10.48 - 19.14
	Non-regular drinker	85.19	233	2.21	0.95	80.86 - 89.52
	Ever used cannabis	14.78	233	2.26	0.97	10.35 - 19.21
	Never used cannabis	85.22	233	2.26	0.97	80.79 - 89.65

Base	Characteristic	%(p)	Sample size	True standard error of p	Deft	95% confidence Interval
Children with conduct disorders	Seen GP in past year	44.71	490	2.56	1.14	39.69 - 49.73
	Not seen GP in past year	55.29	490	2.56	1.14	50.27 - 60.31
	Outpatient in past year	26.84	490	2.03	1.01	22.86 - 30.82
	Not outpatient in past year	73.16	490	2.03	1.01	69.18 - 77.14
	A&E visit in past year	27.29	490	1.96	0.97	23.45 - 31.13
	No A&E visit in past year	72.71	490	1.96	0.97	68.87 - 76.55
	Parental GHQ12 score 0-2	51.28	489	2.27	1.00	46.83 - 55.73
	Parental GHQ12 score 3-12	47.82	489	2.27	1.00	43.37 - 52.27
	No stressful life events	17.05	490	1.71	1.01	13.70 - 20.40
	1+ stressful life events	82.95	490	1.71	1.01	79.60 - 86.30
	Healthy family functioning	57.39	483	2.26	1.00	52.96 - 61.82
	Unhealthy family functioning	42.61	483	2.26	1.00	38.18 - 47.04
	Severe lack of friendship (score 0-2)	8.74	219	1.94	1.01	4.94 - 12.54
	Moderate lack of friendship (score 3-4)	33.99	219	3.35	1.04	27.42 - 40.56
	Little/no lack of friendship (score 5-6)	57.27	219	3.27	0.98	50.86 - 63.68
	Smoker	28.89	217	2.73	0.89	23.54 - 34.24
	Non-smoker	71.11	217	2.73	0.89	65.76 - 76.46
	Regular drinker	13.73	217	2.37	1.01	9.08 - 18.38
	Non-regular drinker	86.27	217	2.37	1.01	81.62 - 90.92
	Ever used cannabis	19.76	215	2.52	0.93	14.82 - 24.70
	Never used cannabis	80.24	215	2.52	0.93	75.30 - 85.18

Table C5 Standard errors and 95% confidence intervals for key characteristics of children within the three broad categories of mental disorders: conduct disorders

Table C6	Standard errors and 95% confidence intervals for key characteristics of children within the three broad categories of mental disorders: hyperkinetic disorders

Base	Characteristic	%(p)	Sample size	True standard error of p	Deft	95% confidence Interval
Children with hyperkinetic disorders	Seen GP in past year	51.98	137	4.32	1.01	43.51 - 60.45
	Not seen GP in past year	48.02	137	4.32	1.01	39.55 - 56.49
	Outpatient in past year	42.68	137	4.38	1.03	34.10 - 51.26
	Not outpatient in past year	57.32	137	4.38	1.03	48.70 - 65.90
	A&E visit in past year	30.80	137	3.66	0.92	23.63 - 37.97
	No A&E visit in past year	69.20	137	3.66	0.92	62.03 - 76.37
	Parental GHQ12 score 0-2	58.02	137	4.03	0.95	50.12 - 65.92
	Parental GHQ12 score 3-12	41.98	137	4.03	0.95	34.08 - 49.88
	No stressful life events	15.71	137	3.29	1.05	9.26 - 22.16
	1+ stressful life events	84.29	137	3.29	1.05	77.84 - 90.74
	Healthy family functioning	63.45	137	3.90	0.94	55.81 - 71.09
	Unhealthy family functioning	36.55	137	3.90	0.94	28.91 - 44.19
	Severe lack of friendship (score 0-2)	11.88	49	4.58	0.98	2.90 - 20.86
	Moderate lack of friendship (score 3-4)	32.76	49	6.54	0.97	19.94 - 45.58
	Little/no lack of friendship (score 5-6)	55.36	49	6.88	0.96	41.88 - 68.84
	Smoker	18.44	49	5.42	0.97	7.82 - 29.06
	Non-smoker	81.56	49	5.42	0.97	70.94 - 92.18
	Regular drinker	14.43	49	4.93	0.97	4.77 - 24.09
	Non-regular drinker	85.57	49	4.93	0.97	75.91 - 95.23
	Ever used cannabis	21.56	48	5.86	0.98	10.07 - 33.05
	Never used cannabis	78.44	48	5.86	0.98	66.95 - 89.93

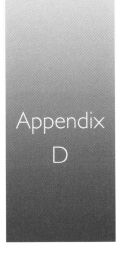

Appendix D

Follow-up findings

D1 Background and aims

A six-month follow-up procedure was incorporated into the study to examine the persistence or chronicity of the three main groups of mental disorders.

The strength of follow-up surveys is "that they allow a focus on chronic or persistent psychiatric disorders.... This is potentially important because a high proportion of otherwise normal children exhibit transient disorders at some time during their development" (Rutter,1989). Emotional and behavioural problems which resolve rapidly and spontaneously are far less relevant for service planning than problems that persist unless help is provided.

A prospective approach to determine the prevalence of persistent disorders, asking informants on two separate occasions about symptoms and resultant impairments was regarded as preferable to asking informants to recall how long symptoms (and resultant impairments) have been present at the time of interview.

D2 Sampling strategy

All parents and all children aged 11 or over from Wave 1 interviews (4 January to 14 February) who agreed to be contacted again, and a sample of teachers, were allocated for follow-up.

The calculation of response was based on the following factors:

- Number of postal sectors selected in the Wave 1 quota of work
- Total number of achieved parent interviews in that quota
- Total number of interviews with the 11-15 year olds, assuming the parent was

interviewed and did not object to the child taking part again
- Response from teachers

Assuming an 80% response from all three possible sources and subsampling teachers by the ratio 1 in 3, we estimated the follow-up survey would yield data from approximately 2100 parents, 900 children and 900 teachers.

D3 Content of interview

The questionnaire designed for the follow-up survey included the following elements:

For parents of all subjects - a repeat of the two-sided Strengths and Difficulties Questionnaire (SDQ).

For young people aged 11-15 - a repeat of the two-sided SDQ.

For teachers: a repeat of the two-sided SDQ plus a few additional questions on any new service provision through schools (e.g. school counselling, advice from educational psychologist).

D4 Response to the follow up procedures

The response to the follow-up procedure was better than expected - approximately 8 in 10 parents and children and 9 in 10 teachers responded.

Table D4.1 Response to follow up survey

	Questionnaires sent out	Questionnaires returned	Response rate
Parents	2797	2234	80%
Children (11-15)	1097	844	77%
Teachers	1037	940	91%

D5   Results

Two approaches were used to analyse the chronicity of disorders. First, the SDQ scores themselves were used to see how far these drifted back to the population mean over the follow-up period. The second method used a specially created SDQ algorithm to try to predict whether the child was still likely to meet diagnostic criteria at follow-up.

The findings from the first method, as judged by serial SDQ scores, are summarised in the Figures D5.1 to D5.5. Four of the graphs deal with symptom scores and one with impact score. All the symptom scores fall with time (both for children with and without disorders). This sort of "attenuation" effect is well-recognised when the same measure is administered a second time, though the reason for this is not clear. In most cases, the gap between the children with and without disorder narrows slightly but not much - this narrowing is most evident for the children with emotional disorders. Overall, symptoms generally persist at a high level, though there is some "normalisation", particularly for emotional symptoms. The graph showing change in impact scores is more dramatic. The normal group does not change at all, the group with emotional symptoms improves markedly and significantly, but the groups with hyperkinesis and conduct disorder seem to get worse (though the change is not significant). So as far as impact is concerned, emotional disorders clearly have a much better prognosis than the externalising disorders. It is curious that emotional symptoms only improve a little while their impact improves a lot, but this may be due to "ceiling" effects on the SDQ emotional symptoms scale. The findings from the second method, as derived from an SDQ algorithm, are summarised in Table D5.1.

The algorithm for predicting persistence was based on finding that the child had elevated symptom and impact scores at both times. It was only possible to apply this algorithm to children who had a disorder plus "potentially informative" SDQs. For example, imagine a child who as part of the initial assessment had parent, teacher and self-report SDQs, and who was independently diagnosed on the basis of the clinical assessment as having a conduct disorder primarily limited to the school setting. Imagine too that the only follow-up SDQ available on the child was a parent SDQ. If the initial parent SDQ was normal (with conduct and impact scores in the normal range), then it would not be possible to use the follow-up SDQ to decide if the child's conduct disorder had persisted. This is because if the follow-up SDQ completed by the parent again shows normal SDQ scores, it is impossible to judge from this whether the school-based conduct disorder had persisted or not. This was an "uninformative" case and was excluded from the analyses summarised in the table above.

The inference which can be reasonably drawn from the SDQ algorithm is that emotional disorders have a better prognosis than conduct or hyperactivity disorders - in line with all previous findings. The extent to which emotional disorders seem to recover over 4-6 months is probably exaggerated. Had the children been reassessed with the complete interview and clinical assessment, it is likely that a higher proportion would still have had a disorder. Even the ones who no longer met the criteria for a disorder would rarely be completely recovered - as the graphs suggest, the most likely outcome is that the child has slipped just below the diagnostic threshold, but still has some continuing symptoms and impact.

D6   Conclusions

- Psychiatric disorders were generally very persistent - few of the initially surveyed children were entirely normal 4-6 months later, and many were still severely affected.
- Persistence varied with the type of disorder, with recovery being more likely for emotional disorders, less likely for hyperkinesis and intermediate for conduct disorders.

Table D5.1 Persistence of mental disorders	
	Persistence
Any ICD-10 disorder	75% (84/112)
Emotional disorder	51% (24/47)
Conduct disorder	74% (51/69)
Hyperkinesis	91% (29/32)

References

Rutter, M., (1989) *Isle of Wight Revisited: Twenty five years of Child Psychiatric Epidemiology* American Academy of Child and Adolescent Psychiatry.

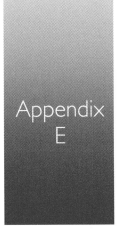

Appendix E

Survey documents

Parent questionnaire... .... 150 - 186

Parent self-completion.. .... 186 - 188

Child questionnaire.. .... 188 - 209

Child self-completion... .... 209 - 218

Teacher questionnaire.. .... 219 - 227

Note

The Strength and Difficulties Questionnaire (SDQ)
- Section D in Parent Questionnaire
- Section CB in Child Questionnaire
- Section B in Teacher Questionnaire

is copyrighted © to Professor Robert Goodman, Department of Child and Adolescent Psychiatry, Institute of Psychiatry, Denmark Hill, London, SE5 8AF

HOUSEHOLD DETAILS

FOR ALL ADDRESSES

Area   Information already entered
Address   Information already entered

INFORMATION COLLECTED FOR ALL PERSONS IN HOUSEHOLD

WhoHere

Who normally lives at this address?

Name

RECORD THE NAME (OR A UNIQUE IDENTIFIER) FOR HOH, THEN A NAME/IDENTIFIER FOR EACH MEMBER OF THE HOUSEHOLD

Sex

Code ...'s sex

(1)   Male
(2)   Female

Age

What was your age last birthday?
98 or more = CODE 97

0..97

IF: AGE < 20
DOB

(As you are under 20, may I just check)
What is your date of birth?
USE 1 FOR DAY OR MONTH NOT KNOWN,
e.g. 1-1-94

IF: AGE >= 16
MarStat

ASK OR RECORD
CODE FIRST THAT APPLIES
Are you

(1)   single, that is, never married?
(2)   married and living with your husband/wife?
(3)   married and separated from your husband/wife?
(4)   divorced?
(5)   or widowed?

IF: AGE 16+ AND MARSTAT=1,3,4 OR 5 AND MORE THAN ONE ADULT IN HOUSEHOLD
LiveWith

ASK OR RECORD
May I just check, are you living with someone in the household as a couple?

(1)   Yes
(2)   No
(3)   SPONTANEOUS ONLY - same sex couple

IF AGE 16+ AND MORE THAN ONE ADULT IN HOUSEHOLD
Hhldr

In whose name is the accommodation owned or rented?

ASK FOR WHOLE GRID, THEN ASK OR RECORD
(1)   This person alone
(3)   This person jointly
(5)   NOT owner/renter

HoHnum

ENTER PERSON NUMBER OF HOH.

HoHprtnr

THE HoH IS (NAME)

ENTER THE PERSON NUMBER OF HOH's SPOUSE/ PARTNER - NO SPOUSE/PARTNER = 11

Nation

What is (PERSON'S NAME) nationality?

(1)   UK, British
(6)   Irish Republic
(36)   Hong Kong
(58)   China
(59)   Other

IF: NATION = OTHER
NatSpec

TYPE IN (MAIN) NATIONALITY

IF: NATION = OTHER
NatCode

PRESS <SPACE BAR> TO ENTER THE CODING FRAME

Cry

In what country was (PERSON'S NAME) born?

(1)   UK, British
(6)   Irish Republic
(36)   Hong Kong
(58)   China
(59)   Other

IF: CRY = OTHER
CrySpec

TYPE IN COUNTRY

IF: CRY = OTHER
CryCode

PRESS <SPACE BAR> TO ENTER THE CODING FRAME

1..138

IF: (CRY <> UK) AND NOT (CRYSPEC = 01)
CameYr

Which year did (PERSON'S NAME) arrive in this country?
(ENTER ALL 4 DIGITS OF YEAR)

IF: (CRY <> UK) AND NOT (CRYSPEC = 01)
IF: (NATION = UK) AND ((CRY = HK) OR (CRY = CHINA))
Citizn

Is (PERSON'S NAME):

(1)   a British Dependent Territories Citizen, or a British National Overseas
(2)   or a Full British Citizen with right of abode in the UK?
(3)   Other/Don't Know

Ethnic

USE SHOW CARD
[*] To which of these groups do you consider you belong?

(1)   White
(2)   Black - Caribbean
(3)   Black - African
(4)   Black - Other Black groups
(5)   Indian
(6)   Pakistani
(7)   Bangladeshi
(8)   Chinese
(9)   None of these

Accommodation and tenure

ASK OR RECORD
Accom

IS THE HOUSEHOLD'S ACCOMMODATION:

N.B. MUST BE SPACE USED BY HOUSEHOLD

(1)   a house or bungalow
(2)   a flat or maisonette
(3)   a room/rooms
(4)   or something else?

IF: ACCOM = HSE
HseType

IS THE HOUSE/BUNGALOW:

(1)   detached
(2)   semi-detached
(3)   or terraced/end of terrace?

IF: ACCOM = FLAT
FltTyp

IS THE FLAT/MAISONETTE:

(1)   a purpose-built block
(2)   a converted house/some other kind of building?

IF: ACCOM = OTHER
AccOth

IS THE ACCOMMODATION A:

(1)   caravan, mobile home or houseboat
(2)   or some other kind of accommodation?

ASK ALWAYS:
Ten1

In which of these ways do you occupy this accommodation?
SHOW CARD 2 MAKE SURE ANSWER APPLIES TO HoH

(1)   Own outright
(2)   Buying it with the help of a mortgage or loan
(3)   Pay part rent and part mortgage (shared ownership)
(4)   Rent it
(5)   Live here rent-free (including rent-free in relative's/friend's property; excluding squatting)
(6)   Squatting

IF: (TEN1 = RENT) OR (TEN1 = RENTF)
Tied

Does the accommodation go with the job of anyone in the household?

(1)   Yes
(2)   No

IF: (TEN1 = RENT) OR (TEN1 = RENTF)
LLord

Who is your landlord?...
CODE FIRST THAT APPLIES

(1) the local authority/council/New Town Development/ Scottish Homes
(2) a housing association or co-operative or charitable trust
(3) employer (organisation) of a household member
(4) another organisation
(5) relative/friend (before you lived here) of a household member
(6) employer (individual) of a household member
(7) another individual private landlord?

IF: (TEN1 = RENT) OR (TEN1 = RENTF)
Furn

Is the accommodation provided: ...

(1)   furnished
(2)   partly furnished (eg carpets and curtains only)
(3)   or unfurnished?

Details of child and interviewed parent

ASK ALWAYS:
Childno

ENTER PERSON NUMBER OF THE SELECTED CHILD

DISPLAY ALWAYS:
ChldAge

Selected child's age

DISPLAY ALWAYS:
ChldDOB

child's DOB

DISPLAY ALWAYS:
ChldSex

child's sex

(1)   Male
(2)   female

ASK ALWAYS:
Adultno

ENTER PERSON NUMBER OF Child's PRIMARY CARE GIVER WHO HAS AGREED TO BE INTERVIEWED

AdltSex

Selected adult's sex

(1)   Male
(2)   female

ASK ALWAYS:
TranSDQ

INTERVIEWER: Code 'YES' if the parent will only be completing a translated version of the strengths and difficulties questionnaire. If you will be proceeding with a full interview with the parent code 'NO'

(1)   Yes, translation only
(2)   No, full interview

Parent interview

General health

GenHlth

[*] How is (CHILD'S) health in general?
Would you say it was ...
RUNNING PROMPT

(1)   very good
(2)   good
(3)   fair
(4)   bad
(5)   or is it very bad?

B2

Is (CHILD'S NAME) registered with a GP?

(1)   Yes
(2)   No

B4

Here is a list of health problems or conditions which some children or adolescents may have.

Please can you tell me whether (CHILD'S NAME) has...
SHOW CARD 3

SET [12] OF
(1)   Asthma
(2)   Eczema
(3)   Hay fever
(4)   Glue ear or otitis media, or having grommets
(5)   Bed wetting
(6)   Soiling pants
(7)   Stomach/digestive problems or abdominal/ tummy pains
(8)   A heart problem
(9)   Any blood disorder
(10)   Epilepsy
(11)   Food allergy
(12)   Some other allergy
(13)   None of these

B4a

Here is another list of health problems or conditions which some children or adolescents may have.
Please can you tell me whether (CHILD'S NAME) has...
SHOW CARD 4

SET [11] OF
(1)   Hyperactivity
(2)   Behavioural problems
(3)   Emotional problems
(4)   Learning difficulties
(5)   Dyslexia
(6)   Cerebral palsy
(7)   Migraine or severe headaches
(8)   The Chronic Fatigue Syndrome or M.E
(9)   Eye/Sight problems
(10)   Speech/or language problems
(11)   Hearing problems
(12)   None of these

B5

And finally, another list of health problems or conditions which some children or adolescents may have.

Please can you tell me whether (CHILD'S NAME) has...
SHOW CARD 5

SET [11] OF
(1)   Diabetes
(2)   Obesity
(3)   Cystic fibrosis
(4)   Spina Bifida
(5)   Kidney, urinary tract problems
(6)   Missing fingers, hands, arms, toes, feet or legs
(7)   Any stiffness or deformity of the foot,leg, fingers, arms or back
(8)   Any muscle disease or weakness
(9)   Any difficulty with co-ordination
(10)   A condition present since birth such as club foot or cleftpalate
(11)   Cancer
(12)   None of these

AnyElse

Does (CHILD'S NAME) have any other health problems?

(1)   Yes
(2)   No

IF: ANYELSE = YES
ElseSpec

What are these other health problems?

HeadInj

Has s/he ever had a head injury with loss of consciousness?

(1)   Yes
(2)   No

IF: HEADINJ = YES
HeadInja
How long is it since s/he had a head injury?

(1) Less than a month ago

(2) At least one month but less than 6 months ago
(3) At least 6 months but less than a year ago
(4) A year ago or more

B7

Has s/he ever had an accident causing broken bones or fractures that is not a head injury?

(1) Yes
(2) No

IF: B7 = YES
B7a

How long is it since s/he had a broken bone?

(1) Less than a month ago
(2) At least one month but less than 6 months ago
(3) At least 6 months but less than a year ago
(4) A year ago or more

B8

Has s/he ever had a burn requiring admission to hospital?

(1) Yes
(2) No

IF: B8 = YES
B8a

How long ago is it since s/he had this burn?

(1) Less than a month ago
(2) At least one month but less than 6 months ago
(3) At least 6 months but less than a year ago
(4) A year ago or more

B9

Has s/he ever had an accidental poisoning requiring admission to hospital?

(1) Yes
(2) No

IF: B9 = YES
B9a

How long ago is it since s/he was accidentally poisoned?

(1) Less than a month ago
(2) At least one month but less than 6 months ago
(3) At least 6 months but less than a year ago
(4) A year ago or more

B10

Has (CHILD'S NAME) ever been so ill that you thought that s/he may die?

(1) Yes
(2) No

IF: B10 = YES
B10a

How long ago was this?

(1) Less than a month ago

(2) At least one month but less than 6 months ago
(3) At least 6 months but less than a year ago
(4) A year ago or more

IF: (CHILD 11+ YEARS AND FEMALE)
B11

Have her periods started yet?

(1) Yes
(2) No

Strengths and difficulties

IntrSDQ

The next section is about (CHILD'S) personality and behaviour this is to give us an overall view of his/her strengths and difficulties - we will be coming back to specific areas in more detail later in the interview.

SectnD

For each item that I am going to read out can you please tell me whether it is 'not true', 'somewhat true' or 'certainly true' for (CHILD'S NAME) - over the past six months

D4

[*] Considerate of other people's feelings
SHOW CARD 6

D5

[*] Restless, overactive, cannot stay still for long
SHOW CARD 6

D6

[*] Often complains of headaches, stomach aches or sickness
SHOW CARD 6

D7

[*] Shares readily with other children (treats,toys, pencils etc)
SHOW CARD 6

D8

[*] Often has temper tantrums or hot tempers
SHOW CARD 6

D9

[*] Rather solitary, tends to play alone
SHOW CARD 6

D10

[*] Generally obedient, usually does what adults request
SHOW CARD 6

D11

[*] Many worries, often seems worried
SHOW CARD 6

D12

[*] Helpful if someone is hurt, upset or feeling ill
SHOW CARD 6

D13

[*] Constantly fidgeting or squirming
SHOW CARD 6

D14

[*] Has at least one good friend
SHOW CARD 6

D15

[*] Often fights with other children or bullies them
SHOW CARD 6

D16

[*] Often unhappy, down-hearted or tearful
SHOW CARD 6

D17

[*] Generally liked by other children
SHOW CARD 6

D18

[*] Easily distracted, concentration wanders
SHOW CARD 6

D19

[*] Nervous or clingy in new situations,easily loses confidence
SHOW CARD 6

D20

[*] Kind to younger children
SHOW CARD 6

D21

[*] Often lies or cheats
SHOW CARD 6

D22

[*] Picked on or bullied by other children
SHOW CARD 6

D23

[*] Often volunteers to help others (parents, teachers, other children)
SHOW CARD 6

D24

[*] Thinks things out before acting
SHOW CARD 6

D25

[*] Steals from home, school or elsewhere

SHOW CARD 6

D26

[*] Gets on better with adults than with other children
SHOW CARD 6

D27

[*] Many fears,easily scared
SHOW CARD 6

D28

[*] Sees tasks through to the end,good attention span?
SHOW CARD 6

D29

[*] SHOW CARD 7
Overall, do you think that your child has difficulties in one or more of the following areas: emotions, concentration, behaviour or getting on with other people?

(5)   No
(6)   Yes: minor difficulties
(7)   Yes: definite difficulties
(8)   Yes: severe difficulties

IF: D29 >= 6
D29a

How long have these difficulties been present?

(1)   Less than a month
(2)   One to five months
(3)   Six to eleven months
(4)   A year or more

IF: D29 >= 6
D29b

Do the difficulties upset or distress your child..
RUNNING PROMPT

(5)   not at all
(6)   only a little
(7)   quite a lot
(8)   or a great deal?

IF: D29 >= 6
D30

Do the difficulties interfere with your child's everyday life in terms of his or her
...home life?
SHOW CARD 8

(5)   not at all
(6)   only a little
(7)   quite a lot
(8)   a great deal

IF: D29 >= 6
D30a

[*] (Do the difficulties interfere with your child's everyday life in terms of his or her)
... friendships?
SHOW CARD 8

(5)   not at all
(6)   only a little

(7)   quite a lot
(8)   a great deal

IF: D29 >= 6
D30b

[*] (Do the difficulties interfere with your child's everyday life in terms of his or her)
... classroom learning?
SHOW CARD 8

(5)   not at all
(6)   only a little
(7)   quite a lot
(8)   a great deal

IF: D29 >= 6
D30c

[*] (Do the difficulties interfere with your child's everyday life in terms of his or her)
... or leisure activities?
SHOW CARD 8

(5)   not at all
(6)   only a little
(7)   quite a lot
(8)   a great deal

IF: D29 >= 6
D31

[*] Do the difficulties put a burden on you or the family as a whole?
SHOW CARD 8

(5)   not at all
(6)   only a little
(7)   quite a lot
(8)   a great deal

Separation anxiety

IntroF

Most children are particularly attached to one person or a few key people, looking to them for security, and turning to them when distressed.
They can be mum and dad, grandparents, favourite teachers, neighbours etc.
INTERVIEWER NOTE: Though children and teenagers can be particularly attached to other people of about the same age (sisters, brothers, friends), aim to identify ADULT attachment figures.

FigName

[*] Who would you say (CHILD'S NAME) was particularly attached to?
 - RECORD THE NAME (OR A UNIQUE IDENTIFIER) FOR EACH PERSON

F1a1

[*] Who are the three most important for (CHILD'S NAME)
IF THREE OR LESS ENTER ALL ATTACHMENT FIGURES

AtHome

Do any of these people live at home with the (CHILD'S NAME)

(1)   Yes
(2)   No

IF: AtHome = Yes
Home

Who are these people who live at home with (CHILD'S NAME) ?

F2intr

This section of the interview is about how much (CHILD'S NAME) worries about being separated from (ATTACHMENT FIGURES). Most children have some worries of this sort, but what I would like to know about is how (CHILD'S NAME) compares with other children of his/her age. I am interested in how s/he is usually - not in the occasional 'clingy day' or 'off day'.

F2

[*] Overall, in the past month, has s/he been particularly worried about being separated from his/her (ATTACHMENT FIGURES)?

(1)   Yes
(2)   No

IF: F2=Yes OR SDQ Emotion score>3
F2a

[*] Over the past month, and compared to with other children of the same age.. has s/he often been worried either about something unpleasant happening to (ATTACHMENT FIGURES), or about losing you/them?
SHOW CARD 9

(5)   No more than other children of the same age
(6)   A little more than other children of the same age
(7)   A lot more than other children of the same age

IF: F2=Yes OR SDQ Emotion score>3
F2b

[*] (Over the past month, and compared with other children of the same age...)
... has s/he often worried that he might be taken away from (ATTACHMENT FIGURES) for example, by being kidnapped, taken to hospital or killed?
SHOW CARD 9

(5)   No more than other children of the same age
(6)   A little more than other children of the same age
(7)   A lot more than other children of the same age

IF: F2=Yes OR SDQ Emotion score>3
AND: AtHome = Yes
F2c

[*] (Over the past month, and compared with other children of the same age...)
... has s/he often not wanted to go to school in case something nasty happened to (ATTACHMENT FIGURES AT HOME) while at school?
SHOW CARD 9

(DO NOT INCLUDE RELUCTANCE TO GO TO
SCHOOL FOR OTHER REASONS, EG. FEAR OF
BULLYING OR EXAMS)

(5)   No more than other children of the same age
(6)   A little more than other children of the same age
(7)   A lot more than other children of the same age

IF: F2=YES OR SDQ EMOTION SCORE>3
F2d

[*] (Over the past month, and compared with other
children of the same age...)
... has s/he worried about sleeping alone?
DNA = CODE 5
SHOW CARD 9

(5)   No more than other children of the same age
(6)   A little more than other children of the same age
(7)   A lot more than other children of the same age

IF: F2=YES OR SDQ EMOTION SCORE>3
AND: ATHOME = YES
F2e

[*] (Over the past month, and compared with other
children of the same age...)
... has s/he often come out of his/her bedroom at night to
check on, or to sleep near (ATTACHMENT FIGURES AT
HOME)?
DNA = CODE 5
SHOW CARD 9

(5)   No more than other children of the same age
(6)   A little more than other children of the same age
(7)   A lot more than other children of the same age

IF: F2=YES OR SDQ EMOTION SCORE>3
F2f

[*] (Over the past month, and compared with other
children of the same age...)
... has s/he worried about sleeping in a strange place?
SHOW CARD 9

(5)   No more than other children of the same age
(6)   A little more than other children of the same age
(7)   A lot more than other children of the same age

IF: F2=YES OR SDQ EMOTION SCORE>3
AND: (ATHOME = YES) AND (CHILD <11 YEARS)
F2g

[*] (Over the past month, and compared with other
children of the same age...)
... has s/he been particularly afraid of being alone in a
room alone at home without(ATTACHMENT FIGURES
AT HOME) even if you or they are close by?
SHOW CARD 9

(5)   No more than other children of the same age
(6)   A little more than other children of the same age
(7)   A lot more than other children of the same age

IF: F2=YES OR SDQ EMOTION SCORE>3
AND: (ATHOME = YES) AND (CHILD 11+ YEARS)
F2h

[*] (Over the past month, and compared with other
children of the same age...)
...s/he been particularly afraid of being alone at home if
(ATTACHMENT FIGURES AT HOME) pop out for a
moment?

SHOW CARD 9

(5)   No more than other children of the same age
(6)   A little more than other children of the same age
(7)   A lot more than other children of the same age

IF: F2=YES OR SDQ EMOTION SCORE>3
F2i

[*] (Over the past month, and compared with other
children of the same age...)
... has s/he had repeated nightmares or bad dreams
about being separated from (ATTACHMENT FIG-
URES)?
SHOW CARD 9

(5)   No more than other children of the same age
(6)   A little more than other children of the same age
(7)   A lot more than other children of the same age

IF: F2=YES OR SDQ EMOTION SCORE>3
F2j

[*] (Over the past month, and compared with other
children of the same age...)
... has s/he had headaches, stomach aches or felt sick
when s/he has to leave (ATTACHMENT FIGURES) or
when s/he knew it was about to happen?
SHOW CARD 9

(5)   No more than other children of the same age
(6)   A little more than other children of the same age
(7)   A lot more than other children of the same age

IF: F2=YES OR SDQ EMOTION SCORE>3
F2k

[*] (Over the past month, and compared with other
children of the same age...)
... has being apart or the thought of being apart from
(ATTACHMENT FIGURES) led to worry,
crying,tantrums,clinginess or misery?
SHOW CARD 9

(5)   No more than other children of the same age
(6)   A little more than other children of the same age
(7)   A lot more than other children of the same age

IF: ANY F2A - F2K = 7
F3

[*] You have told me about (CHILD'S) worries about
separations. Has s/he been like that for at least a
month?

(1)   Yes
(2)   No

IF: ANY F2A - F2K = 7 AND F3 = YES
AND: CHILD 6 + YEARS
F3a

[*] Was s/he like this by the age of 6?

(1)   Yes
(2)   No

IF: ANY F2A - F2K = 7 AND F3 = YES
F4

[*] Thinking still of (CHILD'S) worries about separation,
how much do you think they have upset him/her

RUNNING PROMPT

(5)   not at all
(6)   only a little
(7)   quite a lot
(8)   or a great deal?

F5Intr

I now want to ask you about the extent to which these worries have interfered with his/her day to day life.

IF: ANY F2A - F2K = 7 AND F3 = YES
F5a

[*] Have they interfered with...
... How well s/he gets on with you and the rest of the family?
SHOW CARD 8

(5)   not at all
(6)   only a little
(7)   quite a lot
(8)   a great deal

IF: ANY F2A - F2K = 7 AND F3 = YES
F5b

[*] (Have they interfered with...)
....Making and keeping friends?
SHOW CARD 8

(5)   not at all
(6)   only a little
(7)   quite a lot
(8)   a great deal

IF: ANY F2A - F2K = 7 AND F3 = YES
F5c

[*] (Have they interfered with...)
...learning or class work?
SHOW CARD 8

(5)   not at all
(6)   only a little
(7)   quite a lot
(8)   a great deal

IF: ANY F2A - F2K = 7 AND F3 = YES
F5d

[*] (Have they interfered with...)
...playing, hobbies, sports or other leisure activities?
SHOW CARD 8

(5)   not at all
(6)   only a little
(7)   quite a lot
(8)   a great deal

IF: ANY F2A - F2K = 7 AND F3 = YES
F5e

[*] Have these problems put a burden on you or the family as a whole?
SHOW CARD 8

(5)   not at all
(6)   only a little
(7)   quite a lot
(8)   a great deal

Specific phobias

F6Intr

This section of the interview is about any particular things or situations that (CHILD'S NAME) is PARTICULARLY scared of, even though they aren't really a danger to him/her. I am interested in how s/he is usually - not in the occasional 'off day'.I shall ask you first about particular fears, but will ask later about social fears.

F7

[*] Is (CHILD'S NAME) PARTICULARLY scared about any of the things or situations on this list?
CODE ALL THAT APPLY
SHOW CARD 10

SET [7] OF
(1)   ANIMALS: Insects, spiders, wasps, bees, mice, snakes, birds or any other animal
(2)   Storms, thunder, heights or water
(3)   Blood-injection-Injury - Set off by the sight of blood or injury or by an injection
(4)   Dentists or Doctors
(5)   The dark
(6)   Other specific situations: for example: lifts, tunnels, flying, driving, trains, buses, small enclosed spaces
(7)   Any other specific fear (specify)
(9)   Not particularly scared of anything

IF: ANYOTH IN F7
F7Oth

What is this other fear?
ENTER A SHORT DESRIPTION

IF: F7 = 1 - 7
F7a

[*] Is this fear/are these fears a real nuisance to him/her, or to you, or to anyone else?

(5)   No
(6)   Perhaps
(7)   Definitely

IF: F7A = DEFINITELY OR SDQ EMOTION SCORE > 3
F8

[*] How long (has this fear/the most severe of these fears) been present?

(1)   less than a month
(2)   At least one month but less than 6 months
(3)   Six months or more

IF: F7A = DEFINITELY OR SDQ EMOTION SCORE > 3
F9

[*] When (CHILD'S NAME) comes up against (PHOBIC STIMULUS) or thinks s/he is about to come up against it, does s/he become anxious or upset?
RUNNING PROMPT

(5)   No
(6)   A little
(7)   A Lot

IF: F9 = A LOT
F9a

[*] Does this happen almost every time s/he comes up against (PHOBIC STIMULUS)?

(1)   Yes
(2)   No

IF: F9 = AL_{OT}
F10

[*] How often does this fear of (PHOBIC STIMULUS) result in his/her becoming upset like this ...
IN THE RELEVANT SEASON IF A SEASONAL STIMU-LUS E.G. WASPS

RUNNING PROMPT

(1)   every now and then
(2)   most weeks
(3)   most days
(4)   many times a day?

IF: F7A = DEFINITELY OR SDQ EMOTION SCORE > 3
F11

[*] Does his/her fear lead to (CHILD'S NAME) avoiding (PHOBIC STIMULUS) ...
SHOW CARD 11
RUNNING PROMPT

(5)   No
(6)   A little
(7)   or a lot ?

IF: F11 = AL_{OT}
F11a

[*] How much does this avoidance interfere with his/her everyday life?
SHOW CARD 11
RUNNING PROMPT

(5)   No
(6)   A little
(7)   or a lot ?

IF: F7A = DEFINITELY OR SDQ EMOTION SCORE > 3
F11b

[*] Does s/he recognize that this fear is excessive or unreasonable?
SHOW CARD 12

(5)   No
(6)   Perhaps
(7)   Definitely

IF : F7 = 1-7
AND: F7A = DEFINITELY OR SDQ EMOTION SCORE > 3
F11c

[*] Is s/he upset that s/he has this fear?
SHOW CARD 12

(5)   No
(6)   Perhaps
(7)   Definitely

IF: F7 = 1-7
AND: F7A = DEFINITELY OR SDQ EMOTION SCORE > 3
F12

[*] Has (CHILD'S) fear of (PHOBIC STIMULUS) put a

burden on you or the family as a whole...
RUNNING PROMPT

(5)   not at all
(6)   only a little
(7)   quite a lot
(8)   or a great deal?

Social Phobia

F13intr

I am interested in whether (CHILD'S NAME) is particu-larly afraid of social situations, that is being with a lot of people, or meeting new people, or having to do things in front of other people. This is as compared with other children of his/her age, and is not counting the occa-sional 'off day' or ordinary shyness.

F13

[*] Overall, does (CHILD'S NAME) particularly fear or avoid social situations which involve a lot of people or meeting new people, or doing things in front of other people?

(1)   Yes
(2)   No

F14Intr
Can I just check, has s/he been particularly afraid of any of the following social situations over the last month?

IF: F13 OR SDQ EMOTION SCORE 3+
F14a

[*] (Can I just check, has s/he been particularly afraid of) . . . meeting new people?
SHOW CARD 11

(5)   No
(6)   A little
(7)   A Lot

IF: F13 OR SDQ EMOTION SCORE 3+
F14b

[*] (Can I just check, has s/he been particularly afraid of) . . .meeting a lot of people, such as at a party?
SHOW CARD 11

(5)   No
(6)   A little
(7)   A Lot

IF: F13 OR SDQ EMOTION SCORE 3+
F14c

[*] (Can I just check, has s/he been particularly afraid of) ...eating in front of others?
SHOW CARD 11

(5)   No
(6)   A little
(7)   A Lot

IF: F13 OR SDQ EMOTION SCORE 3+
F14d

[*] (Can I just check, has s/he been particularly afraid of)

. . .speaking in class?
SHOW CARD 11

(5)   No
(6)   A little
(7)   A Lot

IF: F13 OR SDQ EMOTION SCORE 3+
F14e

[*] (Can I just check, has s/he been particularly afraid of)
. . .reading out loud in front of others?
SHOW CARD 11

(5)   No
(6)   A little
(7)   A Lot

IF: F13 OR SDQ EMOTION SCORE 3+
F14f

[*] (Can I just check, has s/he been particularly afraid of)
. . .writing in front of others?
 SHOW CARD 11

(5)   No
(6)   A little
(7)   A Lot

IF: F13 OR SDQ EMOTION SCORE 3+
AND: SEPARATION ANXIETY AND (F14A - F14F)=7
F15

[*] Is (CHILD'S NAME) frightened of these social situations mainly because s/he is worried about being separated from (ATTACHMENT FIGURES) OR are (CHILD'S) fears of social situations still very obvious even when s/he is with them?

(1)   mainly related to his/her fear about being apart from attachment figures
(2)   marked even when attachment figure present

IF: F13 OR SDQ EMOTION SCORE 3+
AND: (F14A -F14F)=7 AND F15=2
F16

[*] Is (CHILD'S NAME) just afraid with adults, or is s/he also afraid in situations that involve a lot of children, or meeting new children?

(1)   Just with adults
(2)   Just with children
(3)   Also with children

IF: F13 OR SDQ EMOTION SCORE 3+
AND: (F14A -F14F)=7 AND F15=2
F17

[*] Outside of these social situations, is (CHILD'S NAME) able to get on well enough with the adults and children s/he knows best?

(1)   Yes
(2)   No

IF: F13 OR SDQ EMOTION SCORE 3+
AND: (F14A -F14F)=7 AND F15=2
F18

[*] Do you think his/her dislike of social situations is because s/he is afraid s/he will act in a way that will be embarrassing or show him/her up?
SHOW CARD 12

(5)   No
(6)   Perhaps
(7)   Definitely

IF: F13 OR SDQ EMOTION SCORE 3+
AND: (F14A -F14F)=7 AND F15=2
AND: ANY (F14D-F14F=6 OR 7)
F18a

[*] Is his/her dislike of social situations related to specific problems with speech, reading or writing?
SHOW CARD 12

(5)   No
(6)   Perhaps
(7)   Definitely

IF: F13 OR SDQ EMOTION SCORE 3+
AND: (F14A -F14F)=7 AND F15=2
F19

[*] How long has this fear of social situations been present?

(1)   Less than a month
(2)   At least one month but less than six months
(3)   Six months or more

IF: F13 OR SDQ EMOTION SCORE 3+
AND: (F14A - F14F)=7 AND F15=2
F20

What age did it begin at..
RUNNING PROMPT

(1)   under six years or
(2)   six years or above?

IF: F13 OR SDQ EMOTION SCORE 3+
AND: (F14A - F14F)=7 AND F15=2
F21

[*] When (CHILD'S NAME) is in one of the social situations s/he fears, or thinks s/he is about to come up against,does s/he become anxious or upset?
RUNNING PROMPT

(5)   No
(6)   A little
(7)   or a lot

IF: F13 OR SDQ EMOTION SCORE 3+
AND: (F14A - F14F)=7 AND F15=2
IF: F21 = ALOT
F22

[*] How often does his/her fear of social situations result in his/her becoming upset like this
RUNNING PROMPT

(1)   many times a day
(2)   most days
(3)   most weeks
(4)   or every now and then?

IF: F13 OR SDQ EMOTION SCORE 3+
AND: (F14A - F14F)=7 AND F15=2

F23

[*] Does his/her fear lead to (CHILD'S NAME) avoiding
social situations...
RUNNING PROMPT

(5) No
(6) A little
(7) or a lot

IF: SocSpCHK = SocFSep
IF: F23 = ALot
F23a

[*] How much does this avoidance interfere with his/her
daily life?
SHOW CARD 11

(5) No
(6) A little
(7) A Lot

IF: F13 or SDQ Emotion score 3+
AND: (F14a - F14f)=7 AND F15=2
F23b

[*] Does s/he recognize that this fear is excessive or
unreasonable?
SHOW CARD 12

(5) No
(6) Perhaps
(7) Definitely

IF: F13 or SDQ Emotion score 3+
AND: (F14a - F14f)=7 AND F15=2
F23c

[*] Is s/he upset about having this fear?
SHOW CARD 12

(5) No
(6) Perhaps
(7) Definitely

IF: F13 or SDQ Emotion score 3+
AND: (F14a - F14f)=7 AND F15=2
F24

[*] Have (CHILD'S) fears put a burden on you or the
family as a whole
RUNNING PROMPT

(5) not at all
(6) only a little
(7) quite a lot
(8) or a great deal?

Panic attacks and agoraphobia

F25Intr

Many children have times when they get very anxious or
worked up about silly little things, but some children get
severe panics that come out of the blue - they just don't
seem to have any trigger at all.

F25

[*] Over the last month has (CHILD'S NAME) had a panic
attack when s/he suddenly became very panicky for no
reason at all, without even a little thing to set him/her off?

(1) Yes
(2) No

F26

[*] Over the last month has (CHILD'S NAME) been very
afraid of, or tried to avoid, the things on this card?
SHOW CARD 13
CODE ALL THAT APPLY

SET [4] OF
(1) Crowds
(2) Public places
(3) Travelling alone (if s/he ever does)
(4) Being far from home
(9) None of the above

IF: F26 = 1 - 4
F27

[*] Do you think this fear or avoidance of (SITUATION) is
because s/he is afraid that if s/he had a panic attack or
something like that, s/he would find it difficult or
embarassing to get away, or would not be able to get the
help s/he needs?

(1) Yes
(2) No

Post Traumatic Stress Disorder (PTSD)

E1

The next section is about events or situations that are
exceptionally stressful, and that would really upset
almost anyone. For example being caught in a burning
house, being abused, being in a serious car crash or
seeing you being mugged at gunpoint.

[*] During (CHILD'S) lifetime has anything like this
happened to him/her?

(1) Yes
(2) No

IF: E1 = Yes
E2

What was it, please describe?
OPEN

IF: E1 = Yes
E4

INTERVIEWER CODE :
DO YOU REGARD THIS AS AN EXCEPTIONALLY
STRESSFUL OR TRAUMATIC EVENT?

(1) Yes
(2) No

IF: E1 = Yes
AND: E4 = Yes
E3

[*] At the time, was (CHILD'S NAME) very distressed or
did his/her behaviour change dramatically?

(1) Yes
(2) No

IF: E1 = YES
AND: E4 = YES
E5

At present, is it affecting (CHILD'S) behaviour, feelings or concentration?

(1)   Yes
(2)   No

IF: E1 = YES
AND: E4 = YES
AND: E5 = YES
E21a

[*] (Over the last month, has CHILD)
. . 'relived' the event with vivid memories (flashbacks) of it?
SHOW CARD 11

(5)   No
(6)   A little
(7)   A Lot

IF: E1 = YES
IF: E4 = YES
IF: E5 = YES
E21b

[*] (Over the last month, has CHILD ...)
.. had repeated distressing dreams of the event?
SHOW CARD 11

(5)   No
(6)   A little
(7)   A Lot

IF: E1 = YES
AND: E4 = YES
AND: E5 = YES
E21c

[*] (Over the last month, has CHILD ...)
.. got upset if anything happened which reminded him/her of it?
SHOW CARD 11

(5)   No
(6)   A little
(7)   A Lot

IF: E1 = YES
AND: E4 = YES
AND: E5 = YES
E21d

[*] (Over the last month, has CHILD ...)
.. tried to avoid thinking or talking about anything to do with the event?
SHOW CARD 11

(5)   No
(6)   A little
(7)   A Lot

IF: E1 = YES
AND: E4 = YES
AND: E5 = YES
E21e

[*] (Over the last month, has CHILD ...)
.. tried to avoid activities places or people that remind

him/her of the event?
SHOW CARD 11

(5)   No
(6)   A little
(7)   A Lot

IF: E1 = YES
AND: E4 = YES
AND: E5 = YES
E21f

[*] (Over the last month, has CHILD ...)
.. blocked out important details of the event from his/her memory?
SHOW CARD 11

(5)   No
(6)   A little
(7)   A Lot

IF: E1 = YES
AND: E4 = YES
AND: E5 = YES
E21g

[*] (Over the last month, has CHILD ...)
.. shown much less interest in activities s/he used to enjoy?
SHOW CARD 11

(5)   No
(6)   A little
(7)   A Lot

IF: E1 = YES
AND: E4 = YES
AND: E5 = YES
E21h

[*] (Over the last month, has CHILD ...)
.. felt cut off or distant from others?
SHOW CARD 11

(5)   No
(6)   A little
(7)   A Lot

IF: E1 = YES
AND: E4 = YES
AND: E5 = YES
E21i

[*] (Over the last month, has CHILD ...)
.. expressed a smaller range of feelings than in the past?
(e.g. no longer able to express loving feelings)
SHOW CARD 11

(5)   No
(6)   A little
(7)   A Lot

IF: E1 = YES
AND: E4 = YES
AND: E5 = YES
E21j

[*] (Over the last month, has (CHILD'S NAME) . .)
.. felt less confidence in the future?
SHOW CARD 11

(5)   No
(6)   A little
(7)   A Lot

IF: E1 = YES
AND: E4 = YES
AND: E5 = YES
E21k

[*] (Over the last month, has CHILD ...)
.. had problems sleeping?
SHOW CARD 11

(5)   No
(6)   A little
(7)   A Lot

IF: E1 = YES
AND: E4 = YES
AND: E5 = YES
E21l

[*] (Over the last month, has CHILD ...)
.. felt irritable or angry?
SHOW CARD 11

(5)   No
(6)   A little
(7)   A Lot

IF: E1 = YES
AND: E4 = YES
AND: E5 = YES
E21m

[*] (Over the last month, has CHILD ...)
.. had difficulty concentrating?
SHOW CARD 11

(5)   No
(6)   A little
(7)   A Lot

IF: E1 = YES
AND: E4 = YES
AND: E5 = YES
E21n

[*] (Over the last month, has CHILD ...)
.. always been on the alert for possible dangers?
SHOW CARD 11

(5)   No
(6)   A little
(7)   A Lot

IF: E1 = YES
AND: E4 = YES
AND: E5 = YES
E21o

[*] (Over the last month, has CHILD ...)
.. jumped at little noises or easily startled in other ways?
SHOW CARD 11

(5)   No
(6)   A little
(7)   A Lot

IF: ANYE21 - E21o = 7
E22

[*] You have told me about how (DEFINITE SYMP-TOMS)
How long after the event did these problems begin?

(1)   within six months
(2)   more than six months after the event

IF: ANYE21 - E21o = 7
E23

How long has s/he been having these problems?

(1)   Less than a month
(2)   At least one month but less than three months
(3)   Three months or more

IF: ANYE21 - E21o = 7
E24

[*] How much have these problems upset or distressed
your child...
RUNNING PROMPT

(5)   not at all
(6)   only a little
(7)   quite a lot
(8)   or a great deal?

IF: ANYE21 - E21o = 7
E25a

[*] Have they interfered with...
how well s/he gets on with you and the rest of the
family?
SHOW CARD 8

(5)   not at all
(6)   only a little
(7)   quite a lot
(8)   a great deal

IF: ANYE21 - E21o = 7
E25b

[*] (Have they interfered with...)
.. making and keeping friends?
SHOW CARD 8

(5)   not at all
(6)   only a little
(7)   quite a lot
(8)   a great deal

IF: ANYE21 - E21o = 7
E25c

[*] (Have they interfered with...)
.. learning or class work?
SHOW CARD 8

(5)   not at all
(6)   only a little
(7)   quite a lot
(8)   a great deal

IF: ANYE21 - E21o = 7
E25d

[*] (Have they interfered with...)
.. playing, hobbies, sports or other leisure activities?
SHOW CARD 8

(5)   not at all

(6) only a little
(7) quite a lot
(8) a great deal

IF: ANYE21 - E21o = 7
E26

[*] Have these problems put a burden on you or the family as a whole. .
RUNNING PROMPT

(5) not at all
(6) only a little
(7) quite a lot
(8) or a great deal?

Compulsions and obsessions

F28Intr

Many young people have some habits or superstitions, such as not stepping on the cracks in the pavement, or having to go through a special goodnight ritual, or needing to wear lucky clothes or have a lucky mascot for exams or football/netball matches. It is also common for children to go through phases when they seem obsessed by one particular subject or activity. I want to ask whether (CHILD'S NAME) has rituals or obsessions that go beyond this.

F28

[*] Overall, does (CHILD'S NAME) have rituals or obsessions that upset him/her, waste a lot of his/her time or interfere with his/her ability to get on with everyday life?

(1) Yes
(2) No

IF: F28=YES OR SDQ EMOTION SCORE >3
F29Intr

Can I just check, over the last month has s/he been doing any of the following things over and over again even though s/he has already done them or doesn't need to do them at all?

IF: F28=YES OR SDQ EMOTION SCORE >3
F29a

[*] (Over the last month has s/he been doing any of the following things over and over again even though s/he has already done them or doesn't need to do them at all)

Excessive cleaning; handwashing, baths, showers, toothbrushing etc. ?
SHOW CARD 11

(5) No
(6) A little
(7) A Lot

IF: F28=YES OR SDQ EMOTION SCORE >3
F29b

[*] (Over the last month has s/he been doing any of the following things over and over again even though s/he has already done them or doesn't need to do them at all)

Other special measures to avoid dirt, germs or poisons?
SHOW CARD 11

(5) No
(6) A little
(7) A Lot

IF: F28=YES OR SDQ EMOTION SCORE >3
F29c

[*] (Over the last month has s/he been doing any of the following things over and over again even though s/he has already done them or doesn't need to do them at all)

Checking: doors, locks, oven, gas taps, electric switches?
SHOW CARD 11

(5) No
(6) A little
(7) A Lot

IF: F28=YES OR SDQ EMOTION SCORE >3
F29d

[*] (Over the last month has s/he been doing any of the following things over and over again even though s/he has already done them or doesn't need to do them at all)

Repeating actions:like going in and out through a door many times in a row, getting up and down from a chair, or anything like this?
SHOW CARD 11

(5) No
(6) A little
(7) A Lot

IF: F28=YES OR SDQ EMOTION SCORE >3
F29e

[*] (Over the last month has s/he been doing any of the following things over and over again even though s/he has already done them or doesn't need to do them at all)

Touching things or people in particular ways?
SHOW CARD 11

(5) No
(6) A little
(7) A Lot

IF: F28=YES OR SDQ EMOTION SCORE >3
F29f

[*] (Over the last month has s/he been doing any of the following things over and over again even though s/he has already done them or doesn't need to do them at all)

Arranging things so they are just so, or exactly symmetrical?
SHOW CARD 11

(5) No
(6) A little
(7) A Lot

IF: F28=YES OR SDQ EMOTION SCORE >3
F29g

[*] (Over the last month has s/he been doing any of the following things over and over again even though s/he

has already done them or doesn't need to do them at all)

Counting to particular lucky numbers or avoiding unlucky numbers?
SHOW CARD 11

(5)   No
(6)   A little
(7)   A Lot

IF: F28=Yᴇs OR SDQ ᴇᴍᴏᴛɪᴏɴ sᴄᴏʀᴇ >3
F31a

[*] Over the last month, has (CHILD'S NAME) been particularly concerned about ...
Dirt, germs or poisons?
SHOW CARD 11

(5)   No
(6)   A little
(7)   A Lot

IF: F28=Yᴇs OR SDQ ᴇᴍᴏᴛɪᴏɴ sᴄᴏʀᴇ >3
F31b

[*] (Over the last month, has (CHILD'S NAME) been particularly concerned about) ... something terrible happening to him/her self or others - illnesses,accidents, fires etc.?
SHOW CARD 11

(5)   No
(6)   A little
(7)   A Lot

IF: F28=Yᴇs OR SDQ ᴇᴍᴏᴛɪᴏɴ sᴄᴏʀᴇ >3
AND CHILD HAS SEPARATION ANXIETY AND F31ʙ = ALᴏᴛ
F32

[*] Is this just part of his/her general concern about separation from (SEPARATION ANIXETY) or is this a serious additional problem in its own right?

(1)   mainly related to separation anxiety
(2)   a problem in it's own right

IF: F28=Yᴇs OR SDQ ᴇᴍᴏᴛɪᴏɴ sᴄᴏʀᴇ >3
AND: ꜰ29A- ꜰ29G = 7 ᴏʀ ꜰ31A - ꜰ31B = 7 ᴏʀ ꜰ32 = 2
F33

[*] You have just told me about (CHILD'S) habits and obsessions. Have they been present on most days for a period of at least two weeks?

(1)   Yes
(2)   No

IF: F28=Yᴇs OR SDQ ᴇᴍᴏᴛɪᴏɴ sᴄᴏʀᴇ >3
AND: ꜰ29A- ꜰ29G = 7 ᴏʀ ꜰ31A - ꜰ31B = 7 ᴏʀ ꜰ32 = 2
F34

[*] Does s/he recognise that these (acts/thoughts) are excessive or unreasonable?

(5)   No
(6)   Perhaps
(7)   Definitely

IF: F28=Yᴇs OR SDQ ᴇᴍᴏᴛɪᴏɴ sᴄᴏʀᴇ >3
AND: ꜰ29A- ꜰ29G = 7 ᴏʀ ꜰ31A - ꜰ31B = 7 ᴏʀ ꜰ32 = 2
F35

[*] Does s/he try not to do them or think about them?

(5)   No
(6)   Perhaps
(7)   Definitely

IF: F28=Yᴇs OR SDQ ᴇᴍᴏᴛɪᴏɴ sᴄᴏʀᴇ >3
AND: ꜰ29A- ꜰ29G = 7 ᴏʀ ꜰ31A - ꜰ31B = 7 ᴏʀ ꜰ32 = 2
F36

[*] Does s/he become upset because s/he has to do or think about these things?

(5)   No,enjoys it
(6)   Neutral, neither enjoys it or becomes upset
(7)   Sometimes/somewhat upset
(8)   Upset a great deal

IF: F28=Yᴇs OR SDQ ᴇᴍᴏᴛɪᴏɴ sᴄᴏʀᴇ >3
AND: ꜰ29A- ꜰ29G = 7 ᴏʀ ꜰ31A - ꜰ31B = 7 ᴏʀ ꜰ32 = 2
F37

[*] Do these (acts/thoughts) use up at least an hour a day on average?

(1)   Yes
(2)   No

IF: F28=Yᴇs OR SDQ ᴇᴍᴏᴛɪᴏɴ sᴄᴏʀᴇ >3
AND: ꜰ29A- ꜰ29G = 7 ᴏʀ ꜰ31A - ꜰ31B = 7 ᴏʀ ꜰ32 = 2
F38a

[*] Have these acts/thoughts interfered with ...
.. how well s/he gets on with you and the rest of the family?
SHOW CARD 8

(5)   not at all
(6)   only a little
(7)   quite a lot
(8)   a great deal

IF: F28=Yᴇs OR SDQ ᴇᴍᴏᴛɪᴏɴ sᴄᴏʀᴇ >3
AND: ꜰ29A- ꜰ29G = 7 ᴏʀ ꜰ31A - ꜰ31B = 7 ᴏʀ ꜰ32 = 2
F38b

[*] (Have these acts/thoughts interfered with ...)
... making and keeping friends?
SHOW CARD 8

(5)   not at all
(6)   only a little
(7)   quite a lot
(8)   a great deal

IF: F28=Yᴇs OR SDQ ᴇᴍᴏᴛɪᴏɴ sᴄᴏʀᴇ >3
AND: ꜰ29A- ꜰ29G = 7 ᴏʀ ꜰ31A - ꜰ31B = 7 ᴏʀ ꜰ32 = 2
F38c

[*] (Have these acts/thoughts interfered with ...)
...learning or class work?
SHOW CARD 8

(5)   not at all
(6)   only a little
(7)   quite a lot
(8)   a great deal

IF: F28=Yᴇs OR SDQ ᴇᴍᴏᴛɪᴏɴ sᴄᴏʀᴇ >3
AND: ꜰ29A- ꜰ29G = 7 ᴏʀ ꜰ31A - ꜰ31B = 7 ᴏʀ ꜰ32 = 2
F38d

[*] (Have these acts/thoughts interfered with ...)
...playing, hobbies, sports or other leisure activities?
SHOW CARD 8

(5)   not at all
(6)   only a little
(7)   quite a lot
(8)   a great deal

IF: F28=YES OR SDQ EMOTION SCORE >3
AND: F29A- F29G = 7 OR F31A - F31B = 7 OR F32 = 2
F38e

[*] Have these problems put a burden on you or the
family as a whole?
SHOW CARD 8

(5)   not at all
(6)   only a little
(7)   quite a lot
(8)   a great deal

Generalised anxiety
F39

[*] Does (CHILD'S NAME) ever worry?

(1)   Yes
(2)   No

IF: F39 = YES
F39a

[*] From now on I am going to concentrate on general
worrying (that is apart from his/her (SPECIFIC ANXIE-
TIES) that you have already told me about).
Over the last six months, has s/he worried so much
about so many things that it has really upset him/her or
interfered with his/her life?

(5)   No
(6)   Perhaps
(7)   Definitely

IF: F39 = YES
AND: F39A=6 OR 7 OR SDQ EMOTION SCORE > 3
F40a

[*] Over the last 6 months, and by comparison with
other children of the same age, has (CHILD'S NAME)
worried about: Past behaviour: Did I do that wrong?
Have I upset someone? Have they forgiven me?

(5)   No more than other children of the same age
(6)   A little more than other children of the same
       age
(7)   A lot more than other children of the same age

IF: F39 = YES
AND: F39A=6 OR 7 OR SDQ EMOTION SCORE > 3
F40b

[*] (Over the last 6 months, and by comparison with
other children of the same age, has (CHILD'S NAME)
worried about:) School work,homework or examinations

(5)   No more than other children of the same age
(6)   A little more than other children of the same
       age
(7)   A lot more than other children of the same age

IF: F39 = YES
AND: F39A=6 OR 7 OR SDQ EMOTION SCORE > 3
F40c

[*] (Over the last 6 months, and by comparison with
other children of the same age, has (CHILD'S NAME)
worried about:) Disasters: Burglaries, muggings, fires,
bombs etc.

(5)   No more than other children of the same age
(6)   A little more than other children of the same age
(7)   A lot more than other children of the same age

IF: F39 = YES
AND: F39A=6 OR 7 OR SDQ EMOTION SCORE > 3
F40d

[*] (Over the last 6 months, and by comparison with
other children of the same age, has (CHILD'S NAME)
worried about:) His/her own health

(5)   No more than other children of the same age
(6)   A little more than other children of the same age
(7)   A lot more than other children of the same age

IF: F39 = YES
AND: F39A=6 OR 7 OR SDQ EMOTION SCORE > 3
F40e

[*] (Over the last 6 months, and by comparison with
other children of the same age, has (CHILD'S NAME)
worried about:) Bad things happening to others: family
friends, pets, the world..

(5)   No more than other children of the same age
(6)   A little more than other children of the same age
(7)   A lot more than other children of the same age

IF: F39 = YES
AND: F39A=6 OR 7 OR SDQ EMOTION SCORE > 3
F40f

[*] (Over the last 6 months, and by comparison with
other children of the same age, has (CHILD'S NAME)
worried about:) The future: e.g. getting a job, boy/
girlfriend, moving out

(5)   No more than other children of the same age
(6)   A little more than other children of the same age
(7)   A lot more than other children of the same age

IF: F39 = YES
AND: F39A=6 OR 7 OR SDQ EMOTION SCORE > 3
F40g

[*] Has s/he worried about anything else?

(1)   Yes
(2)   No

IF: F39 = YES
AND: F39A=6 OR 7 OR SDQ EMOTION SCORE > 3
AND: F40G = YES
F40ga

[*] What else has s/he worried about?

IF: F39 = YES
AND: F39A=6 OR 7 OR SDQ EMOTION SCORE > 3
AND: F40G = YES
F40gb

[*] How much does s/he worry about this

(5)   No more than other children of the same age
(6)   A little more than other children of the same age
(7)   A lot more than other children of the same age

IF:TWO OF F40A - F40GB = 7
GenWCHK

INTERVIEWER CHECK: Are there two or more specific worries (SPECIFIC WORRIES) over and above those which have already been mentioned in earlier sections?

(1)   Yes
(2)   No

IF: GENWCHK = YES
F42

[*] Over the last six months has s/he worried excessively on more days than not?

(1)   Yes
(2)   No

IF: (GENWCHK = YES) AND (F42 = YES)
F43

[*] Does s/he find it difficult to control the worry?

(1)   Yes
(2)   No

IF: (GENWCHK = YES) AND (F42 = YES)
F44

[*] Does worrying lead to him /her being restless, feeling keyed up, tense or on edge, or being unable to relax?

(1)   Yes
(2)   No

IF: (GENWCHK = YES) AND (F42 = YES)
AND: F44 = YES
F44a

[*] Has this been true for more days than not in the last six months?

(1)   Yes
(2)   No

IF: (GENWCHK = YES) AND (F42 = YES)
F45

[*] Does worrying lead to him/her feeling tired or 'worn out' more easily?

(1)   Yes
(2)   No

IF: (GENWCHK = YES) AND (F42 = YES)
AND: F45 = YES
F45a

[*] Has this been true for more days than not in the last six months?

(1)   Yes
(2)   No

IF: (GENWCHK = YES) AND (F42 = YES)
F46

[*] Does worrying lead to difficulties in concentrating or his/her mind going blank?

(1)   Yes
(2)   No

IF: (GENWCHK = YES) AND (F42 = YES)
IF: F46 = YES
F46a

[*] Has this been true for more days than not in the last six months?

(1)   Yes
(2)   No

IF: (GENWCHK = YES) AND (F42 = YES)
F47

[*] Does worrying make him/her irritable?

(1)   Yes
(2)   No

IF: (GENWCHK = YES) AND (F42 = YES)
IF: F47 = YES
F47a

[*] Has this been true for more days than not in the last six months?

(1)   Yes
(2)   No

IF: (GENWCHK = YES) AND (F42 = YES)
F48

[*] Does worrying lead to muscle tension?

(1)   Yes
(2)   No

IF: (GENWCHK = YES) AND (F42 = YES)
IF: F48 = YES
F48a

[*] Has this been true for more days than not in the last six months?

(1)   Yes
(2)   No

IF: (GENWCHK = YES) AND (F42 = YES)
F49

[*] Does worrying interfere with his/her sleep, leading to difficulty in falling or staying asleep, or to restless,unsatisfying sleep?

(1)   Yes
(2)   No

IF: (GENWCHK = YES) AND (F42 = YES)
IF: F49 = YES
F49a

[*] Has this been true for more days than not in the last six months?

(1)   Yes
(2)   No

IF: (GenWCHK = YES) AND (F42 = YES)
F50

[*] Overall, how upset and distressed is (CHILD'S NAME) as a result of all his/her various worries ...
RUNNING PROMPT

(5)   not at all
(6)   only a little
(7)   quite a lot
(8)   or a great deal?

IF: (GenWCHK = YES) AND (F42 = YES)
F51Intr

I now want to ask you about the extent to which these worries have interfered with his/her day to day life.

IF: (GenWCHK = YES) AND (F42 = YES)
F51a

[*] Have they interfered with ...How well s/he gets on with you and the rest of the family?
SHOW CARD 8

(5)   not at all
(6)   only a little
(7)   quite a lot
(8)   a great deal

IF: (GenWCHK = YES) AND (F42 = YES)
F51b

[*] (Have they interfered with ...)
making and keeping friends?
SHOW CARD 8

(5)   not at all
(6)   only a little
(7)   quite a lot
(8)   a great deal

IF: (GenWCHK = YES) AND (F42 = YES)
F51c

[*] (Have they interfered with ...)
learning or class work?
SHOW CARD 8

(5)   not at all
(6)   only a little
(7)   quite a lot
(8)   a great deal

IF: (GenWCHK = YES) AND (F42 = YES)
F51d

[*] (Have they interfered with ...)
playing, hobbies, sports or other leisure activities?
SHOW CARD 8

(5)   not at all
(6)   only a little
(7)   quite a lot
(8)   a great deal

IF: (GenWCHK = YES) AND (F42 = YES)
F52

[*] SHOW CARD 8
Have these worries put a burden on you or the family as a whole...

RUNNING PROMPT

(5)   not at all
(6)   only a little
(7)   quite a lot
(8)   or a great deal?

Depression

DepIntr

This next section of the interview is about (CHILD'S) mood.

G1

[*] In the past month, have there been times when (CHILD'S NAME) has been very sad, miserable, unhappy or tearful?

(1)   Yes
(2)   No

IF: G1 = YES
G3

[*] Was there a period when s/he was really miserable nearly every day?

(1)   Yes
(2)   No

IF: G1 = YES
G4

[*] During this period, was s/he really miserable for most of the day? (i.e.for more hours than not)

(1)   Yes
(2)   No

IF: G1 = YES
G5

[*] During this period, could s/he be cheered up...
RUNNING PROMPT

(1)   easily
(2)   with difficulty/only briefly
(3)   or not at all?

IF: G1 = YES
G6

[*] Can you tell me how long that period lasted?

(1)   less than two weeks
(2)   two weeks or more

G8

[*] In the past month, have there been times when (CHILD'S NAME) has been very grumpy or irritable in a way that was out of character for him/her?

(1)   Yes

(2)   No

IF: G8 = YES
G10

[*] Was there a period when s/he was really irritable nearly everyday?

(1)   Yes
(2)   No

IF: G8 = YES
G11

[*] During this period, was s/he really irritable for most of the day?

(1)   Yes
(2)   No

IF: G8 = YES
G12

[*] Was the irritability improved by particular activities, friends coming around or anything else...
RUNNING PROMPT

(1)   easily
(2)   with difficulty/only briefly
(3)   or not at all?

IF: G8 = YES
G13

[*] Can you tell me how long that period lasted?

(1)   less than two weeks
(2)   two weeks or more

G15

[*] In the past month, has there been a time when (CHILD'S NAME) lost interest in everything, or nearly everything, s/he normally enjoys doing?

(1)   Yes
(2)   No

IF: G15 = YES
G17

[*] Was there a period when s/he was lacking in interest nearly every day?

(1)   Yes
(2)   No

IF: G15 = YES
G18

[*] During this period, was s/he lacking in interest for most of each day? (i.e.for more hours than not)

(1)   Yes
(2)   No

IF: G15 = YES
G19

[*] Can you tell me how long this loss of interest lasted?

(1)   less than two weeks

---

(2)   two weeks or more

IF: G15 = YES
AND: G4=YES AND G3 =YES OR: G10=YES OR **G11=YES**
G20

[*] Was this loss of interest present during the same period when s/he was really miserable/irritable for most of the time?

(1)   Yes
(2)   No

IF: G3 AND G4=YES OR G10 AND G11=YES OR **G17=YES**
G21a

[*] During that time when s/he was (feeling DE-PRESSED/IRRITABLE/A LACK OF INTEREST) did s/he lack energy and seem tired all the time?

(1)   Yes
(2)   No

IF: G3 AND G4=YES OR G10 AND G11=YES OR **G17=YES**
G21ba

[*] During this time when s/he was was s/he eating much more or much less than normal?

(1)   Yes
(2)   No

IF: G3 AND G4=YES OR G10 AND G11=YES OR **G17=YES**
G21b

[*] (During this time when s/he was (feeling DE-PRESSED/IRRITABLE/A LACK OF INTEREST)
. . . did s/he either lose or gain a lot of weight?

(1)   Yes
(2)   No

IF: G3 AND G4=YES OR G10 AND G11=YES OR **G17=YES**
G21c

[*] (During this time when s/he was (feeling DE-PRESSED/IRRITABLE/A LACK OF INTEREST)
. . . did s/he find it hard to get to sleep?

(1)   Yes
(2)   No

IF: G3 AND G4=YES OR G10 AND G11=YES OR **G17=YES**
G21d

[*] (During this time when s/he was (feeling DE-PRESSED/IRRITABLE/A LACK OF INTEREST)
. . .did s/he sleep too much?

(1)   Yes
(2)   No

IF: G3 AND G4=YES OR G10 AND G11=YES OR **G17=YES**
G21e

[*] (During this time when s/he was (feeling DE-PRESSED/IRRITABLE/A LACK OF INTEREST)
. . . was s/he agitated or restless much of the time?

(1)   Yes
(2)   No

IF: G3 AND G4=YES OR G10 AND G11=YES OR G17=YES
G21f

[*] (During this time when s/he was (feeling DE-PRESSED/IRRITABLE/A LACK OF INTEREST)?
.. did s/he feel worthless or unnecessarily guilty much of the time?

(1)   Yes
(2)   No

IF: G3 AND G4=YES OR G10 AND G11=YES OR G17=YES
G21g

[*] (During this time when s/he was (feeling DE-PRESSED/IRRITABLE/A LACK OF INTEREST))
.. did s/he find it unusually hard to concentrate or to think things out?

(1)   Yes
(2)   No

IF: G3 AND G4=YES OR G10 AND G11=YES OR G17=YES
G21h

[*] (During this time when s/he was (feeling DE-PRESSED/IRRITABLE/A LACK OF INTEREST))
. . . did s/he think about death a lot?

(1)   Yes
(2)   No

IF: G3 AND G4=YES OR G10 AND G11=YES OR G17=YES
G21k

[*] Over the whole of his/her lifetime has s/he ever tried to harm himself/herself or kill himself/herself?

(1)   Yes
(2)   No

IF: G3 AND G4=YES OR G10 AND G11=YES OR G17=YES
AND: G21k = Yes
G21j

[*] (During this time when s/he was (feeling DE-PRESSED/IRRITABLE/A LACK OF INTEREST))
. . . did s/he ever try to harm himself/herself or kill himself/herself?

(1)   Yes
(2)   No

IF: G3 AND G4=YES OR G10 AND G11=YES OR G17=YES
G21i

[*] (During this time when s/he was (feeling DE-PRESSED/IRRITABLE/A LACK OF INTEREST))

. . . did s/he ever talk about harming himself/herself or killing himself/herself?

(1)   Yes
(2)   No

IF: G3 AND G4=YES OR G10 AND G11=YES OR G17=YES
G22

[*] You have told me about (CHILD'S NAME) (feeling DEPRESSED/IRRITABLE/A LACK OF INTEREST).
Overall, how upset and distressed is (CHILD'S NAME) as a result of this.
RUNNING PROMPT

(5)   not at all
(6)   only a little
(7)   quite a lot
(8)   or a great deal?

IF: G3 AND G4=YES OR G10 AND G11=YES OR G17=YES
G23Intr

I also want to ask you about the extent to (feeling DEPRESSED/IRRITABLE/A LACK OF INTEREST) has interfered with his/her day to day life.

IF: G3 AND G4=YES OR G10 AND G11=YES OR G17=YES
G23a

[*] Has this interfered with ... how well s/he gets on with you and the rest of your family?
SHOW CARD 8

(5)   not at all
(6)   only a little
(7)   quite a lot
(8)   a great deal

IF: G3 AND G4=YES OR G10 AND G11=YES OR G17=YES
G23b

[*] (Has this interfered with ...) making and keeping friends?
SHOW CARD 8

(5)   not at all
(6)   only a little
(7)   quite a lot
(8)   a great deal

IF: G3 AND G4=YES OR G10 AND G11=YES OR G17=YES
G23c

[*] (Has this interfered with ...) learning or class work?
SHOW CARD 8

(5)   not at all
(6)   only a little
(7)   quite a lot
(8)   a great deal

IF: G3 AND G4=YES OR G10 AND G11=YES OR G17=YES
G23d

[*] (Has this interfered with ...) playing, hobbies, sports or other leisure activities?
SHOW CARD 8

(5)   not at all
(6)   only a little
(7)   quite a lot
(8)   a great deal

IF: G3 AND G4=YES OR G10 AND G11=YES OR G17=YES
G24

[*] Has (CHILD'S) (DEPRESSED/IRRITABLE/A LACK OF INTEREST) put a burden on you or the family as a whole...
RUNNING PROMPT

(5)   not at all
(6)   only a little
(7)   quite a lot
(8)   or a great deal?

IF: G3 AND G4=NO OR G10 AND G11=NO OR G17=NO
G25

Over the past month, has s/he talked about deliberately harming or hurting himself/herself?

(1)   Yes
(2)   No

IF: G3 AND G4=NO OR G10 AND G11=NO OR G17=NO
G26

Over the past month, has s/he ever tried to harm or hurt himself/herself?

(1)   Yes
(2)   No

IF: G3 AND G4=NO OR G10 AND G11=NO OR G17=NO
G27

Over the whole of his/her lifetime, has s/he ever tried to harm or hurt himself/herself?

(1)   Yes
(2)   No

Attention and activity

AttnIntr

This section of the interview is about concentration and activity. I am going to ask you about (CHILD'S) activity and concentration over the past six months.
Nearly all children are overactive or lose concentration at times,but what I would like to know is how (CHILD'S NAME) compares with other children of his/her age.? I am interested in how s/he is usually - not in the occasional 'off day'.

H1

[*] Allowing for his/her age, do you think that (CHILD'S NAME) definitely has some problems with overactivity or poor concentration?

(1)   Yes
(2)   No

IF: H1=YES OR SDQ HYPERACTIVITY SCORE = 6+
H2Intr

I would now like to go through some more detailed questions about how (CHILD'S NAME) has usually been over the last six months? I will start with questions about how active s/he has been

IF: H1=YES OR SDQ HYPERACTIVITY SCORE = 6+
H2a

[*] Over the last 6 months, and compared with other children of is/her age... Does s/he often fidget?
SHOW CARD 9

(5)   No more than other children of the same age
(6)   A little more than other children of the same age
(7)   A lot more than other children of the same age

IF: H1=YES OR SDQ HYPERACTIVITY SCORE = 6+
H2b

[*] (Over the last 6 months, and compared with other children of his/her age..) Is it hard for him/her to stay sitting down for long?
SHOW CARD 9

(5)   No more than other children of the same age
(6)   A little more than other children of the same age
(7)   A lot more than other children of the same age

IF: H1=YES OR SDQ HYPERACTIVITY SCORE = 6+
H2c

[*] (Over the last 6 months, and compared with other children of his/her age..) Does s/he run or climb about when s/he shouldn't?
SHOW CARD 9

(5)   No more than other children of the same age
(6)   A little more than other children of the same age
(7)   A lot more than other children of the same age

IF: H1=YES OR SDQ HYPERACTIVITY SCORE = 6+
H2d

[*] (Over the last 6 months, and compared with other children of his/her age..) Does s/he find it hard to play or take part in other leisure activities without making a noise?
SHOW CARD 9

(5)   No more than other children of the same age
(6)   A little more than other children of the same age
(7)   A lot more than other children of the same age

IF: H1=YES OR SDQ HYPERACTIVITY SCORE = 6+
H2e

[*] (Over the last 6 months, and compared with other children of his/her age..) If s/he is rushing about, does s/he find it hard to calm down when someone asks him/her to?
SHOW CARD 9

(5)   No more than other children of the same age
(6)   A little more than other children of the same age
(7)   A lot more than other children of the same age

IF: H1=YES OR SDQ HYPERACTIVITY SCORE = 6+
H3Intr

The next few questions are about impulsiveness
Over the past six months and compared with other
children of his/her age.
SHOW CARD 9

IF: H1=YES OR SDQ HYPERACTIVITY SCORE = 6+
H3a

[*] (Over the past 6 months and compared with other
children of his/her age.) Does s/he often blurt out an
answer before s/he had heard the question properly?
SHOW CARD 9

(5)   No more than other children of the same age
(6)   A little more than other children of the same
        age
(7)   A lot more than other children of the same age

IF: H1=YES OR SDQ HYPERACTIVITY SCORE = 6+
H3b

[*] (Over the past 6 months and compared with other
children of his/her age.) Is it hard for him/her to wait his/
her turn?
SHOW CARD 9

(5)   No more than other children of the same age
(6)   A little more than other children of the same
        age
(7)   A lot more than other children of the same age

IF: H1=YES OR SDQ HYPERACTIVITY SCORE = 6+
H3c

[*] (Over the past 6 months and compared with other
children of his/her age.) Does s/he often butt in on other
people's conversations or games?
SHOW CARD 9

(5)   No more than other children of the same age
(6)   A little more than other children of the same
        age
(7)   A lot more than other children of the same age

IF: H1=YES OR SDQ HYPERACTIVITY SCORE = 6+
H3d

[*] (Over the past 6 months and compared with other
children of his/her age.) Does s/he often go on talking
even if s/he has been asked to stop or no one is
listening?
SHOW CARD 9

(5)   No more than other children of the same age
(6)   A little more than other children of the same
        age
(7)   A lot more than other children of the same age

IF: H1=YES OR SDQ HYPERACTIVITY SCORE = 6+
H4Intr

The next set of questions are about attention.
Over the past 6 months and compared with other
children his/her age...

IF: H1=YES OR SDQ HYPERACTIVITY SCORE = 6+
H4a

[*] (Over the past 6 months and compared with other
children of his/her age.) Does s/he often make careless
mistakes or fail to pay attention to what s/he is supposed
to be doing?
SHOW CARD 9

(5)   No more than other children of the same age
(6)   A little more than other children of the same age
(7)   A lot more than other children of the same age

IF: H1=YES OR SDQ HYPERACTIVITY SCORE = 6+
H4b

[*] (Over the past 6 months and compared with other
children of his/her age.) Does s/he often seem to lose
interest in what s/he is doing?
SHOW CARD 9

(5)   No more than other children of the same age
(6)   A little more than other children of the same age
(7)   A lot more than other children of the same age

IF: H1=YES OR SDQ HYPERACTIVITY SCORE = 6+
H4c

[*] (Over the past 6 months and compared with other
children of his/her age.) Does s/he often not listen to
what people are saying to him/her?
SHOW CARD 9

(5)   No more than other children of the same age
(6)   A little more than other children of the same age
(7)   A lot more than other children of the same age

IF: H1=YES OR SDQ HYPERACTIVITY SCORE = 6+
H4d

[*] (Over the past 6 months and compared with other
children of his/her age.) Does s/he often not finish a job
properly?
SHOW CARD 9

(5)   No more than other children of the same age
(6)   A little more than other children of the same age
(7)   A lot more than other children of the same age

IF: H1=YES OR SDQ HYPERACTIVITY SCORE = 6+
H4e

[*] (Over the past 6 months and compared with other
children of his/her age.) Is it often hard for him/her to get
himself/herself organised to do something?
SHOW CARD 9

(5)   No more than other children of the same age
(6)   A little more than other children of the same age
(7)   A lot more than other children of the same age

IF: H1=YES OR SDQ HYPERACTIVITY SCORE = 6+
H4f

[*] (Over the past 6 months and compared with other
children of his/her age.) Does s/he often try to get out of
things s/he would have to think about, such as home-
work?
SHOW CARD 9

(5)   No more than other children of the same age
(6)   A little more than other children of the same age
(7)   A lot more than other children of the same age

IF: H1=YES OR SDQ HYPERACTIVITY SCORE = 6+
H4g

[*] (Over the past 6 months and compared with other children of his/her age.) Does s/he often lose things s/he needs for school or games?
SHOW CARD 9

(5)   No more than other children of the same age
(6)   A little more than other children of the same age
(7)   A lot more than other children of the same age

IF: H1=Yes OR SDQ Hyperactivity score = 6+
H4h

[*] (Over the past 6 months and compared with other children of his/her age.) Is s/he easily distracted?
SHOW CARD 9

(5)   No more than other children of the same age
(6)   A little more than other children of the same age
(7)   A lot more than other children of the same age

IF: H1=Yes OR SDQ Hyperactivity score = 6+
H4i

[*] (Over the past 6 months and compared with other children of his/her age.) Is s/he often forgetful?
SHOW CARD 9

(5)   No more than other children of the same age
(6)   A little more than other children of the same age
(7)   A lot more than other children of the same age

IF: H1=Yes OR SDQ Hyperactivity score = 6+
H5a

[*] Could you tell me if (CHILD'S) teacher has complained, over the past 6 months of him/her being fidgety,restless or overactive
SHOW CARD 11

(5)   No
(6)   A little
(7)   A Lot

IF: H1=Yes OR SDQ Hyperactivity score = 6+
H5b

[*] (Could you tell me if (CHILD'S) teacher has complained over the last six months of problems with...)
Poor concentration or being easily distracted?
SHOW CARD 11

(5)   No
(6)   A little
(7)   A Lot

IF: H1=Yes OR SDQ Hyperactivity score = 6+
H5c

[*] (Could you tell me if (CHILD'S) teacher has complained over the last six months of problems with...)
Acting without thinking about what s/he was doing, frequently butting in, or not waiting his/her turn?
SHOW CARD 11

(5)   No
(6)   A little
(7)   A Lot

IF: H1=Yes OR SDQ Hyperactivity score = 6+
IF: TWO OF (H2A-H2E) or (H3A-H3D) or (H4A-H4I) or (H5A-H5C) = 7
H7

[*] You have told me about (CHILD'S) difficulties with some aspects of activity and concentration. Have they been there for much of his/her life?

(1)   Yes
(2)   No

IF: H1=Yes OR SDQ Hyperactivity score = 6+
IF: TWO OF (H2A-H2E) or (H3A-H3D) or (H4A-H4I) or (H5A-H5C) = 7
H8

[*] What age did they start at?
IF 'ALWAYS' OR SINCE BIRTH, ENTER 00
ENTER AGE

0..15

IF: H1=Yes OR SDQ Hyperactivity score = 6+
IF: TWO OF (H2A-H2E) or (H3A-H3D) or (H4A-H4I) or (H5A-H5C) = 7
H9

[*] Thinking still of (CHILD'S) difficulties with activity and attention, how much do you think they have upset or distressed him/her
SHOW CARD 8
RUNNING PROMPT

(5)   not at all
(6)   only a little
(7)   quite a lot
(8)   or a great deal?

IF: H1=Yes OR SDQ Hyperactivity score = 6+
IF: TWO OF (H2A-H2E) or (H3A-H3D) or (H4A-H4I) or (H5A-H5C) = 7
H10Intr

I also want to ask you about the extent to which these difficulties have interfered with his/her day to day life.
SHOW CARD 8

IF: H1=Yes OR SDQ Hyperactivity score = 6+
IF:TWO OF (H2A-H2E) or (H3A-H3D) or (H4A-H4I) or (H5A-H5C) = 7
H10a

[*] Have they interfered with ... how well s/he gets on with you and the rest of the family?
SHOW CARD 8

(5)   not at all
(6)   only a little
(7)   quite a lot
(8)   a great deal

IF: H1=Yes OR SDQ Hyperactivity score = 6+
IF: TWO OF (H2A-H2E) or (H3A-H3D) or (H4A-H4I) or (H5A-H5C) = 7
H10b

[*] (Have they interfered with ...)
.. making and keeping friends?
SHOW CARD 8

(5)   not at all
(6)   only a little
(7)   quite a lot
(8)   a great deal

IF: H1=Yes OR SDQ Hyperactivity score = 6+

IF: TWO OF (*H2A-H2E*) OR (*H3A-H3D*) OR (*H4A-H4I*) OR
(*H5A-H5C*) = 7
H10c

[*] (Have they interfered with ...)
.. learning or class work?
SHOW CARD 8

(5)   not at all
(6)   only a little
(7)   quite a lot
(8)   a great deal

IF: H1=YES **OR SDQ** HYPERACTIVITY SCORE = 6+
IF: TWO OF (*H2A-H2E*) OR (*H3A-H3D*) OR (*H4A-H4I*) OR
(*H5A-H5C*) = 7
H10d

[*] (Have they interfered with ...)
.. playing, hobbies, sports or other leisure activities?
SHOW CARD 8

(5)   not at all
(6)   only a little
(7)   quite a lot
(8)   a great deal

IF: H1=YES **OR SDQ** HYPERACTIVITY SCORE = 6+
IF: TWO OF (*H2A-H2E*) OR (*H3A-H3D*) OR (*H4A-H4I*) OR
(*H5A-H5C*) = 7
H11

[*] Have these problems put a burden on you or the
family as a whole?
RUNNING PROMPT

(5)   not at all
(6)   only a little
(7)   quite a lot
(8)   or a great deal?

Awkward and troublesome behaviour

AwkIntr

This next section of the interview is about behaviour.
All children can be awkward and difficult at times, but
once again what I would like to know is how (CHILD'S
NAME) compares with other children of the same age.

I'm going to ask you first about (CHILD'S) awkward
behaviour over the past six months, things like, not
doing what s/he is told, being irritable, having temper
outbursts, or deliberately annoying other people.

I am interested in how s/he is usually, and not just on
the occasional 'off days'.

I1

[*] Overall, how do you think (CHILD'S NAME) compares with other children of his/her age as far as this
sort of awkward behaviour is concerned, is s/he.....
RUNNING PROMPT

(1)   less troublesome than average
(2)   about average
(3)   or more troublesome than average

IF: I1=3 (MORE TROUBLESOME**) OR SDQ** CONDUCT SCORE 3+
I2Intr

Some children are awkward or annoying with just one
person - perhaps with yourself or just one brother or
sister. Other children are troublesome with a range of
adults or children. The following questions are about
how (CHILD'S NAME) is in general, and not just with
one person.

IF: I1=3 (MORE TROUBLESOME**) OR SDQ** CONDUCT SCORE 3+
I2a

[*] Over the last six months and compared with other
children of the same age. Has s/he often had severe
temper outbursts?
SHOW CARD 9

(5)   No more than other children of the same age
(6)   A little more than other children of the same age
(7)   A lot more than other children of the same age

IF: I1=3 (MORE TROUBLESOME**) OR SDQ** CONDUCT SCORE 3+
I2b

[*] (Over the last six months and compared with other
children of the same age.) Has s/he often argued with
grown-ups?
SHOW CARD 9

(5)   No more than other children of the same age
(6)   A little more than other children of the same age
(7)   A lot more than other children of the same age

IF: I1=3 (MORE TROUBLESOME**) OR SDQ** CONDUCT SCORE 3+
I2c

[*] (Over the last six months and compared with other
children of the same age.) Has s/he often taken no
notice of rules, or refused to do as s/he is told?
SHOW CARD 9

(5)   No more than other children of the same age
(6)   A little more than other children of the same age
(7)   A lot more than other children of the same age

IF: I1=3 (MORE TROUBLESOME**) OR SDQ** CONDUCT SCORE 3+
I2d

[*] (Over the last six months and compared with other
children of the same age.) Has s/he often seemed to do
things to annoy other people on purpose?
SHOW CARD 9

(5)   No more than other children of the same age
(6)   A little more than other children of the same age
(7)   A lot more than other children of the same age

IF: I1=3 (MORE TROUBLESOME**) OR SDQ** CONDUCT SCORE 3+
I2e

[*] (Over the last six months and compared with other
children of the same age.) Has s/he often blamed others
for his/her own mistakes or bad behaviour?
SHOW CARD 9

(5)   No more than other children of the same age
(6)   A little more than other children of the same age
(7)   A lot more than other children of the same age

IF: I1=3 (MORE TROUBLESOME**) OR SDQ** CONDUCT SCORE 3+
I2f

[*] (Over the last six months and compared with other
children of the same age.) Was s/he often touchy and
easily annoyed?

SHOW CARD 9

(5) No more than other children of the same age
(6) A little more than other children of the same age
(7) A lot more than other children of the same age

IF: I1=3 (MORE TROUBLESOME) OR SDQ CONDUCT SCORE 3+
I2g

[*] (Over the last six months and compared with other children of the same age.) Was s/he often angry and resentful?
SHOW CARD 9

(5) No more than other children of the same age
(6) A little more than other children of the same age
(7) A lot more than other children of the same age

IF: I1=3 (MORE TROUBLESOME) OR SDQ CONDUCT SCORE 3+
I2h

[*] (Over the last six months and compared with other children of the same age.) Was s/he often spiteful?
SHOW CARD 9

(5) No more than other children of the same age
(6) A little more than other children of the same age
(7) A lot more than other children of the same age

IF: I1=3 (MORE TROUBLESOME) OR SDQ CONDUCT SCORE 3+
I2i

[*] (Over the last six months and compared with other children of the same age.) Has s/he often tried to get his/her own back on people?
SHOW CARD 9

(5) No more than other children of the same age
(6) A little more than other children of the same age
(7) A lot more than other children of the same age

IF: I1=3 (MORE TROUBLESOME) OR SDQ CONDUCT SCORE 3+
I3

Could you also tell me if (CHILD'S) teacher has complained over the last six months of problems with this same kind of awkward behaviour or disruptiveness in class?
SHOW CARD 11

(5) No
(6) A little
(7) A Lot

IF: I2A - I2I = 7
I4

[*] You have told me about (CHILD'S) awkward behaviour.
Has it been there for much of his/her life?

(1) Yes
(2) No

IF: I2A - I2I = 7
I5

What age did it start at?

0..15

IF: I2A - I2I = 7
I6Intr

I also want to ask you about the extent to which it has interfered with ...
SHOW CARD 8

IF: I2A - I2I = 7
I6a

[*] (Has it interfered with...) how well s/he gets on with you and the rest of the family?
SHOW CARD 8

(5) not at all
(6) only a little
(7) quite a lot
(8) a great deal

IF: I2A - I2I = 7
I6b

[*] (Has it interfered with...)
...making and keeping friends?
SHOW CARD 8

(5) not at all
(6) only a little
(7) quite a lot
(8) a great deal

IF: I2A - I2I = 7
I6c

[*] (Has it interfered with...)
...learning or class work?
SHOW CARD 8

(5) not at all
(6) only a little
(7) quite a lot
(8) a great deal

IF: I2A - I2I = 7
I6d

[*] (Has it interfered with...)
... playing, hobbies, sports or other leisure activities?
SHOW CARD 8

(5) not at all
(6) only a little
(7) quite a lot
(8) a great deal

IF: I2A - I2I = 7
I7

[*] Have these problems put a burden on you or the family as a whole?
RUNNING PROMPT

(5) not at all
(6) only a little
(7) quite a lot
(8) or a great deal?

IF: I1=3 (MORE TROUBLESOME) OR SDQ CONDUCT SCORE=3+
I8Intr

I'm now going to ask about behaviour that sometimes gets children into trouble, including dangerous, aggressive or antisocial behaviour. Please answer according to how s/he has been over the last year - I'm switching to the past 12 months for this set of questions. As before, I am interested in how s/he is usually, and not just in occasional 'off days'.

IF: I1=3 (MORE TROUBLESOME) OR SDQ CONDUCT SCORE=3+
I8a

[*] Has s/he often told lies in order to get things or favours from others, or to get out of having to do things s/he is supposed to do?
SHOW CARD 12

(5)   No
(6)   Perhaps
(7)   Definitely

IF: I1=3 (MORE TROUBLESOME) OR SDQ CONDUCT SCORE=3+
AND: I8A = DEF
I8aa

[*] Has this been going on for the last 6 months?

(1)   Yes
(2)   No

IF: I1=3 (MORE TROUBLESOME) OR SDQ CONDUCT SCORE=3+
I8b

[*] Has s/he often started fights?
(other than with brothers or sisters)
SHOW CARD 12

(5)   No
(6)   Perhaps
(7)   Definitely

IF: I1=3 (MORE TROUBLESOME) OR SDQ CONDUCT SCORE=3+
AND: I8B = DEF
I8ba

[*] Has this been going on for the last 6 months?

(1)   Yes
(2)   No

IF: I1=3 (MORE TROUBLESOME) OR SDQ CONDUCT SCORE=3+
I8c

[*] Has s/he often bullied or threatened people?
SHOW CARD 12

(5)   No
(6)   Perhaps
(7)   Definitely

IF: I1=3 (MORE TROUBLESOME) OR SDQ CONDUCT SCORE=3+
AND: I8C = DEF
I8ca

[*] Has this been going on for the last 6 months?

(1)   Yes
(2)   No

IF: I1=3 (MORE TROUBLESOME) OR SDQ CONDUCT SCORE=3+
I8d

[*] Has s/he often stayed out after dark much later than

s/he was supposed to?
SHOW CARD 12

(5)   No
(6)   Perhaps
(7)   Definitely

IF: I1=3 (MORE TROUBLESOME) OR SDQ CONDUCT SCORE=3+
AND: I8D = DEF
I8da

[*] Has this been going on for the last 6 months?

(1)   Yes
(2)   No

IF: I1=3 (MORE TROUBLESOME) OR SDQ CONDUCT SCORE=3+
I8e

[*] Has s/he stolen from the house, or from other people's houses, from shops or school? (Do not include things of trivial value)
SHOW CARD 12

(5)   No
(6)   Perhaps
(7)   Definitely

IF: I1=3 (MORE TROUBLESOME) OR SDQ CONDUCT SCORE=3+
IF: I8E = DEF
I8ea

[*] Has this been going on for the last 6 months?

(1)   Yes
(2)   No

IF: I1=3 (MORE TROUBLESOME) OR SDQ CONDUCT SCORE=3+
I8f

[*] Has s/he run away from home more than once or ever stayed away all night without your permission?
SHOW CARD 12

(5)   No
(6)   Perhaps
(7)   Definitely

IF: I1=3 (MORE TROUBLESOME) OR SDQ CONDUCT SCORE=3+
IF: I8F = DEF
I8fa

[*] Has this been going on for the last 6 months?

(1)   Yes
(2)   No

IF: I1=3 (MORE TROUBLESOME) OR SDQ CONDUCT SCORE=3+
I8g

[*] Has s/he often played truant ('bunked off') from school?
SHOW CARD 12

(5)   No
(6)   Perhaps
(7)   Definitely

IF: I1=3 (MORE TROUBLESOME) OR SDQ CONDUCT SCORE=3+ 1
IF: I8G = DEF
I8ga

[*] Has this been going on for the last 6 months?

(1)   Yes
(2)   No

IF: CHILD = 13+ YEARS AND I8G = DEF
I9

[*] Did s/he start playing truant ('bunking off') from school before s/he was 13?

(1)   Yes
(2)   No

IF: ANY (I2A-I2I=7) OR ANY(I8A - I8G=7)
I10Intr

May I now ask you about a list of less common but potentially more serious behaviours. I have to ask everyone all these questions even when they are not likely to apply. Have any of the following happened even once in the past year?

SHOW CARD 8

IF: ANY (I2A-I2I=7) OR ANY(I8A - I8G=7)
I10a

Has s/he used a weapon or anything that could seriously hurt someone?

(1)   Yes
(2)   No

IF: ANY (I2A-I2I=7) OR ANY(I8A - I8G=7)
IF: I10A = YES
I10aa

Has this happened in the past six months?

(1)   Yes
(2)   No

IF: ANY (I2A-I2I=7) OR ANY(I8A - I8G=7)
I10b
[*] Has s/he really hurt someone or been physically cruel to them? (e.g. ties up, cuts or burns victim)?

(1)   Yes
(2)   No

IF: ANY (I2A-I2I=7) OR ANY(I8A - I8G=7)
IF: I10B = YES
I10ba

[*] Has this happened in the past six months?

(1)   Yes
(2)   No

IF: ANY (I2A-I2I=7) OR ANY(I8A - I8G=7)
I10c

[*] Has s/he been really cruel on purpose to animals and birds?

(1)   Yes
(2)   No

IF: ANY (I2A-I2I=7) OR ANY(I8A - I8G=7)
IF: I10C = YES

I10ca

[*] Has this happened in the past six months?

(1)   Yes
(2)   No

IF: ANY (I2A-I2I=7) OR ANY(I8A - I8G=7))
I10d

[*] Has s/he deliberately started a fire? (has to be with the intention of causing severe damage. Do not include campfires, burning individual matches or pieces of paper)

(1)   Yes
(2)   No

IF: ANY (I2A-I2I=7) OR ANY(I8A - I8G=7)
IF: I10D = YES
I10da

Has this happened in the past six months?

(1)   Yes
(2)   No

IF: ANY (I2A-I2I=7) OR ANY(I8A - I8G=7)
I10e

Has s/he deliberately destroyed someone else's property? (Exclude setting fire to things or very minor acts, eg. destroying sister's drawing. Include acts such as smashing car windows or school vandalism)

(1)   Yes
(2)   No

IF: ANY (I2A-I2I=7) OR ANY(I8A - I8G=7)
IF: I10E = YES
I10ea

Has this happened in the past six months?

(1)   Yes
(2)   No

IF: ANY (I2A-I2I=7) OR ANY(I8A - I8G=7)
I10f

Has s/he been involved in stealing from someone in the street?

(1)   Yes
(2)   No

IF: ANY (I2A-I2I=7) OR ANY(I8A - I8G=7)
IF: I10F = YES
I10fa

Has this happened in the past six months?

(1)   Yes
(2)   No

IF: ANY (I2A-I2I=7) OR ANY(I8A - I8G=7)
I10g

Has s/he tried to force someone to have sexual activity against their will?

(1)   Yes

(2)   No

IF: ANY (I2A-I2I=7) OR ANY(I8A - I8G=7)
IF: I10G = YES
I10ga

Has this happened in the past six months?

(1)   Yes
(2)   No

IF: ANY (I2A-I2I=7) OR ANY(I8A - I8G=7)
I10h

Has s/he broken into a house, any other building, or a car?

(1)   Yes
(2)   No

IF: ANY (I2A-I2I=7) OR ANY(I8A - I8G=7)
IF: I10H = YES
I10ha

Has this happened in the past six months?

(1)   Yes
(2)   No

IF: ANY (I2A-I2I=7) OR ANY(I8A - I8G=7)
I11

Could you also tell me if (CHILD'S) teacher has complained over the last six momths of problems with any of these same kinds of behaviour?

(1)   Yes
(2)   No

IF: ANY (I8A-I8G=7) OR ANY (I10AA - I10HA=YES)
I13Intr

You have told me about (CHILD'S) troublesome behaviour. I also want to ask you about the extent to which this behaviour has interfered with his/her day to day life

IF: ANY (I8A-I8G=7) OR ANY (I10AA - I10HA=YES)
I13a

Have this interfered with... how well s/he gets on with you and the rest of the family ?
SHOW CARD 8

(5)   not at all
(6)   only a little
(7)   quite a lot
(8)   a great deal

IF: ANY (I8A-I8G=7) OR ANY (I10AA - I10HA=YES)
I13b

(Have this interfered with...)
making and keeping friends
SHOW CARD 8

(5)   not at all
(6)   only a little
(7)   quite a lot
(8)   a great deal

IF: ANY (I8A-I8G=7) OR ANY (I10AA - I10HA=YES)

I13c

(Have this interfered with...)
earning or class work?
SHOW CARD 8

(5)   not at all
(6)   only a little
(7)   quite a lot
(8)   a great deal

IF: ANY (I8A-I8G=7) OR ANY (I10AA - I10HA=YES)
I13d

(Have this interfered with...)
playing, hobbies, sports or other leisure activities?
SHOW CARD 8

(5)   not at all
(6)   only a little
(7)   quite a lot
(8)   a great deal

IF: ANY (I8A-I8G=7) OR ANY (I10AA - I10HA=YES)
I14

Have these problems put a burden on you or the family as a whole
RUNNING PROMPT

(5)   not at all
(6)   only a little
(7)   quite a lot
(8)   or a great deal?

Less common disorders

LessIntr

This next section is about a variety of different aspects of (CHILD'S) behaviour and development.

I15a

[*] In his/her first three years of life, was there anything that seriously worried you about...
the way his/her speech developed?

(1)   Yes
(2)   No

I15b

[*] (In his/her first three years of life, was there anything that seriously worried you about...)
how s/he got on with other people?

(1)   Yes
(2)   No

I15c

[*] (In his/her first three years of life, was there anything that seriously worried you about...)
any odd rituals or unusual habits that were very hard to interrupt?

(1)   Yes
(2)   No

IF: ((I15A = YES) OR (I15B = YES)) OR (I15C = YES)

I15aa

[*] Has this/Have all of these now cleared up completely?

(1)   some continuing problems
(2)   completely cleared up

I16

[*] Coming back to the present, does s/he have any tics or twitches that s/he can't seem to control?

(1)   Yes
(2)   No

I17

[*] Have you been concerned about him/her being too thin or dieting too much?

(1)   Yes
(2)   No

I18

[*] Apart from the things you have already told me about, are there any other aspects of (CHILD'S) psychological development that really concern you?

(1)   Yes
(2)   No

I19

[*] Apart from the things you have already told me about, are there any other aspects of (CHILD'S) psychological development that really concern his/her teachers?

(1)   Yes
(2)   No
(3)   Don't know

Significant problems

IF: SIGNIFICANT PROBLEM HAS BEEN IDENTIFIED (I.E. CHILD HAS SYMPTOMS AND THESE ARE CAUSING AN IMPACT OR BURDEN) IN ONE OR MORE AREA.

Intro

You have told me about (LIST OF SIGNIFICANT PROBLEMS) I'd now like to hear a bit more about these difficulties in your own words.

TypNow

INTERVIEWER: if you prefer to take notes by hand rather than typing the details during the interview just type 'later' in the response box - but please remember to come back and complete the question befor transmission.
WILL YOU BE TYPING IN THE ANSWERS NOW OR LATER

(1)   Now
(2)   Later

SigProb

LIST OF PROBLEMS

INTERVIEWER: Please try and cover all areas of difficulty, but it is a good idea to let the parent choose which order to cover them in, starting with the area that concerns them most.

Use the suggested prompts written below and on the prompt card.

1.   Description of the problem?
2.   How often does the problem occur?
3.   How severe is the problem at its worst?
4.   How long has it been going on for?
5.   Is the problem interfering with the child's quality of life? If so, how?
6.   WHERE APPROPRIATE,record what the family think the problem is due to, and what they have done about it.

Anxiety

Does (CHILD'S NAME) experience any of the following symptoms when he/she feels anxious, nervous or tense ?
INDIVIDUAL PROMPT

SET [7] OF
(1)   Heart racing or pounding?
(2)   Hands sweating or shaking?
(3)   Feeling dizzy?
(4)   Difficulty getting his/her breath?
(5)   Butterflies in stomach?
(6)   Dry mouth?
(7)   Nausea or feeling as though s/he wanted to be sick?
(8)   OR are you not aware of him/her having any of the above?

Use of services for significant problem(s)

IF: SIGNIFICANT PROBLEM HAS BEEN IDENTIFIED (I.E. CHILD HAS SYMPTOMS AND THESE ARE CAUSING AN IMPACT OR BURDEN) IN ONE OR MORE AREA.

Family

Have you spoken to family or friends about any of the difficulties we have just been talking about?

(1)   Yes
(2)   No

Profess

Have you spoken to a professional about them?

(1)   Yes
(2)   No

IF: PROFESS = YES
ProfWho

Which of these areas did the professional come from?
SHOW CARD 14
CODE ALL THAT APPLY

SET [6] OF
(1)   Primary healthcare (eg. GP, health visitor)
(2)   Specialist healthcare (eg. Paediatrician, child guidance)
(3)   Social services (eg. social worker)
(4)   Education (eg. teacher, educational psychologist, school counsellor)
(5)   Alternative therapist

(6)   Other

IF: PROFESS = YES
Treat

What sort of help, advice or treatment did they give?
PLEASE ENTER A BRIEF DESCRIPTION

Impact

IF: SIGNIFICANT PROBLEM HAS BEEN IDENTIFIED (I.E. CHILD HAS SYMPTOMS AND THESE ARE CAUSING AN IMPACT OR BURDEN) IN ONE OR MORE AREA.

J2Intr

I now want to ask you about the impact of some of (CHILD'S) difficulties that you have just been telling me about.

IF: PARENT HAS A PARTNER LIVING AT HOME WITH THEM.
J2a

[*] (Sorry if these questions do not apply to you - but we have to ask everyone them....)
Has (CHILD'S) difficulties made your relationship with your partner
RUNNING PROMPT

(1)   Stronger
(2)   more strained
(3)   or has it made no difference?

IF: J2 = No
J3

[*] Do you believe that (CHILD'S) difficulties put a strain on your previous relationship and was part of the reason that relationship broke up...
RUNNING PROMPT
SHOW CARD 15a

(1)   to a great extent
(2)   to some extent
(3)   or not at all?
(4)   SPONTANEOUS: No previous relationship
(5)   SPONTANEOUS: Problems started since relationship broke up

J4

[*] Have (CHILD'S) difficulties made your relationship with your other children (including step-children and any who no longer live at home).....
RUNNING PROMPT

(1)   Stronger
(2)   More difficult
(3)   or has it made no difference?
(4)   SPONTANEOUS: No other children

IF: J4 < NoOTH
J5

[*] Have (CHILD'S) difficulties made his/her relationship with your other children (including step-children and any who no longer live at home).....
RUNNING PROMPT

(1)   Stronger
(2)   More difficult

(3)   or has it made no difference?
(4)   SPONTANEOUS: No other children

J6

[*] Has (CHILD'S) difficulties caused any problems with other members of your family (including family members in other households)?

(1)   Yes
(2)   No

J7

[*] Has (CHILD'S) difficulties caused any problems with your relationship with your friends?

(1)   Yes
(2)   No

J8

Thinking about your own leisure and social activities, has (CHILD'S) difficulties disrupted these..
RUNNING PROMPT
SHOW CARD 15

(5)   to a great extent
(6)   to some extent
(7)   or not at all?

J9

[*] Have these difficulties kept you from doing things socially with (CHILD'S NAME)

RUNNING PROMPT
SHOW CARD 15

(5)   to a great extent
(6)   to some extent
(7)   or not at all?

J10
[*] Are you embarrassed about his/her difficulties?

(1)   Yes
(2)   No

J11

[*] Have you felt others disapprove of you or avoid you because of his/her difficulties?

(1)   Yes
(2)   No

J12a

[*] I now want to ask you how (CHILD'S) problems have affected you.
Would you say they have made you...
Worried?
SHOW CARD 15

(5)   to a great extent
(6)   to some extent
(7)   or not at all

J12b

[*] (Would you say they have made you...)
depressed?
SHOW CARD 15

(5)   to a great extent
(6)   to some extent
(7)   or not at all

J12c

[*] (Would you say they have made you...) tired?
SHOW CARD 15

(5)   to a great extent
(6)   to some extent
(7)   or not at all

J12d

[*] (Would you say they have made you...)
or physically ill?
SHOW CARD 15

(5)   to a great extent
(6)   to some extent
(7)   or not at all

IF: (J12A-J12D=5 OR 6)
J13

Have you been to see a doctor because you felt
(worried/ill/depressed/tired) coping with (CHILD'S
NAME)

(1)   Yes
(2)   No

IF: (J12A-J12D=5 OR 6)
AND: J13 = YES
J14

Were you prescribed any medicine for this?

(1)   Yes
(2)   No

IF: (J12A-J12D=5 OR 6)
J15

[*] Did it make you drink more alcohol?

(1)   Yes
(2)   No
(3)   Don't drink

IF: (J12A-J12D=5 OR 6)
J16

[*] Did it make you smoke more?

(1)   Yes
(2)   No
(3)   Don't smoke

Stressful life events

StrsIntr

I would now like to ask about things that may have
happened or problems that you or (CHILD'S NAME) may

have faced during his/her life.

K1

Since (CHILD'S NAME) was born have you had a
separation due to marital difficulties or broken off a
steady relationship?

(1)   Yes
(2)   No

K2

Since (CHILD'S NAME) was born have you (or your
partner) had a major financial crisis, such as losing the
equivalent of 3 months income?

(1)   Yes
(2)   No

K3

Since (CHILD'S NAME) was born have you (or your
partner) had a problem with the police involving a court
appearance?

(1)   Yes
(2)   No

K4

At any stage in his/her life has s/he ever had serious
illness which required a stay in hospital

(1)   Yes
(2)   No

K5

(At any stage in his/her life)......
Has s/he ever been in a serious accident or badly hurt
in an accident?

(1)   Yes
(2)   No

K6

Now turning to things that have happened to (CHILD'S
NAME) At any stage in his/her life has a parent, brother
or sister of his/hers died?

(1)   Yes
(2)   No

IF: K6 = YES
K6a

ASK OR RECORD
How many have died?
0..5

K7

At any stage in his/her life has a close friend of his/her
died?

(1)   Yes
(2)   No

IF: K7 = YES

K7a

ASK OR RECORD
How many of his/her close friends have died?
0...5

K8

In the PAST YEAR has a grandparent of his/her died?

(1)   Yes
(2)   No

IF: K8 = YES
K8a

ASK OR RECORD
How many of (CHILD'S) grandparents have died?
0..5

K9

In the PAST YEAR has a pet of his/hers died?

(1)   Yes
(2)   No

IF: K9 = YES
K9a

ASK OR RECORD
How many of his/her pets have died?
0..5

IF: CHILD = 13+ YEARS
K10

In the PAST YEAR has (CHILD'S NAME) broken off a
steady relationship with a girl/boy friend?

(1)   Yes
(2)   No

Use of services - general

GPChk

In the past 12 months has (CHILD'S NAME) or have
you or any member of your household talked to a GP or
a family doctor for any reason at all, on his/her behalf
apart from immunisation, child surveillance or development tests?
INCLUDE ASTHMA CLINIC

(1)   Yes
(2)   No

IF: GPCHK = YES
GPVis

About how many times has (CHILD'S NAME) seen the
GP in those 12 months?

(1)   Once
(2)   Twice
(3)   Three
(4)   Four or more

AccEm

Has (CHILD'S NAME) had to visit an Accident and
Emergency department in the last 12 months?

(1)   Yes
(2)   No

IF: AccEm = YES
AEVis

How many seperate visits has (CHILD'S NAME) made
to an Accident and Emergency department in those 12
months?

(1)   Once
(2)   Twice
(3)   Three
(4)   Four or more

InPat

Has (CHILD'S NAME) been in hospital as an in-patient,
overnight or longer, for treatment or tests in the past 12
months?

(1)   Yes
(2)   No

IF: INPAT = YES
InPatVis

How many separate stays has (CHILD'S NAME) been in
hospital as an in-patient in those 12 months

(1)   Once
(2)   Twice
(3)   Three
(4)   Four or more

HospClin

(Apart from seeing your own doctor/when (CHILD'S
NAME) stayed in hospital or seeing an optician or
dentist) In the past 12 months, has (CHILD'S NAME)
been to a hospital or clinic or anywhere else for treatment or check-ups?

(1)   Yes
(2)   No

IF: HOSPCLIN = YES
OutIn

In the past 12 months, on how many separate occasions
has (CHILD'S NAME) been for out-patient or day patient
visits in the past year?

(1)   Once
(2)   Twice
(3)   Three
(4)   Four or more

VisHome

Here is a list of people who visit children and their
families in their homes to give them help and support
when they need it. Have any of these people visited you
to talk about behavioural or emotional problems of
(CHILD'S NAME) in the past year?
SHOW CARD 16

(1)   Yes
(2)   No

SpecSch

Does (CHILD'S NAME) attend a special school or a special unit of an ordinary school?

(1) Yes
(2) No

IF: SPECSCH = YES
BehEm

Is this for ...
INDIVIDUAL PROMPT
behavioural and emotional problems?

(1) Yes
(2) No

IF: SPECSCH = YES
LearnD

learning difficulties?

(1) Yes
(2) No

IF: SPECSCH = YES
SpecOth

or some other reason?

(1) Yes
(2) No

IF: SPECSCH = YES
IF: SPECOTH = YES
OthReas

What is the other reason?

STRING[60]

Police

In the past 12 months has (CHILD'S NAME) ever been in trouble with the police?

(1) Yes
(2) No

IF: POLICE = YES
PolNum

In the past 12 months, on how many occasions has (CHILD'S NAME) been in trouble with the police?
ENTER NO. OF OCCASIONS

0..99

SocSer

In the past 12 months has (CHILD'S NAME) or have you or any member of your household talked to a social worker or someone from social services/ for any reason at all, on his/her behalf?

(1) Yes
(2) No

Strengths

PIntro

I have been asking you a lot of questions about difficulties and problems. I now want to ask you about your child's good points or strengths.

PersIty

[*] In terms of what sort of person (CHILD'S NAME) is, what would you say are the best things about him/her?

OPEN

PersNo

INTERVIEWER: Did the parent mention any qualities?

(1) Yes
(2) No

Quality

[*] Can you tell me some things which (CHILD'S NAME) does which really please you?

OPEN

QualNo

INTERVIEWER: Did the parent mention any things that really please them about (CHILD'S NAME)

(1) Yes
(2) No

RewardA

[*] How often do you reward good behaviour or doing something well by...
giving encouragement or praise?
SHOW CARD 17

(1) Never
(2) Seldom
(3) Sometimes
(4) Frequently

RewardB

[*] (How often do you reward good behaviour or doing something well by...)
giving (CHILD'S NAME) treats, such as extra pocket money, staying up late or a special outing?
SHOW CARD 17

(1) Never
(2) Seldom
(3) Sometimes
(4) Frequently

RewardC

[*] (How often do you reward good behaviour or doing something well by...)
giving (CHILD'S NAME) favourite things?
SHOW CARD 17

(1) Never
(2) Seldom
(3) Sometimes
(4) Frequently

PunishA

[*] All children are naughty at sometime. How often do you punish (CHILD'S NAME) when s/he misbehaves or does something wrong by...
sending him/her to his/her room?
SHOW CARD 17

(1)   Never
(2)   Seldom
(3)   Sometimes
(4)   Frequently

PunishB

[*] (All children are naughty at sometime. How often do you punish (CHILD'S NAME) when s/he misbehaves or does something wrong by...)
...'grounding'/keeping him/her in?
SHOW CARD 17

(1)   Never
(2)   Seldom
(3)   Sometimes
(4)   Frequently
(5)   SPONTANEOUS: Too young to go out on his/ her own

PunishC

[*] (All children are naughty at sometime. How often do you punish (CHILD'S NAME) when s/he misbehaves or does something wrong by...)
... shouting or yelling at him/her?
SHOW CARD 17

(1)   Never
(2)   Seldom
(3)   Sometimes
(4)   Frequently

PunishD

[*] (All children are naughty at sometime. How often do you punish (CHILD'S NAME) when s/he misbehaves or does something wrong by...)
... smacking him/her with your hand?
SHOW CARD 17

(1)   Never
(2)   Seldom
(3)   Sometimes
(4)   Frequently

PunishE

[*] (All children are naughty at sometime. How often do you punish (CHILD'S NAME) when s/he misbehaves or does something wrong by...)
.... hitting him/her with a strap or something else?
SHOW CARD 17

(1)   Never
(2)   Seldom
(3)   Sometimes
(4)   Frequently

PunishF

[*] (All children are naughty at sometime. How often do you punish (CHILD'S NAME) when s/he misbehaves or does something wrong by...)
... shaking him/her?

SHOW CARD 17

(1)   Never
(2)   Seldom
(3)   Sometimes
(4)   Frequently

Education level (interviewed parent)

SchLeft

At what age did you finish your continuous full-time education at school or college?
NEVER WENT TO SCHOOL=01
STILL AT SCHOOL/EDUCATIONAL COLLEGE=99

0..99

AnyQuals
Have you got any qualifications of any sort?

(1)   Yes
(2)   No

IF: AnyQuals = Yes
HiQuals

Please look at this card and tell me whether you have passed any of the qualifications listed. Look down the list and tell me the first one you come to that you have passed
SHOW CARD 18

(1)   Degree level qualification
(2)   Teaching qualification
       or HNC/HND,BEC/TEC Higher,
       BTEC Higher
(3)   'A'Levels/SCE Higher
       or ONC/OND/BEC/TEC not higher
       or City & Guilds Advanced Final Level
(4)   'O'Level passes (Grade A-C if
        after 1975)
       or City & Guilds Craft/Ord level
       or GCSE (Grades A-C)
(5)   CSE Grades 2-5
       GCE 'O'level (Grades D & E if
        after 1975)
       GCSE (Grades D,E,F,G)
       NVQs
(6)   CSE ungraded
(7)   Other qualifications (specify)
(8)   No qualifications

IF: AnyQuals = Yes
IF: HiQuals = Other
OthQuals

What other qualification do you have?
INTERVIEW CHECK THAT THIS QUALIFICATION CANNOT BE CODED AT (HIQUALS)
- IF NOT PLEASE ENTER A SHORT DESCRIPTION OR TITLE

Employment status (interviewed parent)

IF: ALL interviewed adults
Wrking

Did you do any paid work in the 7 days ending Sunday the (DATE), either as an employee or as self-employed?

(1)   Yes
(2)   No

IF: WRKING = No
AND: MEN AGED 16-64 AND WOMEN AGED 16-62
SchemeET

Were you on a government scheme for employment training?

(1)   Yes
(2)   No

IF: WRKING = No
AND: SCHEMEET = No
JbAway

Did you have a job or business that you were away from?

(1)   Yes
(2)   No
(3)   Waiting to take up a new job/business already obtained

IF: WRKING = No
AND: SCHEMEET = No
AND: JBAWAY = No OR JBAWAY = WAITING
OwnBus

Did you do any unpaid work in that week for any business that you own?

(1)   Yes
(2)   No

IF: WRKING = No
AND: SCHEMEET = No
AND: JBAWAY = No OR JBAWAY = WAITING
AND: OWNBUS = No
RelBus

...or that a relative owns?

(1)   Yes
(2)   No

IF: NOT IN EMPLOYMENT I.E. No TO ALL QUESTIONS ABOVE ON WORK
Looked

Thinking of the 4 weeks ending Sunday the (DATE), were you looking for any kind of paid work or govern-ment training scheme at any time in those 4 weeks?

(1)   Yes
(2)   No

IF: NOT IN EMPLOYMENT I.E. No TO ALL QUESTIONS ABOVE ON WORK
AND: LOOKED = YES
StartJ

If a job or a place on a government scheme had been available in the week ending Sunday the (DATE), would you have been able to start within 2 weeks?

(1)   Yes
(2)   No

IF: NOT IN EMPLOYMENT I.E. No TO ALL QUESTIONS ABOVE ON WORK

AND: LOOKED = No OR STARTJ = No
YInAct

What was the main reason you did not seek any work in the last 4 weeks/would not be able to start in the next 2 weeks?

(1)   Student
(2)   Looking after the family/home
(3)   Temporarily sick or injured
(4)   Long-term sick or disabled
(5)   Retired from paid work
(6)   None of these

IF: UNEMPLOYED OR ECONOMICALLY INACTIVE
Everwk

Have you ever had a paid job, apart from casual or holiday work?

(1)   Yes
(2)   No

IF: UNEMPLOYED OR ECONOMICALLY INACTIVE
AND: EVERWK = YES
DtJbL

When did you leave your last PAID job?
FOR DAY NOT GIVEN....ENTER 15 FOR DAY
FOR MONTH NOT GIVEN....ENTER 6 FOR MONTH

IF:ALL ECONOMICALLY INACTIVE EXCEPT THOSE UNEMPLOYED WHO HAVE NEVER WORKED AND ARE NOT WAITING TO TAKE UP A JOB

IndD

CURRENT OR LAST JOB
What did the firm/organisation you worked for mainly make or do (at the place where you worked)?
DESCRIBE FULLY - PROBE MANUFACTURING or PROCESSING or DISTRIBUTING ETC. AND MAIN GOODS PRODUCED, MATERIALS USED, WHOLE-SALE or RETAIL ETC.

OccT

JOBTITLE   CURRENT OR LAST JOB

What was your (main) job (in the week ending Sunday XX) ?

OccD

CURRENT OR LAST JOB
What did you mainly do in your job?

CHECK SPECIAL QUALIFICATIONS/TRAINING NEEDED TO DO THE JOB

Stat

Were you working as an employee or were you self-employed?

(1)   Employee
(2)   Self-employed

IF: STAT = EMP
Manage

Did you have any managerial duties, or were you

supervising any other employees?
ASK OR RECORD

(1) Manager
(2) Foreman/supervisor
(3) Not manager/supervisor

IF: Sᴛᴀᴛ **= E**ᴍᴘ
EmpNo

How many employees were there at the place where you worked?

(1) 1-24
(2) 25 or more

IF: Sᴛᴀᴛ **= S**ᴇʟꜰ**E**ᴍᴘ
Solo

Were you working on your own or did you have employees?

(1) on own/with partner(s) but no employees
(2) with employees

IF: Sᴛᴀᴛ **= S**ᴇʟꜰ**E**ᴍᴘ
IF: Sᴏʟᴏ **= W**ɪᴛʜ**E**ᴍᴘ
SENo

How many people did you employ at the place where you worked?

(1) 1-24
(2) 25 or more

FtPtWk

In your (main) job were you working:

(1) full time
(2) or part time?

Partner's employment status

The employment status section is repeated for interviewed parent's partner (where applicable).

State benefits

Benefits

Looking at the card, are you at present receiving any of these state benefits in your own right, that is, were you the named recipient?
SHOW CARD 19
CODE ALL THAT APPLY

SET [9] OF
(1) Child Benefit
(2) One Parent Benefit
(3) Guardian's Allowance
(4) Invalid Care Allowance
(5) Retirement pension (National Insurance) or old person's pension
(6) Widow's pension or allowance (National Insurance)
(7) War disablement pension
(8) Severe disablement allowance (and related allowances)

(9) Disability working allowance
(10) None of these

CareBen

And looking at this card, are you at present receiving any of the state benefits shown on this card - either in your own name, or on behalf of someone else in the household?
SHOW CARD 20
CODE ALL THAT APPLY

SET [3] OF
(1) Care component of disability living allowance
(2) Mobility allowance of disability living allowance
(3) Attendance Allowance
(4) None of these

IncBen

Now looking at this card, are you at present receiving any of these benefits in your own right, that is where you are the named recipient?
SHOW CARD 21
CODE ALL THAT APPLY

SET [6] OF
(1) Jobseekers Allowance
(2) Income support
(3) Family credit (not received in a lump sum)
(4) Incapacity allowance
(5) Statutory sick pay
(6) Industrial injury disablement benefit
(7) None of these

IF: QSᴇʟᴇᴄᴛ.**A**ᴅʟᴛ**S**ᴇx **= FEMALE**
Matern

Are you receiving either of the things shown on this card, in your own right?
SHOW CARD 22
CODE ALL THAT APPLY

SET [2] OF
(1) Maternity Allowance
(2) Statutory Maternity Pay from your employer or former employer
(3) None of these

Other

In the last 6 months have you received any of the things shown on this card, in your own right?
SHOW CARD 23
CODE ALL THAT APPLY

SET [5] OF
(1) Family credit, paid in a lump sum
(2) A grant from the Social Fund for funeral expenses
(3) Grant from the Social Fund for maternity expenses
(4) A Community Care grant from the Social Fund
(5) Any National Insurance or State benefit not mentioned earlier
(6) None of these

Income

IncKind

(In addition to these)
This card shows a number of (other) possible sources of income. Can you tell me which different kinds of income you personally receive?
CODE ALL THAT APPLY
SHOW CARD 24

SET [7] OF
(1)   Earned income/salary
(2)   Income from self-employment
(3)   Pension from a former employer
(4)   Interest from savings, building society, invest-
       ment dividends from shares etc.
(5)   Other kinds of regular allowances from outside
       the household (e.g. alimony, annuity, educa-
       tional grant)
(6)   Any other source
(7)   None of these
(9)   Refused

IF: OTHER IN INCKIND
IncOther

What is this other source of income?

IF: INCKIND = 1-7
GrossInc

Could you please look at this card and tell me which group represents your own personal gross income from all sources mentioned?
By gross income, I mean income from all sources before deductions for income tax, National Insurance etc.
ENTER GROUP NO. OR CODE 23 FOR REFUSAL
SHOW CARD 25

(1)   Less than 1000
(2)   1,000 to 1,999
(3)   2,000 to 2,999
(4)   3,000 to 3,999
(5)   4,000 to 4,999
(6)   5,000 to 5,999
(7)   6,000 to 6,999
(8)   7,000 to 7,999
(9)   8,000 to 8,999
(10)   9,000 to 9,999
(11)   10,000 to 10,999
(12)   11,000 to 11,999
(13)   12,000 to 12,999
(14)   13,000 to 13,999
(15)   14,000 to 14,999
(16)   15,000 to 17,499
(17)   17,500 to 19,999
(18)   20,000 to 24,999
(19)   25,000 to 29,999
(20)   30,000 to 39,999
(21)   40,000 or more
(22)   No source of income
(23)   Refused

IF: INCKIND = 1-7
HHldInc

INCOME SECTION - PARENT INTERVIEW
Could you look at this card again and tell me which group represents your household's gross income from all sources mentioned.

ASK OR RECORD
IF SINGLE PERSON HOUSEHOLD RECORD GROUP NO.AT INDIVIDUAL
INCOME.

ENTER GROUP NO. OR CODE 23 FOR REFUSAL
SHOW CARD 25

PARENT SELF-COMPLETION QUESTIONNAIRE

SCIntr

I would now like to you to take the computer and answer the next set of questions yourself.

PCGSc

INTERVIEWER: RESPONDENTS SHOULD SELF-COMPLETE. OFFER TO READ THE QUESTIONS FROM THE PRINTED SCRIPT BUT THE RESPOND-ENTS SHOULD STILL TYPE THE ANSWERS INTO THE LAPTOP THEMSELVES IF AT ALL POSSIBLE

(1)   Complete self-completion by respondent
(2)   Questions read from script by the interviewer
(3)   Section read and entered by interviewer

SCTest

This question is just to help you to get used to answering the questions in this section.
I like using computers
PRESS 1 for STRONGLY AGREE
PRESS 2 for AGREE
PRESS 3 for DISAGREE
PRESS 4 for STRONGLY DISAGREE

(1)   Strongly agree
(2)   Agree
(3)   Disagree
(4)   Strongly disagree

HthIntr

We would like to know how your health has been in general, over the past few weeks. Please answer ALL the questions by entering the number next to the answer which describes how you have been feeling recently
THE QUESTION WILL ALWAYS APPEAR AT THE TOP OF THE SCREEN
PRESS <ENTER> TO MOVE ON TO THE FIRST QUESTION

GH1

Have you recently been able to concentrate on whatever you're doing?
ENTER THE NUMBER NEXT TO YOUR ANSWER

(1)   Better than usual
(2)   Same as usual
(3)   Less than usual
(4)   Much less than usual

GH2

Have you recently lost much sleep over worry?

(1)   Not at all

(2)   No more than usual
(3)   Rather more than usual
(4)   Much more than usual

GH3

Have you recently felt that you are playing a useful part in things?

(1)   More so than usual
(2)   Same as usual
(3)   Less so than usual
(4)   Much less useful

GH4

Have you recently felt capable of making decisions about things?

(1)   More so than usual
(2)   Same as usual
(3)   Less so than usual
(4)   Much less capable

GH5

Have you recently felt constantly under strain?

(1)   Not at all
(2)   No more than usual
(3)   Rather more than usual
(4)   Much more than usual

GH6

Have you recently felt you couldn't overcome your difficulties?

(1)   Not at all
(2)   No more than usual
(3)   Rather more than usual
(4)   Much more than usual

GH7

Have you recently been able to enjoy your normal day-to-day activities?

(1)   More so than usual
(2)   Same as usual
(3)   Less so than usual
(4)   Much lessthan usual

GH8

Have you recently been able to face up to your problems?

(1)   More so than usual
(2)   Same as usual
(3)   Less able than usual
(4)   Much less able

GH9

Have you recently been feeling unhappy and depressed?

(1)   Not at all
(2)   No more than usual
(3)   Rather more than usual
(4)   Much more than usual

GH10

Have you recently been losing confidence in yourself?

(1)   Not at all
(2)   No more than usual
(3)   Rather more than usual
(4)   Much more than usual

GH11

Have you recently been thinking of yourself as a worthless person?

(1)   Not at all
(2)   No more than usual
(3)   Rather more than usual
(4)   Much more than usual

GH12

Have you recently been feeling reasonably happy, all things considered?

(1)   More so than usual
(2)   Same as usual
(3)   Less so than usual
(4)   Much lessthan usual

FamIntr

We would like to know how your family gets on together.

Please answer ALL the next set of questions by pressing
1 for STRONGLY AGREE
2 for AGREE
3 for DISAGREE
4 for STRONGLY DISAGREE
THE QUESTION WILL ALWAYS APPEAR AT THE TOP OF THE SCREEN
PRESS <ENTER> TO MOVE TO THE NEXT QUESTION

FF1

Planning family activities is difficult because we misunderstand each other

(1)   Strongly agree
(2)   Agree
(3)   Disagree
(4)   Strongly disagree

FF2

In times of crisis we can turn to each other for support

(1)   Strongly agree
(2)   Agree
(3)   Disagree
(4)   Strongly disagree

FF3

We cannot talk to each other about the sadness we feel

(1)   Strongly agree
(2)   Agree
(3)   Disagree
(4)   Strongly disagree

FF4

Individuals are accepted for what they are

(1)   Strongly agree
(2)   Agree
(3)   Disagree
(4)   Strongly disagree

FF5

We avoid discussing our fears and concerns

(1)   Strongly agree
(2)   Agree
(3)   Disagree
(4)   Strongly disagree

FF6

We can express feelings to each other

(1)   Strongly agree
(2)   Agree
(3)   Disagree
(4)   Strongly disagree

FF7

There is lots of bad feeling in the family

(1)   Strongly agree
(2)   Agree
(3)   Disagree
(4)   Strongly disagree

FF8

We feel accepted for what we are

(1)   Strongly agree
(2)   Agree
(3)   Disagree
(4)   Strongly disagree

FF9

Making decisions is a problem for our family

(1)   Strongly agree
(2)   Agree
(3)   Disagree
(4)   Strongly disagree

FF10

We are able to make decisions on how to solve problems

(1)   Strongly agree
(2)   Agree
(3)   Disagree
(4)   Strongly disagree

FF11

We don't get along well together

(1)   Strongly agree
(2)   Agree
(3)   Disagree
(4)   Strongly disagree

FF12

We confide in each other

(1)   Strongly agree
(2)   Agree
(3)   Disagree
(4)   Strongly disagree

SCExit

Thank you. that is the end of this section.
Please pass the computer back to the interviewer
INTERVIEWER:

IF: PCGSc = SCAccept
PHowCmp

INTERVIEWER: Did the parent complete the whole of this section as a self-completion?

(1)   Yes
(2)   No

ParEnd

THIS IS THE END OF THE PARENT INTERVIEW

CHILD INTERVIEW
(Face to face interview with 11-15 year olds)

ChldNow

INTERVIEWER: Do you want to interview the child now?

(1)   Yes
(2)   No

Friendships

CA1

Do you have any friends?

(1)   Yes
(2)   No

IF: CA1 = Yes
CA2

[*] How much time do you spend together...
RUNNING PROMPT

(1)   all of your spare time
(2)   some of your spare time
(3)   a little of your spare time
(4)   or not at all?

IF: CA1 = Yes
CA4

[*] How often do friends come to your house..
RUNNING PROMPT

(1)   all or most of the time
(2)   some of the time
(3)   or a little time
(4)   or not at all?

IF: CA1 = YES
CA5

[*] How often do you go to your friend's home..
RUNNING PROMPT

(1) all or most of the time
(2) some of the time
(3) a little time
(4) or not at all?

IF: CA1 = YES
CA6

[*] Can you confide in any of your friends such as sharing a secret or telling them private things?
SHOW CARD 1

(1) Definitely
(2) Sometimes
(3) Not at all

IF: CA1 = YES
CA10

[*] (Can I just check) Do you have a 'best' friend or a special friend?

(1) Yes
(2) No

CA15
Over the past 12 months have you belonged to any teams, clubs or other groups with an adult in charge?
INCLUDE CLUBS SUCH AS SCOUTS/GUIDES OR SCHOOL CLUBS

(1) Yes
(2) No

Strengths and difficulties

IntrSDQ

The next section is about your personality and behaviour this is to give us an overall view of your strengths and difficulties - we will be coming back to specific areas in more detail later in the interview.

SectnB

For each item that I am going to read out can you please tell me whether it is 'not true', 'somewhat true' or 'certainly true' for you
SHOW CARD 2

CB4

[*] I try to be nice to other people, I care about their feelings
SHOW CARD 2

(5) Not true
(6) Somewhat true
(7) Certainly true

CB5

[*] I am restless, I cannot stay still for long
SHOW CARD 2

(5) Not true
(6) Somewhat true
(7) Certainly true

CB6

[*] I get a lot of headaches,stomach aches or sickness
SHOW CARD 2

(5) Not true
(6) Somewhat true
(7) Certainly true

CB7

[*] I usually share with others(food, games, pens etc.)
SHOW CARD 2

(5) Not true
(6) Somewhat true
(7) Certainly true

CB8

[*] I get very angry and often lose my temper
SHOW CARD 2

(5) Not true
(6) Somewhat true
(7) Certainly true

CB9

[*] I am usually on my own, I generally play alone or keep to myself
SHOW CARD 2

(5) Not true
(6) Somewhat true
(7) Certainly true

CB10

[*] I usually do as I am told
SHOW CARD 2

(5) Not true
(6) Somewhat true
(7) Certainly true

CB11

[*] I worry a lot
SHOW CARD 2

(5) Not true
(6) Somewhat true
(7) Certainly true

CB12

[*] I am helpful if someone is hurt, upset or feeling ill
SHOW CARD 2

(5) Not true
(6) Somewhat true
(7) Certainly true

CB13

[*] I am constantly fidgeting or squirming

SHOW CARD 2

(5)   Not true
(6)   Somewhat true
(7)   Certainly true

CB14

[*] I have at least one good friend
SHOW CARD 2

(5)   Not true
(6)   Somewhat true
(7)   Certainly true

CB15

[*] I fight a lot. I can make other people do what I want
SHOW CARD 2

(5)   Not true
(6)   Somewhat true
(7)   Certainly true

CB16

[*] I am often unhappy, down-hearted or tearful
SHOW CARD 2

(5)   Not true
(6)   Somewhat true
(7)   Certainly true

CB17

[*] Other people my age generally like me
SHOW CARD 2

(5)   Not true
(6)   Somewhat true
(7)   Certainly true

CB18

[*] I am easily distracted, I find it difficult to concentrate
SHOW CARD 2

(5)   Not true
(6)   Somewhat true
(7)   Certainly true

CB19

[*] I am nervous in new situations.I easily lose my confidence
SHOW CARD 2

(5)   Not true
(6)   Somewhat true
(7)   Certainly true

CB20

[*] I am kind to younger children
SHOW CARD 2

(5)   Not true
(6)   Somewhat true
(7)   Certainly true

CB21

[*] I am often accused of lying or cheating
SHOW CARD 2

(5)   Not true
(6)   Somewhat true
(7)   Certainly true

CB22

[*] Other children or young people pick on me or bully me
SHOW CARD 2

(5)   Not true
(6)   Somewhat true
(7)   Certainly true

CB23

[*] I often volunteer to help others (parents, teachers, other children)
SHOW CARD 2

(5)   Not true
(6)   Somewhat true
(7)   Certainly true

CB24

[*] I think before I do things
SHOW CARD 2

(5)   Not true
(6)   Somewhat true
(7)   Certainly true

CB25

[*] I take things that are not mine from home, school or elsewhere
SHOW CARD 2

(5)   Not true
(6)   Somewhat true
(7)   Certainly true

CB26

[*] I get on better with adults than with people of my own age
SHOW CARD 2

(5)   Not true
(6)   Somewhat true
(7)   Certainly true

CB27

[*] I have many fears,I am easily scared
SHOW CARD 2

(5)   Not true
(6)   Somewhat true
(7)   Certainly true

CB28

[*] I finish the work I'm doing, my attention is good
SHOW CARD 2

(5)   Not true

(6)   Somewhat true
(7)   Certainly true

CB29

[*] Overall, do you think that you have difficulties in one or more of the following areas: emotions,concentration, behaviour or getting on with other people?
SHOW CARD 3

(5)   No
(6)   Yes: minor difficulties
(7)   Yes: definite difficulties
(8)   Yes: severe difficulties

IF: CB29 = 7 OR 8
Cb29a

[*] How long have these difficulties been present?

(1)   Less than a month
(2)   One to five months
(3)   Six to eleven months
(4)   A year or more

IF: CB29 = 7 OR 8
Cb29b

[*] Do the difficulties upset or distress you..
RUNNING PROMPT
SHOW CARD 4

(5)   not at all
(6)   only a little
(7)   quite a lot
(8)   or a great deal?

IF: CB29 = 7 OR 8
CB30

[*] Do the difficulties interfere with your everyday life in terms of your
...home life?
SHOW CARD 4

(5)   not at all
(6)   only a little
(7)   quite a lot
(8)   a great deal

IF: CB29 = 7 OR 8
Cb30a

[*] (Do the difficulties interfere with your everyday life in terms of your)
... friendships?
SHOW CARD 4

(5)   not at all
(6)   only a little
(7)   quite a lot
(8)   a great deal

IF: CB29 = 7 OR 8
Cb30b

[*] (Do the difficulties interfere with your everyday life in terms of your)
... classroom learning?
SHOW CARD 4

(5)   not at all

(6)   only a little
(7)   quite a lot
(8)   a great deal

IF: CB29 = 7 OR 8
Cb30c

[*] (Do the difficulties interfere with your everyday life in terms of your)
... leisure activities?
SHOW CARD 4

(5)   not at all
(6)   only a little
(7)   quite a lot
(8)   a great deal

IF: CB29 = 7 OR 8
Cb31

[*] Do the difficulties make it harder for those around you such as your family, friends and teachers?
SHOW CARD 4

(5)   not at all
(6)   only a little
(7)   quite a lot
(8)   a great deal

Separation anxiety

CIntroF

Most (TEENAGERS/YOUNG PEOPLE are particularly attached to one person or a few key people, looking to them for security, and turning to them when distressed. They can be mum and dad, grandparents, favourite teachers, neighbours etc.

FigNamC

[*] Who are you particularly attached to?

(INTERVIEWER PLEASE NOTE: Though children and teenagers can be particularly attached to other people of the same age for eg. sisters, brothers or friends aim to identify ADULT attachment figures).
- RECORD THE NAME (OR A UNIQUE IDENTIFIER) FOR EACH PERSON

CF1a1

[*] Who are the three most important to you
RECORD BY ENTERING THE NUMBER OF THE ATTACHMENT FIGURE CHOOSE 3 ONLY - IF THREE OR LESS ENTER ALL ATTACHMENT FIGURES

AtHomeC

Do any of these people live at home with you?
ASK OR RECORD

(1)   Yes
(2)   No

IF: AtHomeC = Yes
HomeC

Which of the people live at home with you?
RECORD BY ENTERING THE NUMBER OF THE

ATTACHMENT FIGURE
ASK OR RECORD

CF2intr

This section of the interview is about how much you worry about being separated from (ATTACHMENT FIGURES). Most (TEENAGERS/YOUNG PEOPLE) have some worries of this sort, but what I would like to know about is how you compare with others of your own age. I am interested in how you are usually - not in the occasional 'off day'.

CF2

[*] Overall, in the past month, have you been particularly worried about being separated from your (ATTACH-MENT FIGURES)?

(1)   Yes
(2)   No

IF: CF2=YES OR SDQ(CHILD) EMOTION SCORE = 6+
CF2a

[*] Thinking about the past month and comparing yourself with other people of your age have you often been worried about something unpleasant happening to (ATTACHMENT FIGURES), or about losing them?
SHOW CARD 5

(5)   No more than other children of my age
(6)   A little more than other children of my age
(7)   A lot more than other children of my age

IF: CF2=YES OR SDQ(CHILD) EMOTION SCORE = 6+
CF2b

[*] (Thinking about the past month and comparing yourself with other people of your age..) have you often worried that you might be taken away from (ATTACH-MENT FIGURES) for example, by being kidnapped, taken to hospital or killed?
SHOW CARD 5

(5)   No more than other children of my age
(6)   A little more than other children of my age
(7)   A lot more than other children of my age

IF: CF2=YES OR SDQ(CHILD) EMOTION SCORE = 6+
IF: AtHomeC = YES
CF2c

[*] (Thinking about the past month and comparing yourself with other people of your age..) have you often not wanted to go to school in case something nasty happened to (ATTACHMENT FIGURES AT HOME) while you were at school?
(DO NOT INCLUDE RELUCTANCE TO GO TO SCHOOL FOR OTHER REASONS, EG. FEAR OF BULLYING OR EXAMS)
SHOW CARD 5

(5)   No more than other children of my age
(6)   A little more than other children of my age
(7)   A lot more than other children of my age

IF: CF2=YES OR SDQ(CHILD) EMOTION SCORE = 6+
CF2d

[*] (Thinking about the past month and comparing yourself with other people of your age..) have you

worried about sleeping alone?
IF DNA USE CODE '5' (No more)
SHOW CARD 5

(5)   No more than other children of my age
(6)   A little more than other children of my age
(7)   A lot more than other children of my age

IF: CF2=YES OR SDQ(CHILD) EMOTION SCORE = 6+
IF: AtHomeC = YES
CF2e

[*] (Thinking about the past month and comparing yourself with other people of your age..) have you often come out of your bedroom at night to check on, or to sleep near (ATTACHMENT FIGURES AT HOME)
IF DNA USE CODE '5' (No more)
SHOW CARD 5

(5)   No more than other children of my age
(6)   A little more than other children of my age
(7)   A lot more than other children of my age

IF: CF2=YES OR SDQ(CHILD) EMOTION SCORE = 6+
CF2f

[*] (Thinking about the past month and comparing yourself with other people of your age..) have you worried about sleeping in a strange place?
SHOW CARD 5

(5)   No more than other children of my age
(6)   A little more than other children of my age
(7)   A lot more than other children of my age

IF: CF2=YES OR SDQ(CHILD) EMOTION SCORE = 6+
IF: AtHomeC = YES
CF2h

[*] (Thinking about the past month and comparing yourself with other people of your age..) have you been particularly afraid of being alone if (HomeC[1],HomeC[2], HomeC[3]) pop out for a moment?
SHOW CARD 5

(5)   No more than other children of my age
(6)   A little more than other children of my age
(7)   A lot more than other children of my age

IF: CF2=YES OR SDQ(CHILD) EMOTION SCORE = 6+
CF2i

[*] (Thinking about the past month and comparing yourself with other people of your age..) have you had repeated nightmares or bad dreams about being separated from (ATTACHMENT FIGURES)?
SHOW CARD 5

(5)   No more than other children of my age
(6)   A little more than other children of my age
(7)   A lot more than other children of my age

IF: CF2=YES OR SDQ(CHILD) EMOTION SCORE = 6+
CF2j

[*] (Thinking about the past month and comparing yourself with other people of your age..) have you had headaches, stomach aches or felt sick when you had to leave (ATTACHMENT FIGURES) or when you knew it was about to happen?
SHOW CARD 5

(5) No more than other children of my age
(6) A little more than other children of my age
(7) A lot more than other children of my age

IF: CF2=Y<small>ES</small> OR SDQ (<small>CHILD</small>) E<small>MOTION SCORE</small> = 6+
CF2k

[*] (Thinking about the past month and comparing yourself with other people of your age..) has being apart or the thought of being apart from (ATTACHMENT FIGURES) led to worry, crying, angry outbursts,clinginess or misery?
SHOW CARD 5

(5) No more than other children of my age
(6) A little more than other children of my age
(7) A lot more than other children of my age

IF: ANY(CF2<small>A</small> - CF2<small>K</small> = 7)
CF3

[*] You have told me about your worries about separations. Have you had these for at least a month?

(1) Yes
(2) No

IF: ANY(CF2<small>A</small> - CF2<small>K</small> = 7)
CF3a

Were you like this by the age of 6?

(1) Yes
(2) No

IF: ANY(CF2<small>A</small> - CF2<small>K</small> = 7)
CF4

[*] Thinking still of your worries about separation, how much have they have upset or distressed you
RUNNING PROMPT

(5) not at all
(6) only a little
(7) quite a lot
(8) or a great deal?

IF: ANY(CF2<small>A</small> - CF2<small>K</small> = 7)
CF5Intr

I also want to ask you about the extent to which these worries have interfered with your day to day life.

IF: ANY(CF2<small>A</small> - CF2<small>K</small> = 7)
CF5a

[*] Have they interfered with...
How well you get on with the rest of the family?
SHOW CARD 4

(5) not at all
(6) only a little
(7) quite a lot
(8) a great deal

IF: ANY(CF2<small>A</small> - CF2<small>K</small> = 7)
CF5b

[*] (Have they interfered with...)
....making and keeping friends?
SHOW CARD 4

(5) not at all
(6) only a little
(7) quite a lot
(8) a great deal

IF: ANY(CF2<small>A</small> - CF2<small>K</small> = 7)
CF5c

[*] (Have they interfered with...)
...learning or class work?
SHOW CARD 4

(5) not at all
(6) only a little
(7) quite a lot
(8) a great deal

IF: ANY(CF2<small>A</small> - CF2<small>K</small> = 7)
CF5d

[*] (Have they interfered with...)
...playing, hobbies, sports or other leisure activities?
SHOW CARD 4

(5) not at all
(6) only a little
(7) quite a lot
(8) a great deal

IF: ANY(CF2<small>A</small> - CF2<small>K</small> = 7)
CF5e

[*] Have these worries about separation made it harder for those around you (family, friends or teachers) ?
SHOW CARD 4

(5) not at all
(6) only a little
(7) quite a lot
(8) a great deal

Specific phobia

CF6Intr

This section of the interview is about any particular things or situations that you are particularly scared of, even though they aren't really a danger to you. I am interested in how you are usually - not in the occasional 'off day'. I shall ask you first about particular fears, but will ask later about social fears.

CF7

[*] Are you PARTICULARLY scared about any of the things or situations on this list?
CODE ALL THAT APPLY
SHOW CARD 6

SET [7] OF
(1) ANIMALS: Insects, spiders, wasps, bees, mice, snakes, birds or any other animal
(2) Storms, thunder, heights or water
(3) Blood-injection-Injury Set off by the sight of blood or injury or by an injection
(4) Dentists or Doctors
(5) The dark
(6) Other specific situations: for example: lifts, tunnels, flying, driving, trains, buses, small enclosed spaces
(7) Any other specific fear (specify)

(9)   Not particularly scared of anything

IF: AnyOth IN CF7
CF7Oth

What are these other fears?

IF: CF7 = 1 - 7
CF7a

[*] Is this fear/are these fears a real nuisance to you, or to anyone else?

(5)   No
(6)   Perhaps
(7)   Definitely

IF: CF7 = 1 - 7
AND: (CF7A = 7) OR (SDQ (CHILD) EMOTION SCORE = 6+)
CF8

[*] How long has this fear (the most severe of these fears) been present?

(1)   less than a month
(2)   At least one month but less than 6 months
(3)   Six months or more

IF: CF7 = 1 - 7
AND: (CF7A = 7) OR (SDQ (CHILD) EMOTION SCORE = 6+)
CF9

[*] When you come up against (PHOBIC STIMULUS), or think you are about to come up against it, do you become anxious or upset?
RUNNING PROMPT

(5)   No
(6)   A little
(7)   A Lot

IF: CF7 = 1 - 7
AND: (CF7A = 7) OR (SDQ (CHILD) EMOTION SCORE = 6+)
AND: CF9 = ALot
CF9a

[*] Does this happen almost every time you come up against (PHOBIC STIMULUS)?

(1)   Yes
(2)   No

IF: CF7 = 1 - 7
AND: (CF7A = 7) OR (SDQ (CHILD) EMOTION SCORE = 6+)
AND: CF9 = ALot
CF10

[*] How often does this fear of (PHOBIC STIMULUS) result in you becoming upset like this ...
IN THE RELEVANT SEASON IF A SEASONAL STIMULUS EG. WASPS
RUNNING PROMPT

(1)   many times a day
(2)   most days
(3)   most weeks
(4)   or every now and then?

IF: CF7 = 1 - 7
AND: (CF7A = 7) OR (SDQ (CHILD) EMOTION SCORE = 6+)
CF11

[*] Does your fear lead to you avoiding (PHOBIC STIMULUS)...
RUNNING PROMPT

(5)   No
(6)   A little
(7)   A Lot

IF: CF7 = 1 - 7
AND: (CF7A = 7) OR (SDQ (CHILD) EMOTION SCORE = 6+)
AND: CF11 = ALot
CF11a

[*] How much does this avoidance interfere with your everyday life?
RUNNING PROMPT

(5)   No
(6)   A little
(7)   A Lot

IF: CF7 = 1 - 7
AND: (CF7A = 7) OR (SDQ (CHILD) EMOTION SCORE = 6+)
CF11b

[*] Thinking about it now, do you think your fear is excessive or unreasonable?
SHOW CARD 7

(5)   No
(6)   Perhaps
(7)   Definitely

IF: CF7 = 1 - 7
AND: (CF7A = 7) OR (SDQ (CHILD) EMOTION SCORE = 6+)
CF11c

[*] Are you upset about having this fear?
SHOW CARD 7

(5)   No
(6)   Perhaps
(7)   Definitely

IF: CF7 = 1 - 7
AND: (CF7A = 7) OR (SDQ (CHILD) EMOTION SCORE = 6+)
CF12

[*] Lastly, has your fear of (PHOBIC STIMULUS) made it harder for those around you (family, friends,teachers etc.) ...
RUNNING PROMPT

(5)   not at all
(6)   only a little
(7)   quite a lot
(8)   or a great deal?

Social phobia

CF13intr

I am interested in whether you are particularly afraid of social situations, that is being with a lot of people, meeting new people or having to do things in front of other people.
This is as compared with other (TEENAGERS/YOUNG PEOPLE) of you own age, and is not counting the occasional 'off day' or ordinary shyness.

CF13

[*] Overall, do you particularly fear or avoid social situations which involve a lot of people, meeting new people or doing things in front of other people?

(1)   Yes
(2)   No

IF: CF13 OR SDQ (CHILD) EMOTION SCORE 6+
CF14Intr

Can I just check, have you been particularly afraid of any of the following social situations over the last month?

IF: CF13 OR SDQ (CHILD) EMOTION SCORE 6+
CF14a

[*] Can I just check, have you been particularly afraid of . . . meeting new people?
SHOW CARD 7

(5)   No
(6)   A little
(7)   A Lot

IF: CF13 OR SDQ (CHILD) EMOTION SCORE 6+
CF14b
[*] (Can I just check, have you been particularly afraid of . . .) meeting a lot of people, such as at a party?
SHOW CARD 7

(5)   No
(6)   A little
(7)   A Lot

IF: CF13 OR SDQ (CHILD) EMOTION SCORE 6+
CF14c

[*] (Can I just check, have you been particularly afraid of) . . .eating in front of others?
SHOW CARD 7

(5)   No
(6)   A little
(7)   A Lot

IF: CF13 OR SDQ (CHILD) EMOTION SCORE 6+
CF14d

[*] (Can I just check, have you been particularly afraid of) . . .speaking in class?
SHOW CARD 7

(5)   No
(6)   A little
(7)   A Lot

IF: CF13 OR SDQ (CHILD) EMOTION SCORE 6+
CF14e

[*] (Can I just check, have you been particularly afraid of) . . .reading out loud in front of others?
SHOW CARD 7

(5)   No
(6)   A little
(7)   A Lot

IF: CF13 OR SDQ (CHILD) EMOTION SCORE 6+
CF14f

[*] (Can I just check, have you been particularly afraid of) . . .writing in front of others?
SHOW CARD 7

(5)   No
(6)   A little
(7)   A Lot

IF: CF13 OR SDQ (CHILD) EMOTION SCORE 6+
AND: SEPARATION ANXIETY AND ANY (CF14A - CF14F)=7
CF15

[*] Are your fears of social situations mainly related to you worries about being separated from (ATTACHMENT FIGURES) OR are you still afraid of social situations even when you are with them?

(1)   mainly related to his/her fear of being apart from attachment figures
(2)   marked even when attachment figure present

IF: CF13 OR SDQ (CHILD) EMOTION SCORE 6+
AND: ANY (CF14A - CF14F)=7 AND CF15=2
CF16

[*] Are you just afraid with adults, or are you also afraid in situations that involve a lot of (TEENAGERS/YOUNG PEOPLE), or meeting new people of your age?

(1)   Just with adults
(2)   just with children
(3)   With both children and adults

I IF: CF13 OR SDQ (CHILD) EMOTION SCORE 6+
AND: ANY (CF14A - CF14F)=7 AND CF15=2
CF17

[*] Outside of these social situations, are you able to get on well enough with the adults and (TEENAGERS/YOUNG PEOPLE) you know best?

(1)   Yes
(2)   No

IF: CF13 OR SDQ (CHILD) EMOTION SCORE 6+
AND: ANY (CF14A - CF14F)=7 AND CF15=2
CF18

[*] Is the main reason you dislike social situations because you are afraid you will act in a way that will be embarrassing or show you up?

(5)   No
(6)   Perhaps
(7)   Definitely

IF: CF13 OR SDQ (CHILD) EMOTION SCORE 6+
AND: ANY (CF14A - CF14F)=7 AND CF15=2
AND: ANY (CF14D-CF14F=6 OR 7)
CF18a

[*] Do you dislike social situations because of specific problems with speaking, reading or writing?

(5)   No
(6)   Perhaps
(7)   Definitely

IF: CF13 OR SDQ (CHILD) EMOTION SCORE 6+
AND: ANY (CF14A - CF14F)=7 AND CF15=2
CF19

[*] How long has this fear of social situations been present?

(1)   Less than a month
(2)   At least one month but less than six months
(3)   Six months or more

IF: CF13 OR SDQ (CHILD) EMOTION SCORE 6+
AND: ANY (CF14A - CF14F)=7 AND CF15=2
CF20

[*] What age did it begin at..
RUNNING PROMPT

(1)   under six years or
(2)   six years or above?

IF: CF13 OR SDQ (CHILD) EMOTION SCORE 6+
AND: ANY (CF14A - CF14F)=7 AND CF15=2
CFblush

[*] When you are in one of the social situations you dislike, do you normally... blush (go red) or shake (tremble)?

(1)   Yes
(2)   No

IF: CF13 OR SDQ (CHILD) EMOTION SCORE 6+
AND: ANY (CF14A - CF14F)=7 AND CF15=2
CFSick

[*] (When you are in one of the social situations you dislike, do you normally...)
feel afraid that you are going to be sick (throw up)?

(1)   Yes
(2)   No

IF: CF13 OR SDQ (CHILD) EMOTION SCORE 6+
AND: ANY (CF14A - CF14F)=7 AND CF15=2
CFShort

[*] (When you are in one of the social situations you dislike, do you normally...)
need to rush off to the toilet or worry that you might be caught short?

(1)   Yes
(2)   No

IF: CF13 OR SDQ (CHILD) EMOTION SCORE 6+
AND: ANY (CF14A - CF14F)=7 AND CF15=2
CF21

[*] When you are in one of the social situations you fear, or when you think you are about to be in one, do your become anxious or upset?

(5)   No
(6)   A little
(7)   A Lot

IF: CF13 OR SDQ (CHILD) EMOTION SCORE 6+
AND: ANY (CF14A - CF14F)=7 AND CF15=2
IF: CF21 = ALOT
CF22

[*] How often does this happen

RUNNING PROMPT

(1)   many times a day
(2)   most days
(3)   most weeks
(4)   or every now and then?

IF: CF13 OR SDQ (CHILD) EMOTION SCORE 6+
AND: ANY (CF14A - CF14F)=7 AND CF15=2
CF23

[*] Does your fear lead to you avoiding social situations...
SHOW CARD 7

(5)   No
(6)   A little
(7)   A Lot

IF: CF13 OR SDQ (CHILD) EMOTION SCORE 6+
AND: ANY (CF14A - CF14F)=7 AND CF15=2
IF: CF23 = ALOT
CF23a

[*] How much does this avoidance interfere with your everyday life?
SHOW CARD 7

(5)   No
(6)   A little
(7)   A Lot

IF: CF13 OR SDQ (CHILD) EMOTION SCORE 6+
AND: ANY (CF14A - CF14F)=7 AND CF15=2
CF23b

[*] Thinking about it now, do you think that your fears is excessive or unreasonable?
SHOW CARD 8

(5)   No
(6)   Perhaps
(7)   Definitely

IF: CF13 OR SDQ (CHILD) EMOTION SCORE 6+
AND: ANY (CF14A - CF14F)=7 AND CF15=2
CF23c

[*] Are you upset about having this fear?
SHOW CARD 8

(5)   No
(6)   Perhaps
(7)   Definitely

IF: CF13 OR SDQ (CHILD) EMOTION SCORE 6+
AND: ANY (CF14A - CF14F)=7 AND CF15=2
CF24

[*] Has your fear of social situations made it harder for those around you (family, friends or teachers)
RUNNING PROMPT
SHOW CARD 4

(5)   not at all
(6)   only a little
(7)   quite a lot
(8)   or a great deal?

Panic attacks and agoraphobia

CF25Intr

Many (TEENAGERS/YOUNG PEOPLE) have times when they get very anxious or worked up about silly little things, but some get severe panics that come out of the blue - they just don't seem to have any trigger at all.

CF25

[*] In the last month have you had a panic attack when you suddenly became very panicky for no reason at all, without even a little thing to set you off?

(1)   Yes
(2)   No

IF: CF25 = Yes
CFStart

[*] Can I just check..
Do your panics start very suddenly?

(1)   Yes
(2)   No

IF: CF25 = Yes
CFPeak

[*] Do they reach a peak within a few minutes (up to 10)?

(1)   Yes
(2)   No

IF: CF25 = Yes
CFHowLng

[*] Do they last at least a few minutes?

(1)   Yes
(2)   No

IF: CF25 = Yes
CHeart

[*] When you are feeling panicky, do you also feel... your heart racing, fluttering or pounding away?

(1)   Yes
(2)   No

IF: CF25 = Yes
CFSweat

[*] (When you are feeling panicky, do you also feel...) sweaty?

(1)   Yes
(2)   No

IF: CF25 = Yes
CFTremb

[*] (When you are feeling panicky, do you also feel...) trembly or shaky?

(1)   Yes
(2)   No

IF: CF25 = Yes
CFMouth

[*] (When you are feeling panicky, do you also feel...) that your mouth is dry?

(1)   Yes
(2)   No

IF: CF25 = Yes
CFBreath

[*] (When you are feeling panicky, do you also feel...) that it is hard to get your breath or that you are suffocating?

(1)   Yes
(2)   No

IF: CF25 = Yes
CFChoke

[*] (When you are feeling panicky, do you also feel...) that you are choking?

(1)   Yes
(2)   No

IF: CF25 = Yes
CFPain

[*] (When you are feeling panicky, do you also feel...) pain or an uncomfortable feeling in your chest?

(1)   Yes
(2)   No

IF: CF25 = Yes
CFsick

[*] (When you are feeling panicky, do you also feel...) that you want to be sick (throw up) or that your stomach is turning over?

(1)   Yes
(2)   No

IF: CF25 = Yes
CFDizz

[*] (When you are feeling panicky, do you also feel...) dizzy, unsteady, faint or light-headed?

(1)   Yes
(2)   No

IF: CF25 = Yes
CFunreal

[*] (When you are feeling panicky, do you also feel...) as though things around you were unreal or you were not really there?

(1)   Yes
(2)   No

IF: CF25 = Yes
CFCrazy

[*] (When you are feeling panicky, do you also feel...) afraid that you might lose control, go crazy or pass out?

(1)   Yes
(2)   No

IF: CF25 = Yes
CFDie

[*] (When you are feeling panicky, do you also feel...) afraid you might die?

(1)   Yes
(2)   No

IF: CF25 = Yes
CFCold

[*] (When you are feeling panicky, do you also feel...) hot or cold all over?

(1)   Yes
(2)   No

IF: CF25 = Yes
CFNumb

[*] (When you are feeling panicky, do you also feel...) numbness or tingling feelings in your body?

(1)   Yes
(2)   No

CF26

[*] In the last month have you been very afraid of, or tried to avoid, the things on this card?
CODE ALL THAT APPLY
SHOW CARD 9

SET [4] OF
(1)   Crowds
(2)   public places
(3)   Travelling alone (if you ever do)
(4)   Being far from home
(9)   None of the above

IF: CF26=1-4
CF27

[*] Is this fear or avoidance of (SITUATION) mostly because you are afraid that if you had a panic attack or something like that (such as dizziness or diarrhoea), you would find it difficult or embarassing to get away, or would not be able to get the help you need?

(1)   Yes
(2)   No

Post Traumatic Stress Disorder

CE1

The next section is about events or situations that are exceptionally stressful, and that would really upset almost anyone. For example, being caught in a burning house, being abused, being in a serious car crash or seeing a member of your family or friends being mugged at gun point.

[*] During your lifetime has anything like this happened to you?

(1)   Yes
(2)   No

IF: CE1 = Yes
CE1a

What was it, please describe?

IF: CE1 = Yes
CE1c

DO YOU REGARD THIS AS AN EXCEPTIONALLY STRESSFUL OR TRAUMATIC EVENT?

INTERVIEWER CODE

(1)   Yes
(2)   No

IF: CE1 = Yes
IF: CE1c=Yes
CE1b

[*] At the time, were you very upset or badly affected by it in someway?

(1)   Yes
(2)   No

IF: CE1 = Yes
IF: CE1c = Yes
CE2

[*] At present, is it affecting your behaviour, feelings or concentration?

(1)   Yes
(2)   No

IF: CE1 = Yes
AND: CE2 = Yes
CE2a

[*] Over the last month, have you . .
. . 'relived' the event with vivid memories (flashbacks) of it?
SHOW CARD 7

(5)   No
(6)   A little
(7)   A Lot

IF: CE1 = Yes
AND: CE2 = Yes
CE2b

[*] (Over the last month, have you. .)
.. had a lot of upsetting dreams of the event?
SHOW CARD 7

(5)   No
(6)   A little
(7)   A Lot

IF: CE1 = Yes
AND: CE2 = Yes
CE2c

[*] (Over the last month, have you. .)
.. got upset if anything happened which reminded you of it?
SHOW CARD 7

(5)   No
(6)   A little
(7)   A Lot

IF: CE1 = YES
AND: CE2 = YES
CE2d

[*] (Over the last month, have you. .)
.. tried to avoid thinking or talking about anything to do with the event?
SHOW CARD 7

(5)   No
(6)   A little
(7)   A Lot

IF: CE1 = YES
AND: CE2 = YES
CE2e

[*] (Over the last month, have you. .)
.. tried to avoid activities places or people that remind you of the event?
SHOW CARD 7

(5)   No
(6)   A little
(7)   A Lot

IF: CE1 = YES
AND: CE2 = YES
CE2f

[*] (Over the last month, have you. .)
.. blocked out important details of the event from your memory?
SHOW CARD 7

(5)   No
(6)   A little
(7)   A Lot

IF: CE1 = YES
AND: CE2 = YES
CE2g

[*] (Over the last month, have you. .)
.. shown much less interest in activities you used to enjoy?
SHOW CARD 7

(5)   No
(6)   A little
(7)   A Lot

IF: CE1 = YES
AND: CE2 = YES
CE2h

[*] (Over the last month, have you. .)
.. felt cut off or distant from others?
SHOW CARD 7

(5)   No
(6)   A little
(7)   A Lot

IF: CE1 = YES
IF: CE2 = YES
CE2i

[*] (Over the last month, have you. .)
.. expressed a smaller range of feelings than in the past, e.g. no longer able to express loving feelings?
SHOW CARD 7

(5)   No
(6)   A little
(7)   A Lot

IF: CE1 = YES
AND: CE2 = YES
CE2j

[*] (Over the last month, have you. .)
.. felt less confidence in the future?
SHOW CARD 7

(5)   No
(6)   A little
(7)   A Lot

IF: CE1 = YES
AND: CE2 = YES
CE2k

[*] (Over the last month, have you. .)
.. had problems sleeping?
SHOW CARD 7

(5)   No
(6)   A little
(7)   A Lot

IF: CE1 = YES
AND: CE2 = YES
CE2l

[*] (Over the last month, have you. .)
.. felt irritable or angry?
SHOW CARD 7

(5)   No
(6)   A little
(7)   A Lot

IF: CE1 = YES
AND: CE2 = YES
CE2m

[*] (Over the last month, have you. .)
.. had difficulty concentrating?
SHOW CARD 7

(5)   No
(6)   A little
(7)   A Lot

IF: CE1 = YES
AND: CE2 = YES
CE2n

[*] (Over the last month, have you. .)
.. always been on the alert for possible dangers?
SHOW CARD 7

(5)   No
(6)   A little
(7)   A Lot

IF: CE1 = YES
AND: CE2 = YES
CE2o

[*] (Over the last month, have you. .)
.. jumped at little noises or easily startled in other ways?
SHOW CARD 7

(5) No
(6) A little
(7) A Lot

IF: CE1 = YES
AND: CE2 = YES
AND: ANY (CE2A-CE2O)=7
CE3

[*] You have told me about (TRAUMATIC EVENT)
How long after the event did these problems begin?

(1) within six months
(2) More than six months after the event

IF: CE1 = YES
AND: CE2 = YES
AND: ANY (CE2A-CE2O)=7
CE4

[*] How long have you been having these problems?

(1) Less than a month
(2) At least one month but less than three months
(3) Three months or more

IF: CE1 = YES
AND: CE2 = YES
AND: ANY (CE2A-CE2O)=7
CE5

[*] How much have these problems upset or distressed you...
RUNNING PROMPT

(5) not at all
(6) only a little
(7) quite a lot
(8) or a great deal?

IF: CE1 = YES
AND: CE2 = YES
AND: ANY (CE2A-CE2O)=7
CE6a

[*] Have they interfered with...
how well you get on with the rest of your family?
SHOW CARD 4

(5) not at all
(6) only a little
(7) quite a lot
(8) a great deal

IF: CE1 = YES
AND: CE2 = YES
AND: ANY (CE2A-CE2O)=7
CE6b

[*] (Have they interfered with...)
.. making and keeping friends?
SHOW CARD 4

(5) not at all
(6) only a little
(7) quite a lot
(8) a great deal

IF: CE1 = YES
AND: CE2 = YES
AND: ANY (CE2A-CE2O)=7
CE6c

[*] (Have they interfered with...)
.. learning or class work?
SHOW CARD 4

(5) not at all
(6) only a little
(7) quite a lot
(8) a great deal

IF: CE1 = YES
AND: CE2 = YES
AND: ANY (CE2A-CE2O)=7
CE6d

[*] (Have they interfered with...)
.. playing, hobbies, sports or other leisure activities?
SHOW CARD 4

(5) not at all
(6) only a little
(7) quite a lot
(8) a great deal

IF: CE1 = YES
AND: CE2 = YES
AND: ANY (CE2A-CE2O)=7
CE7

[*] Have these problems made it harder for those around you (family, friends and teachers etc.). .
RUNNING PROMPT

(5) not at all
(6) only a little
(7) quite a lot
(8) or a great deal?

Compulsions and obsessions

CF28Intr

Many young people have some habits or superstitions, such as not stepping on the cracks in the pavement, or having to go through a special goodnight ritual, or having to wear lucky clothes or have a lucky mascot for exams or football/netball matches. It is also common for young people to go through phases when they seem obsessed by one particular subject or activity. I want to ask whether you have rituals or obsessions that go beyond this.

CF28

[*] Overall, do you have rituals or obsessions that upset you, waste a lot of time, or interfere with your ability to get on with everyday life?

(1) Yes
(2) No

IF: CF28=YES OR SDQ (CHILD) EMOTION SCORE = 6+
CF29Intr

Can I just check, over the last month have you been doing any of the following things over and over again even though you have already done them or don't need to do them at all?

IF: CF28=Yes OR SDQ (child) Emotion score = 6+
CF29a

[*] (Over the last month have you been doing any of the following things over and over again even though you have already done them or don't need to do them at all)

Excessive cleaning; handwashing, baths, showers, toothbrushing etc.?
SHOW CARD 7

(5) No
(6) A little
(7) A Lot

IF: CF28=Yes OR SDQ (child) Emotion score = 6+
CF29b

[*] (Over the last month have you been doing any of the following things over and over again even though you have already done them or don't need to do them at all)

Other special measures to avoid dirt, germs or poisons?
SHOW CARD 7

(5) No
(6) A little
(7) A Lot

IF: CF28=Yes OR SDQ (child) Emotion score = 6+
CF29c

[*] (Over the last month have you been doing any of the following things over and over again even though you have already done them or don't need to do them at all)

Checking: doors, locks, oven, gas taps, electric switches?
SHOW CARD 7

(5) No
(6) A little
(7) A Lot

IF: CF28=Yes OR SDQ (child) Emotion score = 6+
CF29d

[*] (Over the last month have you been doing any of the following things over and over again even though you have already done them or don't need to do them at all)
Repeating actions: going in and out of the door many times in a row, or getting up/down from a chair or anything like this?
SHOW CARD 7

(5) No
(6) A little
(7) A Lot

IF: CF28=Yes OR SDQ (child) Emotion score = 6+
CF29e

[*] (Over the last month have you been doing any of the following things over and over again even though you have already done them or don't need to do them at all)

Touching things or people in particular ways?
SHOW CARD 7

(5) No
(6) A little
(7) A Lot

IF: CF28=Yes OR SDQ (child) Emotion score = 6+
CF29f

[*] (Over the last month have you been doing any of the following things over and over again even though you have already done them or don't need to do them at all)

Arranging things so they are just so, or exactly symmetrical?
SHOW CARD 7

(5) No
(6) A little
(7) A Lot

IF: CF28=Yes OR SDQ (child) Emotion score = 6+
CF29g

[*] (Over the last month have you been doing any of the following things over and over again even though you have already done them or don't need to do them at all)

Counting to particular lucky numbers or avoiding unlucky numbers?
SHOW CARD 7

(5) No
(6) A little
(7) A Lot

IF: CF28=Yes OR SDQ (child) Emotion score = 6+
CF31a

[*] Over the last month, have you been thinking over and over again about dirt, germs or poisons?
SHOW CARD 7

(5) No
(6) A little
(7) A Lot

IF: CF28=Yes OR SDQ (child) Emotion score = 6+
CF31b

[*] (Over the last month, have you been thinking over and over again about any of the following) ... Something terrible happening to yourself or others - illnesses,accidents, fires etc.?
SHOW CARD 7

(5) No
(6) A little
(7) A Lot

IF: CF28=Yes OR SDQ (child) Emotion score = 6+
AND: Separation anxiety AND F31b = ALot
CF32

[*] Is this just part of your general concern about being separated from (ATTACHMENT FIGURES) or is this a serious additional problem in its own right?

(1) part of separation anxiety
(2) a problem in it's own right

IF: CF28=Yes OR SDQ (child) Emotion score = 6+
AND: Problem is not part of separation anxiety (CF32=2)
CF33

[*] You have just told me about your habits and obsessions. Have they been present on most days for a period of at least two weeks?

(1)   Yes
(2)   No

*IF: CF28=YES OR SDQ (CHILD) EMOTION SCORE = 6+
AND: PROBLEM IS NOT PART OF SEPARATION ANXIETY
(CF32=2)*
CF34

[*] Does you think that these (acts/thoughts) are
excessive or unreasonable?

(5)   No
(6)   Sometimes
(7)   Definitely

*IF: CF28=YES OR SDQ (CHILD) EMOTION SCORE = 6+
AND: PROBLEM IS NOT PART OF SEPARATION ANXIETY
(CF32=2)*
CF35

[*] Do you try not to do them or think about them?

(5)   No
(6)   Perhaps
(7)   Definitely

*IF: CF28=YES OR SDQ (CHILD) EMOTION SCORE = 6+
AND: PROBLEM IS NOT PART OF SEPARATION ANXIETY
(CF32=2)*
CF36

[*] Do you become upset because you have to do or
think these things?

(5)   No, I enjoy them
(6)   Neutral,I neither enjoy them nor become upset
(7)   Sometimes/somewhat upset
(8)   Upset a great deal

*IF: CF28=YES OR SDQ (CHILD) EMOTION SCORE = 6+
AND: PROBLEM IS NOT PART OF SEPARATION ANXIETY
(CF32=2)*
CF37

[*] Do these (acts/thoughts) use up at least an hour a
day on average?

(1)   Yes
(2)   No

*IF: CF28=YES OR SDQ (CHILD) EMOTION SCORE = 6+
AND: PROBLEM IS NOT PART OF SEPARATION ANXIETY
(CF32=2)*
CF38a

[*] Have these acts/thoughts interfered with ...
.. how well s/he gets on with the rest of your family?
SHOW CARD 4

(5)   not at all
(6)   only a little
(7)   quite a lot
(8)   a great deal

*IF: CF28=YES OR SDQ (CHILD) EMOTION SCORE = 6+
AND: PROBLEM IS NOT PART OF SEPARATION ANXIETY
(CF32=2)*
CF38b

[*] (Have these acts/thoughts interfered with ...)
... making and keeping friends?
SHOW CARD 4

(5)   not at all
(6)   only a little
(7)   quite a lot
(8)   a great deal

*IF: CF28=YES OR SDQ (CHILD) EMOTION SCORE = 6+
AND: PROBLEM IS NOT PART OF SEPARATION ANXIETY
(CF32=2)*
CF38c

[*] (Have these acts/thoughts interfered with ...)
...learning or class work?
SHOW CARD 4

(5)   not at all
(6)   only a little
(7)   quite a lot
(8)   a great deal

*IF: CF28=YES OR SDQ (CHILD) EMOTION SCORE = 6+
AND: PROBLEM IS NOT PART OF SEPARATION ANXIETY
(CF32=2)*
CF38d

[*] (Have these acts/thoughts interfered with ...)
...playing, hobbies, sports or other leisure activities?
SHOW CARD 4

(5)   not at all
(6)   only a little
(7)   quite a lot
(8)   a great deal

*IF: CF28=YES OR SDQ (CHILD) EMOTION SCORE = 6+
AND: PROBLEM IS NOT PART OF SEPARATION ANXIETY
(CF32=2)*
CF38e

[*] Have these acts/thoughts made it harder for those
around you (family, friends or teachers etc.)?
SHOW CARD 4

(5)   not at all
(6)   only a little
(7)   quite a lot
(8)   a great deal

Generalised anxiety

GenAInt

What I want to ask about next is worries. Nearly all
(TEENAGERS/YOUNG PEOPLE) have some worries,
and these are naturally worse on some days than
others, but some (TEENAGERS/YOUNG PEOPLE)
have so many worries for so much of the time that it
makes them really upset or interferes with their lives.

CF40

[*] What I am asking about now is general worrying
(apart from your SPECIFIC ANXIETIES)
Do you ever worry?

(1)   Yes
(2)   No

IF: CF40 = YES
CF40a

[*] Over the last six months, have you worried so much

about so many things that it has really upset you or interfered with your life?

(5) No
(6) Perhaps
(7) Definitely

IF: CF40 = YES
AND: CF40A=6 OR 7 OR SDQ (CHILDS) EMOTION SCORE=6+
CF41a

[*] Thinking of the last 6 months and by comparing yourself with other people of your age, have you worried about: Past behaviour: Did I do that wrong? Have I upset someone? Have they forgiven me?
SHOW CARD 5

(5) No more than other children of my age
(6) A little more than other children of my age
(7) A lot more than other children of my age

IF: CF40 = YES
AND: CF40A=6 OR 7 OR SDQ (CHILDS) EMOTION SCORE=6+
CF41b

[*] (Thinking of the last 6 months and by comparing yourself with other people of your age, have you worried about:) School work,homework or examinations
SHOW CARD 5

(5) No more than other children of my age
(6) A little more than other children of my age
(7) A lot more than other children of my age

IF: CF40 = YES
AND: CF40A=6 OR 7 OR SDQ (CHILDS) EMOTION SCORE=6+
CF41c

[*] (Thinking of the last 6 months and by comparing yourself with other people of your age, have you worried about:) Disasters: Burglaries, muggings, fires, bombs etc.
SHOW CARD 5

(5) No more than other children of my age
(6) A little more than other children of my age
(7) A lot more than other children of my age

IF: CF40 = YES
AND: CF40A=6 OR 7 OR SDQ (CHILDS) EMOTION SCORE=6+
CF41d

[*] (Thinking of the last 6 months and by comparing yourself with other people of your age, have you worried about:) Your own health
SHOW CARD 5

(5) No more than other children of my age
(6) A little more than other children of my age
(7) A lot more than other children of my age

IF: CF40 = YES
AND: CF40A=6 OR 7 OR SDQ (CHILDS) EMOTION SCORE=6+
CF41e

[*] (Thinking of the last 6 months and by comparing yourself with other people of your age, have you

worried about:) Bad things happening to others: family, friends, pets, the world..
SHOW CARD 5

(5) No more than other children of my age
(6) A little more than other children of my age
(7) A lot more than other children of my age

IF: CF40 = YES
AND: CF40A=6 OR 7 OR SDQ (CHILDS) EMOTION SCORE=6+
CF41f

[*] (Thinking of the last 6 months and by comparing yourself with other people of your age, have you worried about:) The future: e.g. getting a job, boy/girlfriend, moving out
SHOW CARD 5

(5) No more than other children of my age
(6) A little more than other children of my age
(7) A lot more than other children of my age

IF: CF40 = YES
AND: CF40A=6 OR 7 OR SDQ (CHILDS) EMOTION SCORE=6+
CF41g

[*] Do you worry about anything else?

(1) Yes
(2) No

IF: CF40 = YES
AND: CF40A=6 OR 7 OR SDQ (CHILDS) EMOTION SCORE=6+
IF: CF41G = YES
CF41ga

[*] What else do you worry about?

IF: CF40 = YES
AND: CF40A=6 OR 7 OR SDQ (CHILDS) EMOTION SCORE=6+
IF: CF41G = YES
CF41gb

[*] How much do you worry about this?
SHOW CARD 5

(5) No more than other children of my age
(6) A little more than other children of my age
(7) A lot more than other children of my age

IF: TWO OF CF41A-CF41GB=7
CF42DV

INTERVIEWER CHECK: Are there two or more specific worries (SPECIFIC WORRIES) over and above those which have already been mentioned in earlier sections?

(1) Yes
(2) No

IF: CF40 = YES
IF: CF42DV = YES
CF43

[*] Over the last six months have you been really worried on more days than not?

(1) Yes
(2) No

IF: CF40 = YES
AND: CF42DV=YES AND CF43=YES
CF44

[*] Do you find it difficult to control the worry?

(1)   Yes
(2)   No

IF: CF40 = YES
AND: CF42DV=YES AND CF43=YES
CF45

[*] Does worrying lead to you being restless, feeling keyed up, tense or on edge, or being unable to relax?

(1)   Yes
(2)   No

IF: CF40 = YES
AND: CF42DV=YES AND CF43=YES
AND: CF45 = YES
CF45a

[*] Has this been true for more days than not in the last six months?

(1)   Yes
(2)   No

IF: CF40 = YES
AND: CF42DV=YES AND CF43=YES
CF46

[*] Does worrying lead to you feeling tired or 'worn out' more easily?

(1)   Yes
(2)   No

IF: CF40 = YES
AND: CF42DV=YES AND CF43=YES
IF: CF46 = YES
CF46a

[*] Has this been true for more days than not in the last six months?

(1)   Yes
(2)   No

IF: CF40 = YES
AND: CF42DV=YES AND CF43=YES
CF47

[*] Does worrying lead to difficulties in concentrating or or your mind going blank?

(1)   Yes
(2)   No

IF: CF40 = YES
AND: CF42DV=YES AND CF43=YES
AND: CF47 = YES
CF47a

[*] Has this been true for more days than not in the last six months?

(1)   Yes
(2)   No

IF: CF40 = YES
AND: CF42DV=YES AND CF43=YES
CF48

[*] Does worrying make you feel irritable?

(1)   Yes
(2)   No

IF: CF40 = YES
AND: CF42DV=YES AND CF43=YES
AND: CF48 = YES
CF48a

[*] Has this been true for more days than not in the last six months?

(1)   Yes
(2)   No

IF: CF40 = YES
AND: CF42DV=YES AND CF43=YES
CF49

[*] Does worrying lead to you feeling tense in your whole body?

(1)   Yes
(2)   No

IF: CF40 = YES
AND: CF42DV=YES AND CF43=YES
AND: CF49 = YES
CF49a

[*] Has this been true for more days than not in the last six months?

(1)   Yes
(2)   No

IF: CF40 = YES
AND: CF42DV=YES AND CF43=YES
CF50

[*] Does worrying interfere with your sleep, making it difficult to fall or stay asleep, or making your sleep restless and unsatisfying?

(1)   Yes
(2)   No

IF: CF40 = YES
AND: CF42DV=YES AND CF43=YES
AND: CF50 = YES
CF50a

[*] Has this been true for more days than not in the last six months?

(1)   Yes
(2)   No

IF: CF40 = YES
AND: CF42DV=YES AND CF43=YES
AND: CF50 = YES
CF51

[*] Overall, how much do your various worries upset and distress you ...
RUNNING PROMPT

(5)   not at all
(6)   only a little
(7)   quite a lot
(8)   or a great deal?

IF: CF40 = YES
AND: CF42DV=YES AND CF43=YES
IF: CF50 = YES
CF52Intr

I now want to ask you about the extent to which these worries have interfered with your day to day life.

IF: CF40 = YES
AND: CF42DV=YES AND CF43=YES
AND: CF50 = YES
CF52a

[*] Have they interfered with ...
how well you get on with the rest of your family?
SHOW CARD 4

(5)   not at all
(6)   only a little
(7)   quite a lot
(8)   a great deal

IF: CF40 = YES
AND: CF42DV=YES AND CF43=YES
IF: CF50 = YES
CF52b

[*] (Have they interfered with ...)
making and keeping friends?
SHOW CARD 4

(5)   not at all
(6)   only a little
(7)   quite a lot
(8)   a great deal

IF: CF40 = YES
AND: CF42DV=YES AND CF43=YES
IF: CF50 = YES
CF52c

[*] (Have they interfered with ...)
learning or class work?
SHOW CARD 4

(5)   not at all
(6)   only a little
(7)   quite a lot
(8)   a great deal

IF: CF40 = YES
AND: CF42DV=YES AND CF43=YES
IF: CF50 = YES
CF52d

[*] (Have they interfered with ...)
playing, hobbies, sports or other leisure activities?
SHOW CARD 4

(5)   not at all
(6)   only a little
(7)   quite a lot
(8)   a great deal

IF: CF40 = YES
AND: CF42DV=YES AND CF43=YES
IF: CF50 = YES

CF53

[*] Have your worries made it harder for those around you (family, friends or teachers etc)
RUNNING PROMPT

(5)   not at all
(6)   only a little
(7)   quite a lot
(8)   or a great deal?

Depression

CDepInt

This next section of the interview is about your mood.

CG1

[*] In the past month, have there been times when you have been very sad, miserable, unhappy or tearful?

(1)   Yes
(2)   No

IF: CG1 = YES
CG3

[*] Over this month was there a period when you were really miserable nearly every day?

(1)   Yes
(2)   No

IF: CG1 = YES
CG4

[*] During the time when you were really miserable were you really miserable for most of the day? (i.e. more hours than not)

(1)   Yes
(2)   No

IF: CG1 = YES
CG5

[*] When you were miserable, could you be cheered up...
RUNNING PROMPT

(1)   easily
(2)   with difficulty/only briefly
(3)   or not at all?

IF: CG1 = YES
CG6

[*] Can you tell me how long that period lasted?

(1)   less than two weeks
(2)   two weeks or more

CG8

[*] In the past month, have there been times when you have been grumpy or irritable in a way that was out of character for you?

(1)   Yes
(2)   No

IF: CG8 = YES
CG10

[*] Over this month, was there a period when you were really irritable nearly every day?

(1)   Yes
(2)   No

IF: CG8 = YES
CG11

[*] During the time when you were grumpy or irritable, were you like this for most of the day? (i.e. more hours than not)

(1)   Yes
(2)   No

IF: CG8 = YES
CG12

[*] Was the irritability improved by particular activities, friends coming around or anything else...
RUNNING PROMPT

(1)   easily
(2)   with difficulty/only briefly
(3)   or not at all?

IF: CG8 = YES
CG13

[*] Can you tell me how long that period lasted?

(1)   less than two weeks
(2)   two weeks or more

CG15

[*] In the past month, has there been a time when you lost interest in everything, or nearly everything, you normally enjoy doing?

(1)   Yes
(2)   No

IF: CG15 = YES
CG17

[*] Over this month, was there a period when you were lacking in interest nearly every day?

(1)   Yes
(2)   No

IF: CG15 = YES
CG18

[*] During these days when you lost interest in things, were you like this for most of each day? (i.e. more hours than not)

(1)   Yes
(2)   No

IF: CG15 = YES
CG19

[*] Can you tell me how long this loss of interest lasted?

(1)   less than two weeks
(2)   two weeks or more

IF: CG15 = YES
IF: (CG3 OR CG4=YES) OR (CG10 OR CG11=YES)
CG20

[*] Was this loss of interest present during the same period when you were really miserable/irritable for most of the time?

(1)   Yes
(2)   No

IF: ((CG10 OR CG11=YES) OR (CG3 OR CG4 = YES)) OR (CG17 = YES)
CG21a

[*] (During that time when you were (IRRITABLE/ DEPRESSED/LACKING INTEREST)...)
did you lack energy and seem tired all the time?

(1)   Yes
(2)   No

IF: ((CG10 OR CG11=YES) OR (CG3 OR CG4 = YES)) OR (CG17 = YES)
CG21b

[*] .... were you eating much more or much less than normal?

(1)   Yes
(2)   No

IF: ((CG10 OR CG11=YES) OR (CG3 OR CG4 = YES)) OR (CG17 = YES)
CG21ba

[*] ...did you either lose or gain a lot of weight?

(1)   Yes
(2)   No

IF: ((CG10 OR CG11=YES) OR (CG3 OR CG4 = YES)) OR (CG17 = YES)
CG21c

[*] ... did you find it hard to get to sleep?

(1)   Yes
(2)   No

IF: ((CG10 OR CG11=YES) OR (CG3 OR CG4 = YES)) OR (CG17 = YES)
CG21d

[*] ... did you sleep too much?

(1)   Yes
(2)   No

IF: ((CG10 OR CG11=YES) OR (CG3 OR CG4 = YES)) OR (CG17 = YES)
CG21e

[*] ...were you agitated or restless much of the time?

(1)   Yes
(2)   No

IF: ((CG10 OR CG11=YES) OR (CG3 OR CG4 = YES)) OR (CG17 = YES)
CG21f

[*] ... did you feel worthless or unnecessarily guilty for much of the time?

(1)   Yes
(2)   No

IF: ((CG10 OR CG11=YES) OR (CG3 OR CG4 = YES))
OR (CG17 = YES)
CG21g

[*] ....did you find it unusually hard to concentrate or to think things out?

(1)   Yes
(2)   No

IF: ((CG10 OR CG11=YES) OR (CG3 OR CG4 = YES))
OR (CG17 = YES))
CG21h

[*] ... did you think about death a lot?

(1)   Yes
(2)   No

IF: ((CG10 OR CG11=YES) OR (CG3 OR CG4 = YES))
OR (CG17 = YES))
CG21k

[*] Over the whole of your lifetime have you ever tried to harm yourself or kill yourself?

(1)   Yes
(2)   No

IF: ((CG10 OR CG11=YES) OR (CG3 OR CG4 = YES))
OR (CG17 = YES))
IF: CG21K = YES
CG21j

(During that time when you were (IRRITABLE/DE-PRESSED/LACKING INTEREST) did you ever try to harm yourself or kill yourself?

(1)   Yes
(2)   No

IF: ((CG10 OR CG11=YES) OR (CG3 OR CG4 = YES))
OR (CG17 = YES))
CG21i

[*] .... did you ever talk about harming yourself or killing yourself?

(1)   Yes
(2)   No

IF: ((CG10 OR CG11=YES) OR (CG3 OR CG4 = YES))
OR (CG17 = YES))
CG22

[*] .... Overall, how upset and distressed are you as a result of this.
RUNNING PROMPT

(5)   not at all
(6)   only a little
(7)   quite a lot
(8)   or a great deal?

IF: ((CG10 OR CG11=YES) OR (CG3 OR CG4 = YES))
OR (CG17 = YES))

CG23Intr

I also want to ask you about the extent to which (IRRITABLE/DEPRESSED/ A LACK OF INTEREST) has interfered with your day to day life.
SHOWCARD 4

IF: ((CG10 OR CG11=YES) OR (CG3 OR CG4 = YES))
OR (CG17 = YES))
CG23a

[*] Has this interfered with ...
how well you get on with the rest of your family?
SHOW CARD 4

(5)   not at all
(6)   only a little
(7)   quite a lot
(8)   a great deal

IF: ((CG10 OR CG11=YES) OR (CG3 OR CG4 = YES))
OR (CG17 = YES))
CG23b

[*] (Has this interfered with ...)
making and keeping friends?
SHOW CARD 4

(5)   not at all
(6)   only a little
(7)   quite a lot
(8)   a great deal

IF: ((CG10 OR CG11=YES) OR (CG3 OR CG4 = YES))
OR (CG17 = YES))
CG23c

[*] (Has this interfered with ...)
learning or class work?
SHOW CARD 4

(5)   not at all
(6)   only a little
(7)   quite a lot
(8)   a great deal

IF: ((CG10 OR CG11=YES) OR (CG3 OR CG4 = YES))
OR (CG17 = YES))
CG23d

[*] (Has this interfered with ...)
playing, hobbies, sports or other leisure activities?
SHOW CARD 4

(5)   not at all
(6)   only a little
(7)   quite a lot
(8)   a great deal

IF: ((CG10 OR CG11=YES) OR (CG3 OR CG4 = YES))
OR (CG17 = YES))
CG24

[*] Has feeling (DEPRESSED/IRRITABLE/A LACK OF INTEREST) made it harder for those around you (family, friends, teachers etc...
RUNNING PROMPT

(5)   not at all
(6)   only a little
(7)   quite a lot
(8)   or a great deal?

IF: ((CG10 OR CG11=YES) OR (CG3 OR CG4 = YES)) OR (CG17 = YES))
CG25

[*] Over the past month have you thought about harming or hurting yourself?

(1)   Yes
(2)   No

IF: ((CG10 OR CG11=YES) OR (CG3 OR CG4 = YES)) OR (CG17 = YES))
CG26

[*] Over the past month, have you ever tried to harm or hurt yourself?

(1)   Yes
(2)   No

IF: ((CG10 OR CG11=YES) OR (CG3 OR CG4 = YES)) OR (CG17 = YES))
CG27

[*] Over the whole of your lifetime, have you ever tried to harm or hurt yourself?

(1)   Yes
(2)   No

Attention and activity

AttnInt

This section of the interview is about concentration and activity.

CH1

[*] Do your teachers complain about you having problems with overactivity or poor concentration?
SHOW CARD 7

(5)   No
(6)   A little
(7)   A Lot

CH2

[*] Do your family complain about you having problems with overactivity or poor concentration?
SHOW CARD 7

(5)   No
(6)   A little
(7)   A Lot

CH3

[*] And what do you think? Do you think you have definite problems with overactivity or poor concentration?
SHOW CARD 7

(5)   No
(6)   A little
(7)   A Lot

Awkward and troublesome behaviour

CI1

This next section is about behaviour that sometimes gets young people into trouble with parents, teachers or other adults. Do your teachers complain about you being awkward or troublesome?
SHOW CARD 7

(5)   No
(6)   A little
(7)   A Lot

CI2

Do your family complain about you being awkward or troublesome?
SHOW CARD 7

(5)   No
(6)   A little
(7)   A Lot

CI3

And what do you think, do you think you are awkward or troublesome?
SHOW CARD 7

(5)   No
(6)   A little
(7)   A Lot

Less common disorders

LessInt

This next section is about a variety of different aspects of behaviour and development.

CI4

Do you have any tics or twitches that you can't seem to control?

(1)   Yes
(2)   No

CI5
Do you have dyslexia or reading difficulties?

(1)   Yes
(2)   No

CI6

Have other people been concerned that you have been dieting too much?

(1)   Yes
(2)   No

CI7

Have you had any out-of-ordinary experiences - such as seeing or hearing things, or having unusual ideas - that have worried or frightened you?

(1)   Yes
(2)   No

Significant problem(s)

IF: SIGNIFICANT PROBLEM HAS BEEN IDENTIFIED (I.E. CHILD HAS SYMPTOMS AND THESE ARE CAUSING AN IMPACT OR BURDEN) IN ONE OR MORE AREA.

CSigInt

You have told me about (LIST OF PROBLEMS)
I'd now like to hear a bit more about these in your own words.

CTypNow

INTERVIEWER: if you prefer to take notes by hand rather than typing the details during the interview just type 'later' in the response boxes - but please remember to come back and complete the question before transmission.
WILL YOU BE TYPING IN THE ANSWERS NOW OR LATER

(1)   Now
(2)   Later

CSigPrb

LIST OF PROBLEMS
INTERVIEWER: Please try and cover all areas of difficulty, but it is a good idea to let the young person choose which order to cover them in, starting with the area that concerns them most.

Use the suggested prompts written below and on the prompt card.

1.   Description of the problem?
2.   How often does the problem occur?
3.   How severe is the problem at its worst?
4.   How long has it been going on for?
5.   Is the problem interfering with the child's quality of life?
       If so, how?
6.   WHERE APPROPRIATE,record what the child thinks the problem is
        due to, and what s/he has done about it.

CAnxity

Do you experience any of the following when you feel anxious, nervous or tense
INDIVIDUAL PROMPT

SET [7] OF
(1)   Heart racing or pounding?
(2)   Hands sweating or shaking?
(3)   Feeling dizzy?
(4)   Difficulty getting my breath?
(5)   Butterflies in stomach?
(6)   Dry mouth?
(7)   Nausea or feeling as though I wanted to be sick?
(8)   or none of the above?

Strengths

SIntro

I have been asking you a lot of questions about difficulties and problems. I now want to ask you about your good points or strengths.

CPerslty

[*] In terms of what sort of person you are, what would you say are the best things about you?

OPEN

CPersNo

INTERVIEWER: Did the child mention any qualities?

(1)   Yes
(2)   No

CQuality

[*] Can you tell me some things you have done that you are really proud of? They could be related to school, sport, music, friends, charity or anything else

CQualNo

INTERVIEWER: Did the child mention any things they are proud of?

(1)   Yes
(2)   No

EndFTF

THIS IS THE END OF THE CHILD'S FACE TO FACE INTERVIEW -
PLEASE CONTINUE WITH THE CHILD'S SELF-COMPLETION

CHILD SELF-COMPLETION

CSCIntr

I would now like you to take the computer and answer the next set of questions yourself

ChldSc

INTERVIEWER: RESPONDENTS SHOULD SELF-COMPLETE.
ENCOURAGE THE CHILD TO COMPLETE THIS SECTION THEMSELVES
IF ABSOLUTELY NECESSARY ADMINISTER AS AN INTERVIEW

(1)   Complete self-completion by respondent
(2)   Section read and entered by interviewer

Confid

Take your time to read each question carefully in turn and answer it as best you can.
REMEMBER THAT WE ARE ONLY INTERESTED IN YOUR OPINION. THIS IS NOT A TEST

SCTest

This question is just to help you to get used to answering the questions in this section.

Do you like using computers?
PRESS 1 for No PRESS 2 for Just a bit PRESS 3 for

Definitely THEN

(1)   No
(2)   Just a bit
(3)   Definitely

Chronic fatigue syndrome (M.E)

C3D1

Over the last month have you been feeling much more tired and worn out than usual?
PRESS 1 for No PRESS 2 for Yes THEN

(1)   No
(2)   Yes

IF: C3D1 = Yes
C3D2

Why do you think this is?
TYPE IN YOUR ANSWER AND THE

IF: C3D1 = Yes
C3D3

How long have you been feeling tired and worn out like this?

(1)   less than 3 months
(2)   3-5 months
(3)   6 months to 5 years
(4)   Over 5 years
(5)   All my life

IF: C3D1 = Yes
C3D4

Do you feel better after resting?

(1)   Not at all
(2)   only a bit
(3)   Definitely better

IF: C3D1 = Yes
C3D5

Does exercise really wipe you out for the next day?

(1)   No
(2)   Yes

IF: C3D1 = Yes
C3D6

Do you suffer from sore throats?

(1)   No
(2)   A bit
(3)   A lot

IF: C3D1 = Yes
C3D7

Do you suffer from painful glands (lumps) in your neck or armpits?

(1)   No
(2)   A bit
(3)   A lot

IF: C3D1 = Yes
C3D8

Do you suffer from painful muscles?

(1)   No
(2)   A bit
(3)   A lot

IF: C3D1 = Yes
C3D9

Do you suffer from pains in you knees, elbows, wrists or other joints?

(1)   No
(2)   A bit
(3)   A lot

IF: C3D1 = Yes
C3D10

Do you suffer from headaches?

(1)   No
(2)   A bit
(3)   A lot

IF: C3D1 = Yes
C3D11

Do you suffer from problems getting to sleep or staying asleep?

(1)   No
(2)   A bit
(3)   A lot

IF: C3D1 = Yes
C3D12

Do you suffer from feeling sick/wanting to throw up?

(1)   No
(2)   A bit
(3)   A lot

IF: C3D1 = Yes
C3D13

Do you suffer from dizziness or poor balance?

(1)   No
(2)   A bit
(3)   A lot

IF: C3D1 = Yes
C3D14

You have told me about feeling more tired and worn-out than usual. Overall, how much has this upset or distressed you?

(1)   Not at all
(2)   only a little
(3)   quite a lot
(4)   a great deal

IF: C3D1 = Yes
C3D15

Has feeling tired and worn-out interfered with ...
How well you get on with the rest of your family?

(1) not at all
(2) only a little
(3) quite a lot
(4) a great deal

IF: C3D1 = Yes
C3D16

(Has feeling tired and worn-out interfered with ...)
making and keeping friends?

(1) not at all
(2) only a little
(3) quite a lot
(4) a great deal

IF: C3D1 = Yes
C3D17

(Has feeling tired and worn-out interfered with ...)
learning or class work?

(1) not at all
(2) only a little
(3) quite a lot
(4) a great deal

IF: C3D1 = Yes
C3D18

(Has feeling tired and worn-out interfered with ...)
playing, hobbies, sports or other leisure activities?

(1) not at all
(2) only a little
(3) quite a lot
(4) a great deal

IF: C3D1 = Yes
C3D19

Has feeling tired and worn-out made it harder for those
around you (family, friends or teachers etc)
RUNNING PROMPT

(1) not at all
(2) only a little
(3) quite a lot
(4) or a great deal?

Awkward and troublesome behaviour

C3A4a

Thinking of the last year, have you often told lies to get
things or favours from others, or to get out of having to
do things you are supposed to do?
ENTER THE NUMBER OF THE ANSWER WHICH
APPLIES TO YOU

(1) No
(2) perhaps
(3) Definitely

IF: C3A4a = Def
C3A4aa

Has this been going on for the last 6 months?

ENTER 1 FOR 'NO' AND 2 FOR 'YES'

(1) No
(2) Yes

C3A4b

Have you often started fights in the past year?
ENTER THE NUMBER OF THE ANSWER WHICH
APPLIES TO YOU

(1) No
(2) perhaps
(3) Definitely

IF: C3A4b = Def
C3A4ba

Has this been going on for the last 6 months?
ENTER 1 FOR 'NO' AND 2 FOR 'YES'

(1) No
(2) Yes

C3A4c

During the past year, have you often bullied or threat-
ened people?
ENTER THE NUMBER OF THE ANSWER WHICH
APPLIES TO YOU

(1) No
(2) perhaps
(3) Definitely

IF: C3A4c = Def
C3A4ca

Has this been going on for the last 6 months?
ENTER 1 FOR 'NO' AND 2 FOR 'YES'

(1) No
(2) Yes

C3A4d

Thinking of the past year, have you often stayed out
later than you were supposed to?
ENTER THE NUMBER OF THE ANSWER WHICH
APPLIES TO YOU

(1) No
(2) perhaps
(3) Definitely

IF: C3A4d = Def
C3A4da

Has this been going on for the last 6 months?
ENTER 1 FOR 'NO' AND 2 FOR 'YES'

(1) No
(2) Yes

C3A4e

Have you stolen valuable things from your house or
other people's houses. shops or school in the past year?
ENTER THE NUMBER OF THE ANSWER WHICH
APPLIES TO YOU

(1)   No
(2)   perhaps
(3)   Definitely

IF: C3A4ᴇ = Dᴇғ
C3A4ea

Has this been going on for the last 6 months?
ENTER 1 FOR 'NO' AND 2 FOR 'YES'

(1)   No
(2)   Yes

C3A4f

Have you run away from home more than once or ever stayed away all night without permission in the past year?
ENTER THE NUMBER OF THE ANSWER WHICH APPLIES TO YOU

(1)   No
(2)   perhaps
(3)   Definitely

IF: C3A4ꜰ = Dᴇғ
C3A4fa

Has this been going on for the last 6 months?
ENTER 1 FOR 'NO' AND 2 FOR 'YES'

(1)   No
(2)   Yes

C3A4g

Thinking of the past year, have you often played truant ('bunked off') from school?

(1)   No
(2)   perhaps
(3)   Definitely

IF: C3A4ɢ = Dᴇғ
C3A4ga

Has this been going on for the last 6 months?
ENTER 1 FOR 'NO' AND 2 FOR 'YES'

(1)   No
(2)   Yes

IF: C3A4ɢ = Dᴇғ
AND: Cʜɪʟᴅ 13+ ʏᴇᴀʀꜱ ᴏʟᴅꜱ
C3A5

Did you start playing truant ('bunking off') from school before you were 13 years old?
ENTER 1 FOR 'NO' AND 2 FOR 'YES'

(1)   No
(2)   Yes

IF: ANY(C3A3ᴀ-C3A3ɢ=Dᴇғ) OR SDQ (ᴄʜɪʟᴅ) Cᴏɴᴅᴜᴄᴛ = 4+
C3A6a

The next few questions are about some other behaviours that sometimes get people into trouble. We have to ask everyone these questions even when they are not likely to apply. In the past year, have you ever used a weapon against another person (e.g. a bat, brick, broken bottle, knife, gun)?

ENTER 1 FOR 'NO' AND 2 FOR 'YES'

(1)   No
(2)   Yes

IF: ANY(C3A3ᴀ-C3A3ɢ=Dᴇғ) OR SDQ (ᴄʜɪʟᴅ) Cᴏɴᴅᴜᴄᴛ = 4+
IF: C3A6ᴀ = Yᴇꜱ
C3A6aa

Has this happened in the last 6 months?
ENTER 1 FOR 'NO' AND 2 FOR 'YES'

(1)   No
(2)   Yes

IF: ANY(C3A3ᴀ-C3A3ɢ=Dᴇғ) OR SDQ (ᴄʜɪʟᴅ) Cᴏɴᴅᴜᴄᴛ = 4+
C3A6b

In the past year, have you really hurt someone or been physically cruel to them, for example, tied up, cut or burned someone?
ENTER 1 FOR 'NO' AND 2 FOR 'YES'

(1)   No
(2)   Yes

IF: ANY(C3A3ᴀ-C3A3ɢ=Dᴇғ) OR SDQ (ᴄʜɪʟᴅ) Cᴏɴᴅᴜᴄᴛ = 4+
IF: C3A6ʙ = Yᴇꜱ
C3A6ba

Has this happened in the last 6 months?
ENTER 1 FOR 'NO' AND 2 FOR 'YES'

(1)   No
(2)   Yes

IF: ANY(C3A3ᴀ-C3A3ɢ=Dᴇғ) OR SDQ (ᴄʜɪʟᴅ) Cᴏɴᴅᴜᴄᴛ = 4+)
C3A6c

Have you been really cruel to animals or birds on purpose in the past year (eg. tied them up, cut or burnt them)?
ENTER 1 FOR 'NO' AND 2 FOR 'YES'

(1)   No
(2)   Yes

IF: ANY(C3A3ᴀ-C3A3ɢ=Dᴇғ) OR SDQ (ᴄʜɪʟᴅ) Cᴏɴᴅᴜᴄᴛ = 4+
IF: C3A6ᴄ = Yᴇꜱ
C3A6ca

Has this happened in the last 6 months?
ENTER 1 FOR 'NO' AND 2 FOR 'YES'

(1)   No
(2)   Yes

IF: ANY(C3A3ᴀ-C3A3ɢ=Dᴇғ) OR SDQ (ᴄʜɪʟᴅ) Cᴏɴᴅᴜᴄᴛ = 4+
C3A6d

Have you deliberately started a fire in the past year?
(DO NOT INCLUDE BURNING INDIVIDUAL MATCHES OR PIECES OF PAPER, CAMP FIRES ETC.)
ENTER 1 FOR 'NO' AND 2 FOR 'YES'

(1)   No
(2)   Yes

IF: (C3A4DV >= 1) OR (QC1INT.QC1SDQ.SCONDUCT > 3)
IF: C3A6D = YES
C3A6da

Has this happened in the last 6 months?
ENTER 1 FOR 'NO' AND 2 FOR 'YES'

(1)   No
(2)   Yes

IF: (C3A4DV >= 1) OR (QC1INT.QC1SDQ.SCONDUCT > 3)
C3A6e

Thinking of the past year, have you deliberately destroyed someone else's property? (eg. smashing car windows or destroying school property
ENTER 1 FOR 'NO' AND 2 FOR 'YES'

(1)   No
(2)   Yes

IF: ANY(C3A3A-C3A3G=DEF) OR SDQ (CHILD) CONDUCT = 4+
IF: C3A6E = YES
C3A6ea

Has this happened in the last 6 months?
ENTER 1 FOR 'NO' AND 2 FOR 'YES'

(1)   No
(2)   Yes

IF: ANY(C3A3A-C3A3G=DEF) OR SDQ (CHILD) CONDUCT = 4+
C3A6f

Have you been involved in stealing from someone in the street?
ENTER 1 FOR 'NO' AND 2 FOR 'YES'

(1)   No
(2)   Yes

IF: ANY(C3A3A-C3A3G=DEF) OR SDQ (CHILD) CONDUCT = 4+
IF: C3A6F = YES
C3A6fa

Has this happened in the last 6 months?
ENTER 1 FOR 'NO' AND 2 FOR 'YES'

(1)   No
(2)   Yes

IF: ANY(C3A3A-C3A3G=DEF) OR SDQ (CHILD) CONDUCT = 4+
C3A6g

During the past year have you tried to force someone into sexual activity against their will?
ENTER 1 FOR 'NO' AND 2 FOR 'YES'

(1)   No
(2)   Yes

IF: ANY(C3A3A-C3A3G=DEF) OR SDQ (CHILD) CONDUCT = 4+
IF: C3A6G = YES
C3A6ga

Has this happened in the last 6 months?
ENTER 1 FOR 'NO' AND 2 FOR 'YES'

(1)   No
(2)   Yes

IF: ANY(C3A3A-C3A3G=DEF) OR SDQ (CHILD) CONDUCT = 4+
C3A6h

Have you broken into a house, any other building or a car in the past year?

(1)   No
(2)   Yes

IF: ANY(C3A3A-C3A3G=DEF) OR SDQ (CHILD) CONDUCT = 4+
AND: C3A6H = YES
C3A6ha

Has this happened in the last 6 months?

(1)   No
(2)   Yes

C3A7

Have you ever been in trouble with the police?

(1)   No
(2)   Yes

IF: ANY(C3A3A-C3A3G=DEF) OR SDQ (CHILD) CONDUCT = 4+
IF: C3A7 = YES
C3A7a

Please type in why you were in trouble with the police.

C3A8a

You have told me about some behaviours that have got you into trouble. How far have these interfered with how well you get on with the rest of your family?

(1)   not at all
(2)   only a little
(3)   quite a lot
(4)   a great deal

IF: (ANY(C3A3A-C3A3G=DEF) OR SDQ (CHILD) CONDUCT = 4+) OR (C3A7 = YES)
C3A8b

You have told me about some behaviours that have got you into trouble. How far have these interfered with making and keeping friends?

(1)   not at all
(2)   only a little
(3)   quite a lot
(4)   a great deal

IF:(ANY(C3A3A-C3A3G=DEF) OR SDQ (CHILD) CONDUCT = 4+) OR (C3A7 = YES)
C3A8c

You have told me about some behaviours that have got you into trouble. How far have these interfered with learning or class work?

(1)   not at all
(2)   only a little
(3)   quite a lot
(4)   a great deal

IF: (ANY(C3A3A-C3A3G=DEF) OR SDQ (CHILD) CONDUCT = 4+) OR (C3A7 = YES)
C3A8d

You have told me about some behaviours that have got you into trouble. How far have these interfered with playing, hobbies, sports or other leisure activities?

(1)   not at all
(2)   only a little
(3)   quite a lot
(4)   a great deal

IF: (ANY(C3A3A-C3A3G=DEF) OR SDQ (CHILD) CONDUCT = 4+) OR (C3A7 = YES)
C3A9

Have your behaviour made it harder for those around you (family, friends or teachers etc.)?

(1)   not at all
(2)   only a little
(3)   quite a lot
(4)   a great deal

Moods and feelings

MoodIntr

These next few questions are about how you might have been acting or feeling recently. For each statement please say whether it was true most of the time, sometimes true or not true about you.

C3C1

(In the past two weeks)
I felt miserable or unhappy?
TYPE 1 for 'Mostly true' 2 for 'Sometimes true' OR 3 for 'Not True'.

(1)   Mostly true
(2)   Sometimes true
(3)   Not true

C3C2

(In the past two weeks)
I didn't enjoy anything at all?
TYPE 1 for 'Mostly true' 2 for 'Sometimes true' OR 3 for 'Not True'.

(1)   Mostly true
(2)   Sometimes true
(3)   Not true

C3C3

(In the past two weeks)
I felt so tired I just sat around and did nothing?
TYPE 1 for 'Mostly true' 2 for 'Sometimes true' OR 3 for 'Not True'.

(1)   Mostly true
(2)   Sometimes true
(3)   Not true

C3C4

(In the past two weeks)
I was very restless?
TYPE 1 for 'Mostly true' 2 for 'Sometimes true' OR 3 for 'Not True'.

(1)   Mostly true
(2)   Sometimes true
(3)   Not true

C3C5

(In the past two weeks)
I felt I was no good any more?
TYPE 1 for 'Mostly true' 2 for 'Sometimes true' OR 3 for 'Not True'.

(1)   Mostly true
(2)   Sometimes true
(3)   Not true

C3C6

(In the past two weeks)
I cried a lot?

(1)   Mostly true
(2)   Sometimes true
(3)   Not true

C3C7

(In the past two weeks)
I found it hard to think properly or concentrate?

(1)   Mostly true
(2)   Sometimes true
(3)   Not true

C3C8

(In the past two weeks)
I hated myself?

(1)   Mostly true
(2)   Sometimes true
(3)   Not true

C3C9

(In the past two weeks)
I was a bad person?

(1)   Mostly true
(2)   Sometimes true
(3)   Not true

C3C10

(In the past two weeks)
I felt lonely?

(1)   Mostly true
(2)   Sometimes true
(3)   Not true

C3C11

(In the past two weeks)
I thought nobody really loved me?

(1)   Mostly true
(2)   Sometimes true
(3)   Not true

C3C12

(In the past two weeks)
I thought I could never be as good as other young people?

(1)   Mostly true
(2)   Sometimes true
(3)   Not true

C3C13

(In the past two weeks)
I did everything wrong?

(1)   Mostly true
(2)   Sometimes true
(3)   Not true

C3C14

What word best describes how you have felt in the past 2 weeks?

Help from others

C3B1

Have you ever felt so unhappy or worried that you have asked people for help?
PRESS 1 for NO, 2 for YES

(1)   No
(2)   Yes

IF: C3B1 = Yes
C3B1a

Who did you ask for help?
ENTER '10' IF YOU DID NOT ASK ANY OF THESE PEOPLE FOR HELP

SET [10] OF
(1)   Mother
(2)   Father
(3)   Brother or Sister
(4)   Special friend
(5)   School Teacher
(6)   School Nurse
(7)   Doctor
(8)   Social worker
(9)   Telephone helpline
(10)   None of these

IF: C3B1 = Yes
C3B1oth

Did you ask anyone else for help?
PRESS 1 for NO, 2 for YES

(1)   No
(2)   Yes

IF: C3B1 = Yes
AND: C3B1oth = Yes
C3B1Spec

Who else did you ask for help?

PLEASE TYPE IN YOUR ANSWER

IF: C3B1 = Yes
AND: C3B1a=1-9 OR C3B1oth = Yes
C3B1b

Were you trying to get practical advice or did you just need someone to talk things over with?

(1)   Practical advice
(2)   Talk things over
(3)   Both,practical advice and to talk things over

IF: C3B1 = No
C3B2

If you ever felt so unhappy or worried that you needed to ask for help, who would you talk to?
ENTER '10' IF YOU WOULD NOT ASK ANY OF THESE PEOPLE FOR HELP

SET [10] OF
(1)   Mother
(2)   Father
(3)   Brother or Sister
(4)   Special friend
(5)   School Teacher
(6)   School Nurse
(7)   Doctor
(8)   Social worker
(9)   Telephone helpline
(10)   None of these

IF: C3B1 = No
C3B2Oth

Is there anyone else you would ask for help?
PRESS 1 for NO, 2 for YES

(1)   No
(2)   Yes

IF: C3B1 = No
IF: C3B2Oth = Yes
C3B2Spec

Who else would you ask for help?

PLEASE TYPE IN YOUR ANSWER

IF: C3B1 = No
IF: (C3B2=1-8)OR (C3B2Oth = Yes)
C3B2a

What sort of help would you expect to get?

(1)   Practical advice
(2)   Talk things over
(3)   Both,practical advice and to talk things over

Smoking

C3E1

Do you smoke cigarettes at all these days?
TYPE 1 FOR 'NO' AND 2 FOR 'YES'

(1)   No
(2)   Yes

C3E2

Now read all the following statements carefully and type in the number next to the one which best describes you.

(1)   I have never smoked
(2)   I have only tried smoking once
(3)   I used to smoke cigarettes but I never smoke now
(4)   I sometimes smoke cigarettes now, but I don't smoke as many as one a week
(5)   I usually smoke between 1 - 6 cigarettes a week
(6)   I usually smoke more than 6 cigarettes a week

IF: C3E2 = NEVER
C3E3

Just to check, read the statements below carefully and type in the number next to the one which best describes you.

(1)   I have never tried smoking a cigarette, not even a puff or two
(2)   I did once have a puff or two of a cigarette, but I never smoke now
(3)   I do sometimes smoke cigarettes

IF: C3E3 = 3
C3E3a

About how many cigarettes a day do you usually smoke?
IF YOU SMOKE LESS THAN 1, ENTER 0

0..98

Drinking

C3F1

Have you ever had a proper alcoholic drink - a whole drink not just a sip ?
PLEASE DO NOT INCLUDE DRINKS LABELLED LOW ALCOHOL

PRESS 1 for 'NO' or 2 for 'YES' THEN PRESS ENTER

(1)   No
(2)   Yes

IF: C3F1 = YES
C3F2

How often do you usually have an alcoholic drink?

(1)   Almost every day
(2)   About twice a week
(3)   About once a week
(4)   About once a fortnight
(5)   About once a month
(6)   Only a few times a year
(7)   I never drink alcohol

IF: C3F1 = YES
C3F3

When did you last have an alcoholic drink?

(1)   Today
(2)   Yesterday

(3)   Some other time during the last week
(4)   One week, but less than two weeks ago
(5)   Two weeks, but less than four weeks ago
(6)   One month, but less than six months ago
(7)   Six months ago or more

Drug use

CanIntr

The next set of questions are about drugs

The first few questions are about marijuana and hashish. Marijuana is also called cannabis, hash, dope, grass, ganja, kif. Marijuana is usually smoked either in cigarettes, called joints, or in a pipe.

C3C1

Have you ever had a chance to try marijuana or hashish? Having a 'chance to try' means that cannabis was available to you if you wanted to use it or not?
PRESS 1 for NO, 2 for YES,

(1)   No
(2)   Yes

C3c2

Have you ever, even once, used cannabis?
PRESS 1 for NO, 2 for YES, 3 for DON'T KNOW

(1)   No
(2)   Yes
(3)   Never heard of cannabis/don't know

IF: C3c2 = YES
C3c3

Have you ever used cannabis more than 5 times in your life?
PRESS 1 FOR NO, 2 FOR YES

(1)   No
(2)   Yes

IF: C3c2 = YES
C3C4

About how old were you the first time you used cannabis, even once?

0..15

IF: C3c2 = YES
C3C5

About how often have you used cannabis in the past year?

(1)   About daily
(2)   2 or 3 times a week
(3)   about once a week
(4)   about once a month
(5)   only a once or twice in past year
(6)   not at all in past year

IF: C3c2 = YES
C3C6

Have you ever been concerned or worried about using cannabis?

(1)   No
(2)   Yes

IF: C3c2 = YES
C3C7

Has using cannabis ever made you feel ill?

(1)   No
(2)   Yes

IF: C3c2 = YES
C3C8

Have you ever felt you wanted to cut down or stop using cannabis?

(1)   No
(2)   Yes

IF: C3c2 = YES
C3C9

Has anyone expressed concern about you using cannabis - for example a friend or relative or teacher

(1)   No
(2)   Yes

C3G2

Have you ever used any other drug?

(1)   No
(2)   Yes

IF: C3G2 = YES
C3G3

Have you ever used inhalants (these are liquids or sprays that people sniff or inhale to get high or make them feel good such as solvents, sprays, glue or amylnitrate)?

(1)   No
(2)   Yes
(3)   Never heard of inhalants/don't know

IF: C3G2 = YES
IF: C3G3 = YES
C3G3a

Have you ever used inhalants more than 5 times in your life?

(1)   No
(2)   Yes

IF: C3G2 = YES
C3G4

Have you ever used ECSTASY?

(1)   No
(2)   Yes
(3)   Never heard of ecstasy/don't know

IF: C3G2 = YES
IF: C3G4 = YES

C3G4a

Have you ever used ectasy more than 5 times in your life?

(1)   No
(2)   Yes

IF: C3G2 = YES
C3G5

Have you ever used AMPHETAMINES (SPEED)

(1)   No
(2)   Yes
(3)   Never heard of amphetamines/don't know

IF: C3G2 = YES
IF: C3G5 = YES
C3G5a

Have you ever used amphetamines (speed) more than 5 times in your life?

(1)   No
(2)   Yes

IF: C3G2 = YES
C3G6

Have you ever used LSD (ACID)?

(1)   No
(2)   Yes
(3)   Never heard of LSD/don't know

IF: C3G2 = YES
IF: C3G6 = YES
C3G6a

Have you ever used LSD (Acid) more than 5 times in your life?

(1)   No
(2)   Yes

IF: C3G2 = YES
C3G7

Have you ever used TRANQUILISERS (VALIUM,TEMAZAPAN)?

(1)   No
(2)   Yes
(3)   Never heard of tranquilisers/don't know

IF: C3G2 = YES
IF: C3G7 = YES
C3G7a

Have you ever used Tranquilisers (valium, temazapan) more than 5 times in your life?

(1)   No
(2)   Yes

IF: C3G2 = YES
C3G8

Have you ever used COCAINE (CRACK)?

(1)   No
(2)   Yes
(3)   Never heard of cocaine/don't know

IF: C3G2 = YES
IF: C3G8 = YES
C3G8a

Have you ever used cocaine (crack) more than 5 times in your life?

(1)   No
(2)   Yes

IF: C3G2 = YES
C3G9

Have you ever used HEROIN (METHADONE)?

(1)   No
(2)   Yes
(3)   Never heard of heroin/don't know

IF: C3G2 = YES
IF: C3G9 = YES
C3G9a

Have you ever used Heroin (methadone) more than 5 times in your life?

(1)   No
(2)   Yes

CSCExit

Thank you. That is the end of this section.
Now please pass the computer back to the interviewer.

CHowCmp

INTERVIEWER: Did the child complete the whole of this section as a self-completion?

(1)   Yes
(2)   No

Dyslexia test

DysTest

INTERVIEWER: Will you be completing the dyslexia test with this child?

(1)   Yes
(2)   No

* British Picture Vocabulary Scale (BPVS-II)

Introduction:
I want you to look at some pictures with me. See all the pictures on this page.
POINT TO EACH OF THE PICTURES IN TRAINING PLATE A. THEN SAY:
I will say something; the I want you to put your finger on the 'ball'.
IF THE CHILD RESPONDS CORRECTLY PRESS <ENTER> TO CONTINUE WITH ANOTHER TRAINING PLATE.
IF CHILD RESPONDS INCORRECTLY DEMONSTRATE THE CORRECT RESPONSE BY POINTING

TO THE BALL AND SAYING:
That was a good try, but this is the 'ball'. Now try again.
Put your finger on the 'ball'. HELP AS NECESSARY UNTIL A CORRECT RESPONSE IS MADE.
Good let's try another one. Put your finger on the 'dog'.

Starting test::
Fine, now I am going to show you some pictures. Each time I will say something, and you will point to the best picture of it. When we go further along, you may not be sure which one to point to, but I want you to look carefully at all the pictures anyway, and choose the one you think is right.
Point to....

* British Ability Scales (BAS-II)

* Word reading scale

Here is a card with a lot of words. Let's see how many you can read. Read them out loud to me. INTERVIEWER: POINT TO THE FIRST WORD FOR THE CHILD.

* Spelling sheet

GIVE THE CHILD THE SPELLING WORKSHEET AND A PENCIL AND ERASER. POINT TO THE LINE OF THE WORKSHEET CORRESPONDING TO THE CHILD'S STARTING ITEM AND SAY: I would like you to spell some words for me. Try as hard as you can to spell every word. Write the first one here. Get ready, listen.

N1392

D

NATIONAL STATISTICS

IN CONFIDENCE

Survey of Development and Well-being of Children and Adolescents

Questionnaire for teachers of children aged 5 and above in primary or secondary schools

Stick Label Here

How to fill in this questionnaire

1. Please read each question carefully.

2. All questions can be answered by putting a tick in the box next to the answer that applies to the child.

	Not true	Somewhat true	Certainly true
For example		✓	

3. Sometimes you are asked to write a number in a box.

For example   Enter number of days ⟶ | 4 |

4. It would help if you could answer all questions as best as you can even if you are not absolutely certain or you think the question seems a little odd.

A1. Compared with an **average** child of the same age, how does he or she fare in the following areas:

	Above average	Average	Some difficulty	Marked difficulty
(a) Reading?	1	2	3	4
(b) Mathematics?	1	2	3	4
(c) Spelling	1	2	3	4

A2. Although "mental age" is a crude measure that cannot take account of a child being better in some areas than others, it would be helpful if you could answer the following question:

In terms of overall intellectual and scholastic ability, roughly what age level is he or she at?

Enter age level ⟶ ☐ **→ Go to Question A3**

A3. During the last term, how many days overall has the child been absent?

Enter number of days ⟶ ☐
If don't know enter "99"
If none enter "00"
→ Go to Question A4

A4. Does the child have officially recognised special needs?

No .... 0 **→ Go to Section B**

Stage 1 (class teacher or form/year tutor has overall responsibility) 1

Stage 2 (SENCO takes the lead in co-ordinating provision and drawing up IEP) 2

Stage 3 (External specialist support enlisted) 3

Stage 4 (Statutory assessment by LEA) 4

Stage 5 (Statement issued by LEA) 5

→ Go to question A5

A5. Are these special needs related to ......

	Yes	No
General learning difficulties?	1	2
Specific learning difficulties?	1	2
Speech and language difficulties?	1	2
Emotional and behavioural difficulties?	1	2
Physical disability/sensory impairment?	1	2
Other (please specify)	1	2

Section B   Strengths and Difficulties Questionnaire

For each item, please tick a box under one of the headings:
Not True, Somewhat True or Certainly True.

	Not true	Somewhat true	Certainly true
Over the past six months:			
B1. Considerate of other people's feelings	1	2	3
B2. Restless, overactive, cannot stay still for long	1	2	3
B3. Often complains of headaches, stomach aches or sickness	1	2	3
B4. Shares readily with other children (treats, toys, pencils etc)	1	2	3
B5. Often has temper tantrums or hot tempers	1	2	3
B6. Rather solitary, tends to play alone	1	2	3
B7. Generally obedient, usually does what adults ask	1	2	3
B8. Many worries, often seems worried	1	2	3
B9. Helpful if someone is hurt, upset or feeling ill	1	2	3
B10. Constantly fidgeting or squirming	1	2	3

For each item, please tick a box under one of the headings:
Not True, Somewhat True or Certainly True.

	Not true	Somewhat true	Certainly true
Over the past six months:			
B11. Has at least one good friend	1	2	3
B12. Often fights with other children or bullies them	1	2	3
B13. Often unhappy, downhearted or tearful	1	2	3
B14. Generally liked by other children	1	2	3
B15. Easily distracted, concentration wanders	1	2	3
B16. Nervous or clingy in new situations, easily loses confidence	1	2	3
B17. Kind to younger children	1	2	3
B18. Often lies or cheats	1	2	3
B19. Picked on or bullied by other children	1	2	3
B20. Often volunteers to help others (parents, teachers, other children)	1	2	3
B21. Thinks things out before acting	1	2	3
B22. Steals from home, school or elsewhere	1	2	3
B23. Gets on better with adults than with other children	1	2	3
B24. Has many fears, easily scared	1	2	3
B25. Sees tasks through to the end, good attention span	1	2	3

B26. Overall, do you think that this child has difficulties in one or more of the following areas: emotions, concentration, behaviour or getting on with other people?

No .... → **Go to Section C**

Yes: minor difficulties ....
Yes: definite difficulties .... → **Go to Question B26(a)**
Yes: severe difficulties ....

(a) How long have these difficulties been present?

Less than a month 1

1 - 5 months 2

6 - 12 months 3

A year or more 4

	Not at all	Only a little	Quite a lot	A great deal
B27. Do the difficulties upset or distress the child?	1	2	3	4
B28. Do the difficulties interfere with the child's everyday life in terms of his or her . . .				
peer relationships?	1	2	3	4
classroom learning?	1	2	3	4
B29. Do the difficulties put a burden on you or the class as a whole?	1	2	3	4

Section C   Emotions

For each item, please tick a box under one of the headings:
Not True, Somewhat True or Certainly True.

	Not true	Somewhat true	Certainly true
C1. Excessive worries	1	2	3
C2. Marked tension or inability to relax	1	2	3
C3. Excessive concern about his/her own abilities, e.g. academic, sporting or social	1	2	3
C4. Particularly anxious about speaking to class or reading aloud	1	2	3
C5. Reluctant to separate from family to come to school	1	2	3
C6. Unhappy, sad or depressed	1	2	3
C7. Has lost interest in carrying out usual activities	1	2	3
C8. Feels worthless or inferior	1	2	3
C9. Concentration affected by worries or misery	1	2	3
C10. Other emotional difficulties eg. marked fears panic attacks, obsessions or compulsions	1 → **Go to C11**	2 → **Go to C10a**	3 → **Go to C10a**

C10a. Please descibe these briefly

Please review your answers to questions C1 to C10 about worries, misery and so on.

If you have ticked 'CERTAINLY TRUE' to any of the questions C1 to C10 - Please go to question C11. If not, go to Section D.

	Not at all	Only a little	Quite a lot	A great deal
C11. Do the difficulties upset or distress the child?	1	2	3	4
C12. Do the difficulties interfere with the child's everyday life in terms of his or her . . .				
peer relationships?	1	2	3	4
classroom learning?	1	2	3	4
C13. Do the difficulties put a burden on you or the class as a whole?	1	2	3	4

C14. Do you have any further comments about this child's emotional state?

Yes   1   → **Go to Question C14a**

No   2   → **Go to Section D**

C14a. If there are serious concerns in this area, please say how long the child has had these problems, and what, if anything, might have triggered them.

Section D   Attention, Activity and Impulsiveness

D1. When s/he is doing something in class that s/he enjoys and is good at, whether reading or drawing or making a model or whatever, how long does s/he typically stay on that task?

Less than 2 minutes 1

2 - 4 minutes 2

5 - 9 minutes 3

10 - 19 minutes 4

20 minutes or more 5

→ **Go to question D2**

Please review your answers to questions D2 to D20 on attention and activity.

If you have ticked 'CERTAINLY TRUE' to any of the questions D2 to D20 - Please go to question D21. If not, go to Section E.

	Not at all	Only a little	Quite a lot	A great deal
D21. Do the difficulties upset or distress the child?	1	2	3	4
D22. Do the difficulties interfere with the child's everyday life in terms of his or her . . .				
peer relationships?	1	2	3	4
classroom learning?	1	2	3	4
D23. Do the difficulties put a burden on you or the class as a whole?	1	2	3	4

D24. Do you have any further comments about this child in relation to attention or activity and impulsiveness?

Yes [1] → **Go to Question D24a**

No [2] → **Go to Section E**

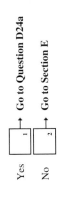

D24a. Please describe. If there are serious concerns in this area, please say how long the child has had these problems, and what, if anything, might have triggered them.

For each item, please tick a box under one of the headings:
Not True, Somewhat true or Certainly true.

	Not true	Somewhat true	Certainly true
D2. Makes careless mistakes	1	2	3
D3. Fails to pay attention	1	2	3
D4. Loses interest in what s/he is doing	1	2	3
D5. Doesn't seem to listen	1	2	3
D6. Fails to finish things s/he starts	1	2	3
D7. Disorganised	1	2	3
D8. Tries to avoid tasks that require thought	1	2	3
D9. Loses things	1	2	3
D10. Easily distracted	1	2	3
D11. Forgetful	1	2	3
D12. Fidgets	1	2	3
D13. Can't stay seated when required to do so	1	2	3
D14. Runs or climbs about when s/he shouldn't	1	2	3
D15. Has difficulty playing quietly	1	2	3
D16. Finds it hard to calm down when asked to do so	1	2	3
D17. Interrupts, blurts out answers to questions	1	2	3
D18. Hard for him/her to wait their turn	1	2	3
D19. Interrupts or butts in on others	1	2	3
D20. Goes on talking if asked to stop	1	2	3

Section E   Awkward and Troublesome Behaviour

For each item, please tick a box under one of the headings:
Not True, Somewhat true or Certainly true.

	Not true	Somewhat true	Certainly true
E1. Temper tantrums or hot tempers	1	2	3
E2. Argues a lot with adults	1	2	3
E3. Disobedient at school	1	2	3
E4. Deliberately does things to annoy others	1	2	3
E5. Blames others for own mistakes	1	2	3
E6. Easily annoyed by others	1	2	3
E7. Angry and resentful	1	2	3
E8. Spiteful	1	2	3
E9. Tries to get his/her own back	1	2	3
E10. Lying or cheating	1	2	3
E11. Starts fights	1	2	3
E12. Bullies others	1	2	3
E13. Plays truant	1	2	3
E14. Uses weapons when fighting	1	2	3
E15. Has been physically cruel, has really hurt someone	1	2	3
E16. Deliberately cruel to animals	1	2	3
E17. Sets fires deliberately	1	2	3

E18. Does (CHILD) steal?

Not true .... 1 → **Go to question E19**

Somewhat true 2

Certainly true .... 3 → **Go to question E18a**

E18a. Please describe this briefly

E19. Does s/he destroy things belonging to others, vandalism?

Not true .... 1 → **Go to question E20**

Somewhat true 2

Certainly true .... 3 → **Go to question E19a**

E19a. Please describe this briefly

E20. Does (CHILD) show unwanted sexualized behaviour towards others?

Not true .... 1 → **Go to question E21**

Somewhat true 2

Certainly true .... 3 → **Go to question E20a**

E20a. Please describe this behaviour

E21. Has (CHILD) been in trouble with the law?

Not true .... 1 → **Go to next page**

Somewhat true 2

Certainly true .... 3 → **Go to question E21a**

E21a. Please describe this briefly

Please review your answers to questions E1 to E21 on awkward and troublesome behaviour.

If you have ticked 'CERTAINLY TRUE' to any of the questions E1 to E21 - Please go to question E22. If not, go to Section F.

	Not at all	Only a little	Quite a lot	A great deal
E22. Do the difficulties upset or distress the child?	1	2	3	4
E23. Do the difficulties interfere with the child's everyday life in terms of his or her . . .				
peer relationships?	1	2	3	4
classroom learning?	1	2	3	4
E24. Do the difficulties put a burden on you or the class as a whole?	1	2	3	4

E25. Do you have any further comments about this child's awkwardness and troublesome behaviour?

Yes ☐1 → **Go to Question E25a**

No ☐2 → **Go to Section F**

E25a. Please describe. If there are serious concerns in this area, please say how long the child h had these problems, and what, if anything, might have triggered them.

Section F   Other Concerns

For each item, please tick a box under one of the headings:
Not True, Somewhat true or Certainly true.

	Not true	Somewhat true	Certainly true
F1. Tics, twitches, involuntary grunts or noises	1	2	3
F2. Diets to excess	1	2	3

F3. Do you have anyother concerns about the child's psychological development?

Yes ☐1 → **Go to question F3a**

No ☐2 → **Go to question F4**

F3a. Please describe this briefly

F4. Do you have any further comments about (CHILD) in general?

Yes ☐1 → **Go to Question F4a**

No ☐2 → **Go to Section G**

F4a. Please describe

Section G   Help from school

G1. During this school year, has s/he had any specific help for emotional or behavioural problems from teachers, educational psychologists, or other professionals working within the school setting.

Yes .... ☐ 1 → **Go to question G1(a)**

No .... ☐ 2 → **END**

G1a. Please describe briefly what sort of help was provided, by whom, and for what:

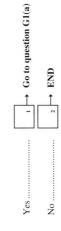

Thank you very much for your help

Please return this questionnaire in the prepaid envelope provided as soon as possible

NATIONAL STATISTICS

ONS
1 Drummond Gate
London
SW1V 2QQ

Glossary of terms

ACORN classification

ACORN is a geodemographic targeting classification, combining geographical and demographic characteristics to distinguish different types of people in different areas in Great Britain. (CACI Information Services, (1993), *ACORN User Guide,* CACI Limited 1994. All Rights Reserved. Source: ONS and GRO(S) (c) Crown Copyright 1991. All Rights Reserved)

Although the ACORN classification has various levels, 6 categories, 17 groups and 54 types, for the purposes of this report, the highest level, i.e. the six broad categories have been chosen for comparative analysis. The ACORN User Guide gives the following description of each category.

A. *Thriving:* wealthy achievers, suburban areas; affluent greys, rural communities; prosperous pensioners, retirement areas.
B. *Expanding:* affluent executives, family areas; well-off workers, family areas.
C. *Rising:* affluent urbanites, town and city areas, prosperous professionals, metropolitan areas; better off executives, inner city areas.
D. *Settling:* comfortable middle agers, mature home owning areas; skilled workers, home owning areas.
E. *Aspiring:* new home owners, mature communities; white collar workers, better-off multi-ethnic areas.
F. *Striving:* older people, less prosperous areas; council estate residents, better off homes; council estate residents, high unemployment; council estate residents, greater hardship, people in multi-ethnic, low-income areas.

Burden of mental disorders

The burden of the child's problem is a measure of the consequences of the symptoms in terms of whether they cause distress to the family by making the parents worried, depressed, tired or physically ill.

Case vignettes

This case vignette approach for analysing survey data uses clinician ratings based on a review of all the information of each subject. This information includes not only the questionnaires and structured interviews but also any additional comments made by the interviewers, and the transcripts of informants' comments to open-ended questions particularly those which ask about the child's significant problems.

Educational level

Educational level was based on the highest educational qualification obtained and was grouped as follows:

Degree (or degree level qualification)

Teaching qualification
HNC/HND, BEC/TEC Higher, BTEC Higher
City and Guilds Full Technological Certificate
Nursing qualifications:
(SRN,SCM,RGN,RM,RHV,Midwife)

A-levels/SCE higher
ONC/OND/BEC/TEC/not higher
City and Guilds Advanced/Final level

GCE O-level (grades A-C if after 1975)
GCSE (grades A-C)
CSE (grade 1)
SCE Ordinary (bands A-C)
Standard grade (levels 1-3)
SLC Lower SUPE Lower or Ordinary

School certificate or Matric
City and Guilds Craft/Ordinary level

GCE O-level (grades D-E if after 1975)
GCSE (grades D-G)
CSE (grades 2-5)
SCE Ordinary (bands D-E)
Standard grade (levels 4-5)
Clerical or commercial qualifications
Apprenticeship
Other qualifications

CSE ungraded

No qualifications

Ethnic Group

Household members were classified into nine groups:

White
Black - Caribbean
Black - African
Black - Other
Indian
Pakistani
Bangladeshi
Chinese
None of these

For analysis purpose these nine groups were subsumed under 5 headings: White, Black, Indian, Pakistani and Bangladeshi and other

Household

The standard definition used in most surveys carried out by ONS Social Survey Division, and comparable with the 1991 Census definition of a household, was used in this survey. A household is defined as a single person or group of people who have the accommodation as their only or main residence and who either share one meal a day or share the living accommodation.
(See E McCrossan *A Handbook for interviewers*. HMSO: London 1985.)

Impact of mental disorders

Impact refers to the consequences of the disorder for the child in terms of social impairment and distress. Social impairment refers to the extent to which the disorder interferes with the child's everyday life in terms of his or her home life, friendships, classroom learning or leisure activities.

Marital status

Two questions were asked to obtain the marital status of the interviewed parent. The first asked: "Are you single, that is never married, married and living with your husband/wife, married and separated from your husband/wife, divorced or widowed?" The second question asked of everyone except those married and living with husband/wife was "May I just check, are you living with someone else as a couple?" The stability of the cohabitation was not assessed.

Mental disorders

The questionnaires used in this survey were based on both the ICD10 and DSM-IV diagnostic research criteria, but this report uses the terms mental disorders as defined by the ICD-10: to imply a clinically recognisable set of symptoms or behaviour associated in most cases with considerable distress and substantial interference with personal functions.

Region

When the survey was carried out there were 14 Regional Health Authorities in England. These were used in the sample design for stratification. Scotland and Wales were treated as two distinct areas. However, for analysis purposes, the postal sectors were allocated to Government Office Regions with Metropolitan counties (GOR2)

1. North East Met
2. North East Non Met
3. North West Met
4. North West Non Met
5. Merseyside
6. Yorks and Humberside Met
7. Yorks and Humberside Non Met
8. East Midlands
9. West Midlands Met
10. West Midlands Non Met

11. Eastern Outer Met
12. Eastern Other
13. London Inner
14. London Outer
15. South East Outer Met
16. South East Other
17. South West
18. Wales 1 - Glamorgan, Gwent
19. Wales 2 - Clwydd, Gwenneyd, Dyfed, Powys
20. Scotland 1 - Highlands, Grampian, Tayside
21. Scotland 2 - Fife, Central, Lothian
22. Scotland 3 - Glasgow Met
23. Scotland 3 - Strathclyde Exc Glasgow
24. Scotland 4 - Borders, Dumfries, Galloway

These 24 codes were collapsed into seven categories and in the tables the two areas of Scotland were grouped together:

1. Inner London
2. Outer London
3. Metropolitan England
4. Non-metropolitan England
5. Wales
6. Glasgow Met
7. Other Scotland

Social class

Based on the Registrar General's *Standard Occupational Classification*, Volume 3 OPCS London: HMSO 1991, social class was as-cribed on the basis of occupation and indus-try:

Descriptive definition	Social class
Professional	I
Managerial and Technical	II
Skilled occupations - non-manual	III non-manual
Skilled occupations - manual	III manual
Partly-skilled	IV
Unskilled occupations	V
Armed Forces	

Social class was not determined where informant (and spouse) had never worked, or was a full-time student or whose occupation was inadequately described.

Tenure

Tenure was assessed by asking two standard questions: how the accommodation was occupied and who was the landlord.

How accommodation was occupied
- Own outright
- Buying it with the help of a mortgage or loan
- Pay part rent and part mortgage (shared ownership)
- Rent it
- Live here rent free (including rent free in relative's or friend's property)
- Squatting

Type of landlord
- Local authority or Council or New Town development or Scottish Homes
- A housing association or co-operative or charitable trust
- Employer (Organisation) of a household member
- Another organisation
- Relative or friend (before living there) of a household member
- Employer (individual(of a household member
- Another individual private landlord

Three types of tenure categories were created:

Owners means bought without mortgage or loan or with a mortgage or loan which has been paid off. Includes co-ownership and shared ownership schemes.

Social sector tenants means rented from local authorities, New Town corporations or commissions or Scottish Homes, and hous-ing associations which include co-operatives and property owned by charitable trusts.

Private renters includes rent from organisa-tions (property company, employer or other organisation) and from individuals (relative, friend, employer or other individual.

Type of accommodation

Four types of accommodation were created:

Detached means a detached house or bungalow
Semi-detached includes a semi-detached whole house or bungalow
Terraced means a terraced or end of terraced whole house or bungalow
Flat/maisonette includes a purpose built flat or maisonette in block, converted flat or maisonette in house, a room in a house or block, a bedsit.

Working status

Working adults

The two categories of working adults include persons who did any work for pay or profit in the week ending the last Sunday prior to interview, even if it was for as little as one hour, including Saturday jobs and casual work (e.g. babysitting, running a mail order club).

Self-employed persons were considered to be working if they worked in their own business, professional practice, or farm for the purpose of making a profit, or even if the enterprise was failing to make a profit or just being set up.

The unpaid 'family worker' (e.g., a wife doing her husband's accounts or helping with the farm or business) was included as working if the work contributed directly to a business, farm or family practice owned or operated by a related member of the same household. (Although the individual concerned may have received no pay or profit, her contribution to the business profit counted as paid work). This only applied when the business was owned or operated by a member of the same household.

Anyone on a Government scheme which was employer based was also 'working last week'

Informants definitions dictated whether they felt they were working full time or part time

Unemployed adults
This category included those who were waiting to take up a job that had already been obtained, those who were looking for work, and people who intended to look for work but prevented by temporary ill-health, sickness or injury.

Economically inactive adults
This category comprised five main categories of people:

"Going to school or college" only applied to people who were under 50 years of age. The category included people following full time educational courses at school or at further education establishments (colleges, university etc). It included all school children (16 years and over).

During vacations, students were still coded as "going to school or college". If their return to college depends on passing a set of exams, you should code on the assumption that they will be passed. If however, they were having a break from full time education, i.e. they were taking a year out, they were not counted as being in full time education.

"Permanently unable to work" only applied to those under state retirement age, i.e. to men aged 16 to 64 and to women aged 16 to 59. Include were people whose inability to work was due to health or emotional problems or disablement.

"Retired" only applied to those who retired from their full-time occupation at approximately the retirement age for that occupation, and were not seeking further employment of any kind.

"Looking after the home or family" covered anyone who was mainly involved in domestic duties, provided this person had not already been coded in an earlier category.

"Doing something else" included anyone for whom the earlier categories were inappropriate.